ANEURYSMS

ANEURYSMS

Editors

Morris D. Kerstein, M.D.

Professor

Peter V. Moulder, M.D.

Professor

Watts R. Webb, M.D.

Professor and Chairman

Department of Surgery
Tulane University School of Medicine
New Orleans, Louisiana

WILLIAMS & WILKINS
Baltimore/London

428 East Preston Street
Baltimore, MD 21202, U.S.A.

Made in the United States of America

Library of Congress Cataloging in Publication Data

Aneurysms.

Includes index.
1. Blood-vessels—Surgery. 2. Aneurysms—Surgery.
I. Kerstein, Morris D. II. Moulder, Peter V.
III. Webb, Watts R. [DNLM: 1. Aneurysm—Surgery—Congresses. WG 580 A597 1981]
RD598.5.A52 1983 617'.413 82-20186
ISBN 0-683-04598-9

Composed and printed at the
Waverly Press, Inc.
Mt. Royal and Guilford Aves.
Baltimore, MD 21202, U.S.A.

This book is dedicated to Margaret, Jane, and Frances.

Preface

Aneurysmal surgery is demanding upon the surgeon for appropriate, safe, perioperative and operative decision making. The purpose of this book is to provide the surgical resident and practicing vascular surgeon a ready reference on the vicissitudes of aneurysmal surgery. The problems in timing and techniques of surgery are unique. The authors hope they have produced a most useful resource for the sophisticated practicing clinician.

Morris D. Kerstein, M.D.
Peter V. Moulder, M.D.
Watts R. Webb, M.D.

Acknowledgments

This was an enjoyable undertaking because of the help of the contributors at a vascular symposium held in New Orleans, Louisiana. Writing is always a sacrifice of personal time, not patient-care time; therefore, the help of the many authors is gratefully acknowledged. Special kudos are directed towards Rye Nelson, John Brand, and Jack Hoover of W.L. Gore and Associates.

Gae Decker-Garrad was the special force in preparation and editing who allowed the book to come to fruition.

Stella Kolb continues patiently as a friend and secretary. Her help is invaluable. Carole Eber's efforts in re-typing the many editions are especially appreciated.

CONTRIBUTORS

Wiley F. Barker, M.D., Professor of Surgery, University of Calfornia at Los Angeles, Los Angeles, California (Chapter 5)
Steven A. Blau, M.D., Assistant Professor of Surgery, Albert Einstein School of Medicine, New York, New York (Chapter 6)
E. Stanley Crawford, M.D., Professor of Surgery, Baylor University College of Medicine, Houston, Texas (Chapter 4)
Giacomo A. DeLaria, M.S., M.D., Assistant Professor of Surgery, Rush Medical College, Chicago, Illinois (Chapter 3)
Ralph A. Deterling, Jr., M.D., Professor of Surgery, Tufts University School of Medicine, Boston, Massachusetts (Chapter 6)
Seymour Glagov, M.D., Professor of Pathology, University of Chicago, School of Medicine, Chicago, Illinois (Chapter 1)
Hushang Javid, M.D., Ph.D., Professor of Surgery, Rush Medical College, Chicago, Illinois (Chapter 3)
Morris D. Kerstein, M.D., Professor of Surgery, Tulane University School of Medicine, New Orleans, Louisiana (Chapter 6; Chapter 8)
Peter V. Moulder, M.D., Professor of Surgery, Tulane University School of Medicine, New Orleans, Louisiana (Chapter 2)
Donald M. Snyder, M.D., Assistant Professor of Surgery, Baylor University College of Medicine, Houston, Texas (Chapter 4)
Edward A. Stemmer, M.D., Professor of Surgery, University of California at Irvine, Irvine, California (Chapter 7)
Thomas F. Sweeney, M.D., Clinical Instructor in Surgery, Yale University School of Medicine, New Haven, Connecticut (Chapter 8)
Christopher K. Zarins, M.D., Professor of Surgery, University of Chicago School of Medicine, Chicago, Illinois (Chapter 1)

Contents

CHAPTER 1

Pathophysiology of Aneurysm Formation

SEYMOUR GLAGOV, M.D.
CHRISTOPHER K. ZARINS, M.D.

Arterial aneurysms are local, irreversible dilatations, outpouchings, or swellings of arterial walls which result in abnormal vessel configurations, alterations in blood flow, and a tendency toward thrombosis and/or rupture. The formation of an aneurysm in a previously normal vessel implies that the arterial wall, at some point in time, was no longer able to maintain its normal configuration or integrity. In more precise terms, the mechanical stress imposed upon the media exceeded its resistance to deformation, disruption, or rupture. In principle, this situation may be due to an abnormal increase in mechanical stress, reduced resistance of the arterial wall to deformation or disruption, or a combination of these influences. Increases in blood pressure or pulse pressure, changes in heart rate or lumen diameter, alterations in branch angles and curvatures, and vibrations distal to critical stenoses may all be associated with long-term increases in medial tensile *stress* (i.e., the tension per unit cross-section of the vessel wall). Reduced medial perfusion, interference with medial cellular metabolism, reduction in medial cellularity, and modifications of matrix composition or mural architecture may all be associated with abnormal increases in medial *strain* (i.e., the deformation associated with a given level of imposed stress). Although there is good evidence to suggest that hemodynamic forces or mechanical displacements may impose greatly increased stresses on arterial walls and result in long-term modifications of vessel wall composition and mechanical properties, most of the findings to date indicate that primary metabolic or structural defects of the media or alterations associated with intimal changes (i.e., atherosclerosis) probably underlie most arterial ectasias and aneurysms. Altered hemodynamic states may, nevertheless, play a significant role. Defects consistent with the preservation of normal arterial wall dimensions and continuity at physiologic levels of medial stress may be sufficiently severe to result in ectasias, aneurysms, and, ultimately, ruptures, when tensile stress is abnormally elevated.

A good deal has been learned in recent years concerning the relationship of structure to function in arterial walls. The aortic media, in particular, has received close attention and data have been forthcoming which indicate that the human abdominal aorta may be especially vulnerable to modifications leading to aneurysmal formation. Findings relating the pathologic anatomy of aortic aneurysms to intimal changes, which may have repercussions on medial nutrition and metabolism and predispose to thrombus formation, have also been forthcoming. In addition, experimental data that tend to link medial disruption and atrophy directly to hyperlipidemia, rather than to atherosclerotic plaque deposition alone, provide new directions for investigating the pathogenesis and natural history of aneurysmal formation. This chapter reviews the relevant features of arterial functional microarchitecture and indicates, from these and other data, the factors which probably underlie the pathogenesis and natural history of the various forms of aneurysmal disease.

MICROARCHITECTURE OF THE AORTIC WALL

The aortic media is a highly organized, mechanically efficient structure consisting of uniform, alternating layers of cells and matrix fibers. On transverse sections of excised and immersion-fixed samples, the fibrous layers appear to contain more or less continuous elastic fiber sheets that appear as wavy lamellae. The cells in such preparations appear to be arrayed obliquely between successive fiber layers and seem to connect the elastic lamellae; in addition, collagen fibers, although abundant, do not appear to be organized in any consistent manner. If, however, aortas are fixed while distended at increasing intraluminal pressures, a somewhat different picture emerges (46). As vessel diameter increases and wall thickness decreases, the wavy elastin lamellae straighten and cells become aligned, not radially, but increasingly in directions that coincide with the curvature of the vessel wall. In transverse sections of straight segments of the aorta, fixed while distended at physiologic distending pressures, this orientation results in the establishment of continuous layers of overlapping cells lying more or less parallel to the straightened elastic lamellae (8). Meanwhile, collagen fibers are also straightened and drawn taut. There is an abrupt decrease in vessel distensibility at diastolic pressure. Further increases in diameter or decreases in wall thickness are minimal as pressures are raised beyond systolic levels. Thus, during the non-physiologic phase of redistention by pressures ranging from zero to diastolic levels, the relatively large changes in aortic radius and wall thickness merely reflect the restoration of cells and fibers to their normal configurations and orientations. The recoiled elastic fiber lamellae are unbending and stretching, and the collagen fibers are becoming aligned and taut. When diastolic pressures are attained, the taut, inextensible collagen fibers resist further extension until the aorta ruptures when the pressure reaches several times the normal level. Thus, the aorta, functioning physiologically at pressures ranging between diastolic and systolic levels, is normally nearly maximally distended. The relatively high elastic modulus of the media at its normal diameter protects the aorta against excessive dilatation at elevated pressures, while the close association and parallel arrangement of elastin and collagen fibers confer a combination of resiliency and tensile strength. Rapid changes in medial stress tend to be distributed uniformly through the compact wall, for elastic fibers are focally shared between adjacent groups of cells within the cell layers and the successive elastic fiber layers are also connected. Medial flaws and defects, therefore, tend *not* to be propagated by the normal range of changes in direction or magnitude of medial stresses, and chances of spontaneous rupture are minimal despite the medial irregularities and disruptions that occur with age.

Tensile Stresses and Medial Structure and Composition

The layers that comprise the aortic media of mammals are of similar thickness and architecture, regardless of species, and the number of layers in the aortic media corresponds closely to the tensile stress normally imposed upon it (47). Thus, for adult mammals, there is a nearly linear relationship between aortic radius at mean blood pressure and the number of its transmedial fibrocellular layers. Since, according to the law of Laplace, the tangential tension imposed on the wall of an aorta is a function of its radius and its distending pressure, and mean pressures are similar for most mammals, the average tension per layer would be expected to be nearly constant and independent of species. Estimates made from a study of several species (47) reveal that each increment of 0.017 mm in aortic radius with increasing species size requires an additional fibrocellular layer. The average tension per aortic layer is about 2,000 dynes/cm.

Although the relationship between radius and the number of medial layers appears to be independent of species or location, the relative proportions of elastin and collagen in the aortic media change with distance from the heart. The thoracic aorta normally contains a greater proportion of elastin than collagen, while the abdominal aorta contains more collagen than elastin (9). Yet, the total scleroprotein concentration (i.e., the sum of the collagen and elastin) does not change with distance from the heart. It has also been demonstrated that the anatomic position along the aorta, at which relative proportions of elastin and collagen reverse, differs from species to species, but is consistent for a given species. It would, therefore, appear that the establishment of the fibrocellular layers and total accumulation of fibrous protein in the aortic media are normally governed by the prevailing tensile stress (3). The relative proportions of elastin and collagen at particular locations may be related to other factors, such as the rate of attenuation of the cyclic tensile stresses associated with cardiac output and hemodynamic modifications. The latter, elastin and collagen levels, results from the steady decrease in cross-section as the major branches occur (33).

Although not as prominent as in the aorta, layers can also be enumerated in the walls of the systemic arteries and the pulmonary artery trunk when these are fully distended (12). Thereafter, a close relationship is once more evident between total estimated medial tension and the number of layers, and the tension per layer is nearly constant for homologous mammalian arteries. Both the total tension and average tension per layer are, however, smaller for branch vessels than for the aorta and correspond to the lower content or fibrous protein compared to smooth muscle in vessels. These vessels may also be expected to undergo considerable changes in diameter in response to neuroendocrine stimulation and changes in peripheral resistance, and during retraction and contraction after injury. Although the static mechanical properties of the aorta outlined above can be demonstrated in vessels devoid of viable smooth muscle, this cannot be assumed to be true of peripheral arteries.

Cohesion and Coordination of Media Structure

In order for an arterial wall to function as a coordinated unit and maintain its integrity in the presence of the varying tensile stresses associated with pressure changes, pulsatile wall motion, and vessel flexion, matrix elements and cells must be closely associated and coordinated. Attachments among the structural components must be sufficiently supple and tenacious to prevent shearing and slippage, which could result in excessive distensibility, aneurysmal dilatation, or rupture. There are at least three modes of interconnection of structural elements in the media (8). Within aortic cell layers, cells are segregated into small groups within which the cells are similarly oriented. Each group is surrounded by a continuous sheath of basal lamina. Running over and into the basal lamina and investing individual cell groups are sheets of interlacing collagen fibrils. Any pull tending to separate the overlapping cells changes the orientation of the surrounding interlacing basketwork of collagen fibrils so that these tighten about the cells, in the fashion of a Chinese finger trap, holding the cell group together and preventing further stretching and slippage. Each cell group is associated with a system of surrounding elastic fibers oriented in the same direction as the cells. Strong focal attachment sites between peripheral dense bodies of the smooth muscle cells and the adjacent elastic fibers form a second mode of bonding. The tenacity of these cell-to-elastin attachment complexes is apparently greater than the cohesiveness of the cell body. Sudden experimental hyperdistention results in focal disruption of cell projections, but preservation of the cell-to-elastin attachments to which they extend. Large collagen fiber bundles are wedged between adjacent elastic fibers and all of the medial structures are embedded in a ubiquitous, fine, and continuous microfibrillar matrix which provides a third means of stress transmission and coordination. Widespread disruption of any of these attachment systems could result in functional inadequacy of the media and yielding, sufficient to form aneurysms.

The structural materials in the walls of major systemic arteries are, in general, organized in a manner similar to that found in the aorta. With the decrease in structural matrix fiber content, however, the prominence of the discrete cell groupings becomes more evident and the component cells in each group are arranged in parallel, which suggests that each group represents a functional subdivision. Preliminary observations reveal that these units are arranged along presumed lines of stress within the arterial media and the size and orientation of each unit appear to correspond to the directional changes in tension, which correspond to modifications in medial geometry (7). The associated elaboration of collagen and elastin fibers would seem, at least in part, to be governed by the magnitude and distribution of the mechanical stresses on the smooth muscle cell groups.

Adaptive Response of the Media

During early growth, as aortic distending pressures and radii increase from fetal to normal adult levels, collagen and elastin accumulations per medial cell increase in proportion to the increase in medial tension. Comparisons between the pulmonary artery trunk and ascending aorta during growth reveal that this adaptation occurs as the diameters of these vessels increase to a comparable degree, while pressure rises in the aorta and falls in the pulmonary circuit (23). The vessels, nearly identical in wall thickness and morphology at birth, subsequently diverge markedly in thickness, medial architecture, and scleroprotein content in keeping with their developing differences in mechanical stress. Experimental hypertension also results in increased cross-sectional area of the aortic media, due to cell proliferation and accumulation of collagen and elastin, and in proportion to the increased medial tension, although the relative proportions of the two fibrous proteins and the number of medial layers are not altered (44). These data suggest that some ideal level of stress (i.e., force per unit cross-sectional area) is maintained by elaboration of suitable quantities of matrix fibers in a fixed proportion. Although this adaptive potential may persist to some degree when maturation is complete, changes related to growth and hypertension may be due to different mechanisms (45). Once established, however, the number of medial layers appears to be fixed. Whether the greater tension per layer which must then prevail places the hypertensive aorta at some functional disadvantage remains to be investigated. In general, elastin turnover differs in rate from collagen turnover and elastic fibers are known to fix lipids and become calcified (23). There is also experimental evidence that cells obtained from thoracic aortic media proliferate more readily in culture than cells derived from abdominal aorta (25). The consequences of these differences with regard to aortic medial adaptability to mechanical stress or to the tendency to develop aneurysms have not been explored, but merit detailed investigation.

Nutrition of the Media

Maintenance of arterial medial microarchitecture, including the growth and continuing differentiation of its cellular functional units and the elaboration, degradation, and accumulation of suitable proportions of matrix fibers by medial smooth muscle cells, would be expected to depend upon the availability of adequate medial nutrition. Thus, information concerning the manner in which tensile stress and medial architecture are related to medial perfusion and its possible limits could provide insights into the train of events which may cause an arterial wall to fail mechanically. The aortic media is normally nourished by diffusion from the endothelial surface and by vasa vasorum, which penetrate into the media from the adventitial side. Diffusion from the lumen is apparently sufficient to nourish the inner 0.5 mm of medial thickness. This zone contains no vasa vasorum and encompasses about 30 medial fibrocellular layers (48). Species large enough to have an aortic media composed of more than 30 layers have aortic medial vasa vasorum beyond the 30th aortic layer. Thus, aortas of small mammals (e.g., rats, rabbits, and small breeds of dogs) have fewer than 30 medial layers and are mainly dependent upon perfusion from the intima, while aortas of large mammals (e.g., pigs, sheep, and large breeds of dogs) have more than 30 medial layers and have medial vasa vasorum beyond the inner avascular zone of 30 layers. The distinction between avascular and vascular aortic medias is apparently already drawn at birth, for animals which are destined to have more than 30 aortic medial layers as adults have more than 30 layers at birth and medial vasa are already present (43). Those aortas which have fewer than 30 layers at birth will not exceed 30 layers at full maturity and do not contain medial vasa at birth.

Two additional features are associated with the presence of medial vasa vasorum. First, although the average tension per aortic medial layer is about 2,000 dynes/cm for mammals, the average tension per medial layer for aortas which contain medial vasa tends to be higher than the mean value, which suggests that the presence of medial vasa somehow permits medial layers to function at a higher level of medial stress (50). The second feature is that in very large mammals (e.g., horses and cattle) the avascular inner zone consistently maintains its orderly lamellar arrangement, while the outer vascularized zone may deviate somewhat from the usual architecture as the animal increases in size during growth (49). Elastic fibers become less evident as smooth muscle cells form increasingly prominent bands, suggesting that functional departures from the usual layered architecture, possibly necessary to tether very large and long aortas, may be dependent upon the presence of medial vasa.

Ectasia and Tortuosity

The considerations outlined above suggest that arterial walls are admirably designed to preserve their dimensions and integrity under normal circumstances and to withstand both sudden and long-term variations in tensile stress. Nevertheless, the aorta, as well as several other major systemic arteries, tend to dilate, elongate, and become less supple with age and to undergo deformations with potentially serious clinical consequences. These changes are probably due to metabolic modifications of medial cells and associated alterations in the concentration, mechanical properties, and organization of the matrix components (4, 16, 21, 24, 27). Although frequently associated with atherosclerosis, the precise nature of the corresponding mechanical changes remains to be defined. Abnormal enlargements of vessels usually include increases in both diameter and length, so that curvatures and configurations are altered and vessels tend to become not only dilated but also tortuous or bowed. With increasing diameters and the establishment of new convexities and concavities, the distribution of tensions is greatly altered, even if blood pressure levels are not greatly changed. Local stresses may, therefore, be augmented at the same time that the aortic wall is becoming less resilient due to changes in compliance. Instead of small defects being bypassed as the result of a well-coordinated distribution of imposed tensions by the structural fibers, flaws are increasingly likely to be propagated and create disruptions. Healing with fibrosis may become the predominant mode of defense rather than the more subtle and mechanically versatile remodeling response which occurs during growth and under normal conditions. A potential vicious circle is, therefore, probable. Chemical and structural alterations in the fibers and the inability of the aortic cells to keep pace and modulate medial fiber composition result both in dilatation and stiffening of the vessel wall. Dilatation results in altered vessel configuration, including tortuosity, with local increases in tensile stress. Since stresses are no longer redistributed and attenuated effectively, due to the associated changes in mechanical properties of the fibers, dilatation and propagation of flaws and disruptions continue. Equilibrium may be reached when sclerosis of the media results in sufficient inextensibility to enable the wall to bear the increased stress without further dilatation, despite the increased radius of curvature and thinning of the wall. Dilatations, whether diffuse or focal, are, however, often not self-limiting. The fibrous reaction which would tend to strengthen the wall appears to lag behind the increased stress in the media associated with dilatation. Concavities of curvatures and obtuse angles at branch points are the sites at which medial tensile stresses are relatively elevated and walls are normally thickest. Stresses are least at acute angle branch points where the media is correspondingly comparatively thin. Depending upon conditions, both locations may be vulnerable to aneurysmal formation—the former because of markedly elevated tension and the latter in relation to its precariously thin wall.

In the sections that follow, we shall attempt to outline the likely pathogenic mechanisms leading to aneurysmal formation in light of the relationships among cell metabolism, medial structure, and composition and the stresses (acute and chronic) that tend to disrupt and distort the vessel wall. In keeping with this approach, arterial aneurysms can be classified according to three principle modes of development. In the most common type, the arterial wall fails to maintain its normal resistance to deformation by the stresses associated with blood flow and pressure. The wall weakens and stretches to form a segmental fusiform or globular enlargement or a focal saccular outpouching. The aneurysmal wall, though it may be attenuated and fibrotic, is continuous with the wall of the adjacent, uninvolved portion of the vessel. Such a lesion is called a true aneurysm. In a second type, overall arterial wall configuration is maintained, but the cohesion among the layers of the media is severely compromised. Entry of blood into medial disruptions results in extensive separation of medial layers by a hematoma—this is a *dissecting aneurysm*, or acute aortic dissection. Finally, local aneurysmal swellings and deformations may arise as the result of the establishment of a communication between the bloodstream and a local periarterial sac by way of a transmural defect—these are *pseudoaneurysms*, or false aneurysms, for the swellings are not attributable to a deformation of the arterial wall, but to a localized absence of the arterial wall and containment of the bloodstream by extra-arterial tissues.

TRUE ANEURYSMS

Special Vulnerability of the Atherosclerotic Human Abdominal Aorta

The abdominal aortic segment, below the level of the renal outflow, is particularly prone to the formation of both true aneurysms and atherosclerotic occlusive disease. Aneurysmal dilatation of the abdominal aortic segment rarely occurs in aortas which do not already show evidence of dilatation elsewhere. Thus, the tendency to overall aortic enlargement or deformation is usually present in patients with atherosclerotic aortic aneurysms and suggests the presence of some general underlying metabolic compromise of the aortic wall which may be more severe in the distal aorta than elsewhere. Some tendency to dilatation is, however, a normal feature of aging in our population, suggesting that special, local factors in the abdominal segment of certain individuals may be of great importance in predisposing to the development of aneurysmal disease.

Nutrition of the Media

Although the relationship between the number of medial layers and the depth of penetration of vasa into the aortic media applies to both the thoracic and abdominal aortic segments in most mammals, the human abdominal aorta is a notable exception (50). Midway between the renal arteries and aortic bifurcation, the adult human aortic media is about 0.7 mm in thickness. For mammals, in general, this thickness would be expected to correspond to about 40 medial layers and such an aortic wall would be expected to include an outer vascularized zone of about 10 layers. Instead, the adult human abdominal aorta contains about 29 layers and is devoid of medial vasa vasorum; thus, each layer is thicker than expected and sustains an average tension of about 3,200 dynes/cm. This dissociation is reminiscent of the situation which occurs in animals exposed to experimentally induced hypertension (40, 44), inasmuch as the thickness and cross-sectional area of the media correspond to the total medial tension, but the number of medial layers does not. In addition, the tension per layer is elevated to the level usually noted in aortic medias with medial vasa. The degree to which these discrepancies among medial tension, medial structure, and medial vasa at this level in man corresponds to maladjustments in the relative quantities of cells and fibers to altered cell metabolism, or to greater cell turnover, has not been determined. The findings do, however, suggest that the increased risk of aneurysmal formation in this location may well be related to such alterations.

Diffuse Intimal Thickening and Atherosclerosis

A zone of intimal fibrocellular thickening develops with age in human aortas (12, 22, 28, 30). Relative to aortic medial thickness, this change appears to increase with distance from the heart, but absolute degrees of thickening may vary in different aortic sites. Although there is evidence that zones of intimal thickening may also be predisposed to increased atherosclerosis, intimal thickening, as such, has not been shown to be a direct precursor of atherosclerosis (41). Intimal thickening may, nevertheless, be considerable and attain or exceed the thickness of the underlying media. Such intimal changes may also have a more or less layered structure resembling (to a variable extent) that of the underlying media, but containing much more abundant collagen. Whatever the causes or adaptive implications of this widespread intimal change, it results in a thicker than normal aortic wall. Such a wall thickness should be associated with a deeper extension of medial vasa toward the intima than is normally present in this location. Although medial vasa vasorum are normally not demonstrable in human branch arteries and may be absent from the abdominal aortic media, adventitial arborizations may be quite prominent. In aortic medias which normally contain medial vasa vasorum, including the human thoracic segment, the zone immediately beyond the 30th medial layer may be considered to be at the limit of perfusion by the medial vasa and just beyond the inner, diffusion-dependent, avascular zone. Ideally then, vasa should proliferate into this precarious marginal zone and into normally avascular abdominal aortic or peripheral artery medias as the intima thickens. In aortic segments which show markedly advanced atherosclerosis with partial occlusion but without aneurysmal formation, vasa vasorum often do penetrate deeply into the media and plaques (14). In such cases, the media may be somewhat thinned, but is usually structurally preserved despite the presence of prominent intimal thickenings or atherosclerosis. When an aneurysm is present, however, the fibrous atrophic wall is usually markedly thinned and devoid of vasa vasorum.

It would seem from these findings that the presence of vasa vasorum in the media, even in the presence of atherosclerosis, may help to maintain a media of normal dimensions, while aneurysmal formation results from the absence or delay of vasal ingrowth in response to intimal thickening or plaque formation. We have already noted that aortas with no medial vasa at birth usually have no medial vasa when fully developed. The human abdominal aortic media, devoid of medial vasa at birth and maturity, may also tend to remain avascular even in the presence of intimal thickening. This tendency may be potentiated by the rapid rate of atherogenesis which prevails in this segment, to a reduced potential for vasal proliferation with increasing age, or to congenital or acquired individual differences in the abundance and location of medial or adventitial vasa. Recent experimental evidence indicates that the presence of hypercholesterolemia retards the healing of medial mechanical injuries (2). Severe injury results in incomplete restitution of the wall, medial atrophy, and aneurysmal formation even in the absence of atherosclerotic plaques. Interference with medial cell metabolism, or recovery by such agents as circulating lipids, catecholamines, or carbon monoxide attributable to smoking, may well be other contributing factors to aneurysmal formation, not only by way of enhancement of atherogenesis but directly by interference with medial metabolism and recovery from injury. As the abdominal aortic media becomes increasingly atrophic, the normally elevated tension per layer increases further. The atrophic media would tend to yield, producing the vicious cycle of dilatation, increased stress, and further atrophy and dilatation. There is also evidence from human material that associated segmental increases in collagenase activity may be related to abdominal aortic aneurysm formation (5). It should also be noted that elastin content decreases and elastase content increases with age in the aorta (19). The recognizable remnant of the arterial wall of an abdominal aortic aneurysm is, indeed, reduced to a fibrous band, often less than 25% of its normal thickness, with markedly reduced cellularity and absence of the fine details of medial organization.

Thrombus Formation

Stagnation of flow in the dilated aneurysmal sac results in a tendency to thrombus formation. Extensive fusiform aneurysms contain multiple layers as fibrocellular intimal thickening or atherosclerotic plaque deposition and may enhance aneurysmal enlargement once the process has begun. There is little evidence to suggest that thrombus deposition precedes or initiates the conditions which lead to local dilatations, although medial thinning below plaques has been demonstrated (10, 17). The lumenal diameter of an abdominal aortic aneurysm depends upon the extent of atherosclerotic plaqueing and deposition of mural thrombus. The wall as a whole may, therefore, be sufficiently thickened by thrombus deposition to be associated with a normal or reduced lumenal diameter, despite the markedly increased external diameter of the aneurysm. It is not clear whether the plaque or its overlying thrombus contribute to resistance of the wall to rupture; for plaques are irregular, often calcified, and easily fractured and the laminated mural thrombus may be irregularly organized, with layers close to the lumen showing little or no organization. Often thrombus appears as a gelatinous, greasy, mummified mass, indicating long-term deposition and decomposition of thrombus components without evidence of organization.

OTHER TRUE ANEURYSMS

We have thus far discussed the anatomic basis for the conservation of vessel integrity, and alluded to some of the conditions which may underlie the formation of true aneurysms in the abdominal aorta. Similar considerations may also be applied to the formation of true aneurysms in other locations, particularly in other portions of the aorta and in peripheral arteries such as the femoral and popliteal. Special local conditions which favor formation of true aneurysms may be operative in other sites. The splenic artery, for example, is the most frequent site of splanchnic artery aneurysm formation. It is also frequently more tortuous and atherosclerotic than other splanchnic vessels in the same individual. In contrast to other vessels, however, splenic artery aneurysms and dysplasias occur most frequently in women and particularly in women who have had multiple pregnancies (6). This phenomenon has been attributed to changes in splenic flow which may occur during pregnancy, but it should also be noted that renal artery dysplasias tend to occur under similar conditions (38) and that the incidence of aortic dissection is also elevated during pregnancy (29). These and other findings suggest hormonal status may modify medial compliance and cohesion by means of a direct hormonal effect on smooth muscle metabolism and/or matrix composition (11, 37). Increased longitudinal stress, due to displacement by the enlarged uterus in the presence of an altered hormonal status, may permit abnormal increases in strain and cause sufficient alteration in medial cohesive structure to result in permanent deformation and/or increased susceptibility to atherosclerosis. When true aneurysms are multiple in the same individual, a generalized metabolic defect or anomaly of arterial medial structure or matrix composition may be suspected but difficult to prove.

In other situations, underlying congenital medial defects have been demonstrated. Their conversion to aneurysms with or without rupture may be potentiated by hypertension, but they occur in the absence of hypertension as well. Typical examples are the aneurysms of the renal arteries in the kidney hilus (20) and the aneurysms which form in relation to the cerebral arteries (40). These aneurysms are situated typically at acute angle branch points where the arterial wall has been shown to be thinnest. The modifications in number, size, and orientation of muscle groupings and matrix fibers which should correspond to changes in configuration at bends and branch points (7) may not be adequate in these areas. Whether such defects are due to congenital malformations or to limitations in the capacity of the vessel wall to remodel as vessels grow and angles change during and after maturation remains to be demonstrated. Finally, dilatations of sufficient magnitude to be characterized as fusiform aneurysms may occur just distal to stenoses or focal compressions. Under experimental conditions, marked increases in arterial wall compliance have been demonstrated beyond constrictions, provided these are associated with bruits (31). This finding suggests that medial organization, cohesion, or composition may have been altered by the associated vibrations. The precise anatomic nature of this change has not been demonstrated.

Syphilitic Aneurysms

Aneurysms of the aorta due to *Treponema pallidum* infection occur mainly in the proximal aorta and are also associated with medial atrophy. The medial changes are, however, somewhat different from those associated with atherosclerosis in the distal aorta. Rather than replacement by a fibrous, avascular band, the syphilitic aortic media shows evidence of irregular atrophy of the outer media with patchy disappearance of elastic fibers and scarification. These changes may be due, in part, to direct penetration by the spirochete, but are most likely to be due to interference with blood supply to the outer media due to focal syphilitic endarteritis of the vasa. The thoracic aorta, largely dependent upon medial vasa for nutrition (48) would, therefore, naturally be expected to be the aortic site at greatest risk. The usual massive involvement of the most proximal ascending portion is probably due to the increased tension at this site associated with ventricular ejection. Thus, the dilatation in syphilitic aortitis is probably due to yielding of a chronically ischemic media at the site of greatest tensile stress. As the lesion evolves, the increasing radius adds further to the tensile stress. The scarification of the media is evidenced by wrinkling of the intima. Atherosclerosis may be potentiated, to some extent, by the intimal irregularities, but the mechanism is not clear. An increased tendency toward plaque deposition probably occurs only late in the development of the dilatation.

Dissecting Aneurysms

Aneurysmal deformations of arteries occur also as a result of hemorrhagic dissection of the media. While true aortic aneurysms consist of gradual, local expansions or outpouchings of weakened vessel walls, the primary event in dissecting aneurysm formation is a precipitous disruption of the media with separation of medial layers in circumferential planes. One or several of the tears may extend to the intima, establishing continuity between the lumen and the disrupted media. When this occurs, blood is considered to enter the media by way of a proximal tear and reenter the lumen by way of a distal tear. Passage may also be established to the adventitial side with catastrophic hemorrhage, or the formation of a massive periarterial hematoma. The extensive longitudinal distribution of the characteristic intramural disruption suggests the underlying defect is a loss or reduction of medial cohesiveness. The presence of a functional defect in medial matrix composition or organization is indicated by several findings. The disease is a feature of the Marfan syndrome as well as other hereditary disorders of matrix fiber metabolism (26). The incidence of dissection is increased in pregnant women and dissection can be induced in experimental animals by administering β-aminoproprionitrile, a compound which interferes with matrix fiber cross-linking (1). The tendency of aortas prone to dissection also to dilate and form true aneurysms in the hereditary disorders suggests that focal or segmental medial weakenings without hemorrhage may also develop on the basis of a general decrease in medial cohesion.

A precipitating role for medial stress is supported by the high frequency with which individuals with acute aortic dissection are hypertensive and the usual occurrence of an acute hypertensive crisis immediately preceding the catastrophic event. Yet, the dissecting aneurysm is not a common complication of hypertension and most hypertensive individuals who are also victims of aortic dissection have no demonstrable metabolic defect. Thus, the basis of the aortic defect remains obscure in most individuals. The associated microscopic medial lesion, cystic medial necrosis, is a degenerative change, disruptive of medial organization (34), which occurs frequently in individuals with aortic dissection but is also noted in many individuals without the disease (13, 35). The presence of such changes may render affected individuals prone to eventual dissection under certain conditions, but the presence of this characteristic medial lesion alone is apparently not sufficient. A combination of extensive medial degenerative involvement, hypertension, and/or some additional mechanical stress to the media may be required before blood gains access to the media and dissects between its layers (36).

Several of the features of aortic microarchitecture outlined above provide leads which may have some bearing on the pathogenesis of the disorder. The predominance of dissecting hematomas in the human thoracic aorta, rather than in the abdominal segment, suggests that interference with medial nutrition may play a role. Vasal supply, essential to thoracic aortic medial nutrition (18), may be inadequate in some individuals, thereby limiting metabolic and biosynthetic adaptation of the media to the increased tensile demands of hypertension. Hypertension may also compress or otherwise interfere with the vasal supply (32). The longitudinal propagation of dissection in the outer layers of the media (i.e., in the region of the potentially ischemic watershed boundary zone between the vascular and avascular portions of the media) tends to support such a hypothesis. Ligation of aortic vasa in experimental animals has actually been shown to cause zonal ischemic necrosis of the media (42); cystic medial necrosis in man may be a morphologic reflection of chronic medial ischemia. Hypertension would be expected to expose the proximal aortic segment to relatively high levels of intramural shearing stress which, under certain conditions (i.e., a sudden further rise in pressure), might exceed the reduced cohesive strength of medial layers—particularly where the media is rendered especially fragile by chronic medial ischemic injury. The transverse intimal-medial disruption, which is thought to provide access of the blood to the media in dissection, commonly occurs in the ascending aorta close to the inner aspect of the arch (i.e., at the site of greatest medial tension). Whether this tear, or the tears in other locations, precede, follow, or occur simultaneously with the extensive medial interlamellar separation is not clear, but a role for disrupted medial vasa as a source of medial hemorrhage must be considered. Extensive aortic hemorrhagic dissection may continue into the major arterial branches, but dissections also originate in major branch arteries without preceding aortic dissection. The medial defect which underlies aortic dissection, therefore, occurs in smaller arteries as well.

Pseudoaneurysms

When an arterial wall is breached and continuity established between the bloodstream and surrounding tissues, fatal hemorrhage may ensue if the defect is large. If the defect is small, the mural defect may seal, due to local retractions or structural readjustments within the vessel wall and formation of a hemostatic plug within the defect. A third possibility is persistence of the defect with local containment of the hemorrhage by the surrounding periarterial tissues, forming a blood-filled cavity in continuity with the vessel lumen. The resulting, localized dilatation resembles an aneurysm inasmuch as it appears as an abnormal outpouching of the wall connected to the circulating bloodstream. Since it is not encompassed by the arterial wall and reflects, instead, a transmural defect in the artery, it is called a false aneurysm, or pseudoaneurysm. Although periarterial tissues, especially in relation to overlying serosal membranes, may provide a surprisingly good barrier and prevent catastrophic hemorrhage, the absence of a wall containing the organized elements of an artery will usually result in progressive enlargement of the pseudoaneurysm as tension in its capsule increases with increasing radius.

Traumatic Aneurysms

Pseudoaneurysms are most commonly formed as a consequence of direct penetrating injuries such as those produced by bullet or knife wounds too large to seal spontaneously but with the hemorrhage contained by surrounding tissues. These may enlarge rapidly and require urgent intervention. In the case of the traumatic thoracic aortic aneurysm which arises from severe crushing chest injuries, transient forces applied to the aorta exceed its bursting strength. Typically, a transverse mural disruption of the descending thoracic aorta occurs just distal to the left subclavian artery. Survival after such an injury is often associated with pseudoaneurysmal formation due to containment of the hemorrhage by the pleura. Other direct blunt injuries of arteries may result in thrombosis or pseudoaneurysmal formation, depending upon the size of the injured vessel. Muscular arteries tend to retract and contract after local disruptive injury. Although a large mural defect may thereby be sealed, flow may also be arrested with formation of a thrombus. In contrast, large elastic arteries are held open by the abundant matrix and will generally not contract or recoil sufficiently to seal an extensive disruptive injury. Pseudoaneurysms, rather than the thrombotic occlusions, are, therefore, likely to occur. Although rupture of an atherosclerotic aneurysm may give rise to a superimposed pseudoaneurysm, it should be noted that most traumatic aneurysms occur in otherwise normal vessels in which cohesive strength of the uninjured portion of the wall is conserved. Thus, despite serious trauma which may result in total local disruption of mural integrity and formation of a pseudoaneurysm, there is no tendency toward splitting or separation between medial layers, or the formation of extended intramural hematomas.

Iatrogenic Aneurysms

Pseudoaneurysms may also be associated with diagnostic or operative procedures. The introduction of catheters for hemodynamic measurements or arteriographic procedures may be followed by persisting blood extravasation through the arterial puncture site after the catheter has been removed, and by formation of a local pseudoaneurysm. Procedures such as transluminal angioplasty may result in arterial wall disruptions and pseudoaneurysmal formation at a site remote from the entering arterial puncture. Catheter penetrations into intimal plaques, however, rarely result in aneurysmal formation unless the underlying media is also penetrated. Plaque disruption and hemorrhage are more likely to result in lumenal narrowing and thrombus formation. Pseudoaneurysms may also develop in association with vascular grafting procedures, particularly at anastomotic sites. Sutures used to perform the anastomosis may fatigue and break, and this effect may be potentiated if mismatched compliance of vessel and prosthesis causes excessive motion at the anastomotic site. Unlike the strong, healed tissue bond which forms when the edges of a transected artery have been approximated and sutured together, the seal between a prosthetic graft and an artery is dependent almost entirely upon the integrity of the sutures, even after many years. Silk sutures, which developed fatigue fractures after several years due to motion at the suture line with each heart beat, have now been replaced by more durable braided Dacron sutures. Infection at graft anastomoses have the same grave implications as mycotic aneurysms formed by embolization of infected material and may become sites of pseudoaneurysmal formation when the infected arterial wall disintegrates. It should be noted, however, that sites of vessel wall injury, or the occurrence of abnormal pressure and flow patterns, are particularly prone to infection. It is, therefore, not only exposure of the operative site and presence of accumulations of blood which favor bacterial localization and persistence of infection at anastomoses, but also local hemodynamic disturbances and the presence of foreign prosthetic material.

Endarterectomy might be expected to predispose to aneurysmal formation, for in addition to removal of intimal plaque, the entire media may be removed leaving only an adventitial tube to contain arterial blood pressure. Yet, aneurysmal formation under such conditions is rare. In experimental tests performed on human iliac artery segments, tensile strength was not diminished by endarterectomy (15, 39). In the long term, however, there is a distinct loss of distensibility, as the perivascular healing process results in the production of a relatively rigid fibrous tube.

SUMMARY

1. The mammalian arterial wall normally functions in a manner which tends to maintain medial tensile stress at a constant level for homologous vessels. The arterial media resists excessive dilatation and disruption and remains resilient, due to the composition of its matrix and the organization and cohesion of its structural units. Medial cells are responsible for the maintenance of medial matrix composition and medial organization in relation to modifications in medial stress.

2. There are essentially three modes of arterial wall alteration which may result in abnormal dilatations and outpouchings: a) chronic failure of the wall as a whole, extensively or locally, to maintain suitable thickness and composition for the stresses imposed (true aneurysms); b) loss or reduction of cohesion among the structural elements of the media, with resultant sudden splitting and separation of its structural units under increased stress (dissecting aneurysms); and c) penetration of blood through the arterial wall and into the surrounding tissues to form a local extravascular sac continuous with the bloodstream (pseudoaneurysms).

3. Dissociations among imposed mechanical stress, matrix composition and organization, media cell metabolism, and media nutrition probably underlie the development of most acquired true abdominal aortic aneurysms, for these are associated with overall dilatation of the aorta, atherosclerosis, and medial atrophy.

4. The human abdominal aorta appears to be at a functional disadvantage. Mammalian aortic walls of comparable thickness are furnished with medial vasa vasorum, but the human abdominal aorta is not. The tension per medial layer is much higher than in other mammalian arteries without medial vasa. In addition, aortic intimal thickening and atherosclerosis are most severe in the abdominal portion. Recent experimental data suggest that hyperlipidemia may inhibit the medial cellular response to stress and injuries, even in the absence of atherosclerotic plaques.

5. Syphilitic aneurysms occur in the thoracic aorta where medial vasa are normally abundant. Dilatations at this level are large and associated with patchy focal losses of matrix fibers, altered matrix organization, and scarring. Endarteritis involving the vasa may play a major role in this patchy atrophy, which ultimately leads to medial mechanical insufficiency and massive dilatation.

6. Dissecting aneurysms appear to be the result of rapid and sudden failures of interlamellar mural cohesion, probably due to an extensive, medial metabolic defect and mechanical tensile stresses which cause the mural cohesive defect to proceed to disruption. Initiation of disruption, primarily in the thoracic aorta and near the arch, suggests vasal supply and local mechanical stress may be important pathogenic factors. Intimal-medial disruptions may be secondary. Inadequacy of vasal supply may play a role by rendering the medial watershed zone between intimal diffusion and medial vasa supply ischemic. Disrupted vasa may also be a source of intramural hemorrhage.

7. In contrast to true aneurysms, either atherosclerotic or syphilitic, which appear to result from a chronic incapacity of the media to sustain normal or elevated medial tensions, pseudoaneurysms result from transmural interruptions of the arterial wall with local containment of the circulating blood by periarterial and serosal tissues. Continuity between the bloodstream and the newly formed periarterial blood space may be maintained for some time, but there is no encompassing arterial wall. Tissue support is, therefore, usually insufficient and the aneurysms continue to enlarge. Most pseudoaneurysms result from trauma or from

defects related to investigative procedures or complications of operative procedures. Pseudoaneurysms may also complicate true aneurysms.

References

1. Barron, M. V., Simpson, C. F., and Miller, E. S. Lathyrism: a review. *Q. Rev. Biol. 49:* 101–128, 1974.
2. Bomberger, R. A., Zarins, C. K., and Glagov, S. Medial injury and hyperlipidemia in development of aneurysms or atherosclerotic plaques. *Surg. Forum 31:* 338–340, 1980.
3. Burton, A. C. Relation of structure to function of the tissues of the wall of blood vessels. *Physiol. Rev. 4:* 619–642, 1954.
4. Busby, D. E., and Burton, A. C. The effect of age on the elasticity of the major brain arteries. *Can. J. Physiol. Pharmacol. 3:* 185–202, 1965.
5. Busuttil, R. W., Abou-Zamzam, A. M., and Machleder, H. I. Collagenase activity of the human aorta. *Arch. Surg. 115:* 1373–1378, 1980.
6. Busuttil, R. W., and Brin, B. J. The diagnosis and management of visceral artery aneurysms. *Surgery 88:* 619–824, 1980.
7. Clark, J. M., and Glagov, S. The smooth muscle facicle: arterial medial unit of structure and function. *Fed. Proc. 36(3):* 393, 1977.
8. Clark, J. M., and Glagov, S. Structural integration of the arterial wall. I. Relationships and attachments of medial smooth muscle cells in normally distended and hyperdistended aortas. *Lab. Invest. 40:* 587–602, 1979.
9. Cleary, E. G. Correlative and comparative study of the non-uniform arterial wall. Thesis, University of Sydney, 1963.
10. Crawford, T., and Levene, C. I. Medial thinning in atheroma. *J. Pathol. Bacteriol. 66:* 19–23, 1953.
11. Fischer, G. M., and Swain, M. L. Influence of contraceptive and other sex steroids on aortic collagen and elastin. *Exp. Mol. Pathol. 33:* 15–24, 1980.
12. Glagov, S. Hemodynamic risk factors: mechanical stress, mural architecture, medial nutrition and the vulnerability of arteries to atherosclerosis. In *Pathogenesis of Atherosclerosis*, edited by R. W. Wissler and J. C. Gear. Williams & Wilkins, Baltimore, 1972.
13. Gore, I., and Hirst, A. E., Jr. Dissecting aneurysm of the aorta. Clinical-pathologic correlations. *Cardiovasc. Clin. 2:* 239–260, 1973.
14. Gottfried, M., Yao, J., and Glagov, S. Vasa vasorum, mural tension and ultra structural organization of human atherosclerotic arteries. *Fed. Proc. 37:* 933–934, 1978.
15. Gryska, P. F. The physical properties of arteries after endarterectomy. *Surgery 113:* 227–229, 1961.
16. Hamlin, C. R., Luschin, J. H., and Kohn, R. R. Aging of collagen: comparative rates in four mammalian species. *Exp. Gerontol. 15:* 393–398, 1980.
17. Hartman, J. D. Structural changes within the media of coronary arteries related to intimal thickening. *Am. J. Pathol. 89:* 13–34, 1977.
18. Heistad, D. D., Marcus, M. L., Law, E. G., Armstrong, M. L., Ehrhardt, J. C., and Abboud, F. M. Regulation of blood flow to the aortic media in dogs. *J. Clin. Invest. 61:* 133–140, 1978.
19. Hornebeck, W., Adnet, J. J., and Robert, L. Age dependent variation of elastin and elastase in aorta and human breast cancers. *Exp. Gerontol. 13:* 293–298, 1978.
20. Hubert, J. P., Pairolero, P. C., and Kazmier, F. J. Solitary renal artery aneurysm. *Surgery 88:* 557–564, 1980.
21. Kanabrocki, E. L., Fels, I. G., and Kaplan, E. Calcium, cholesterol, and collagen levels in human aortas. *Am. J. Pathol. 90:* 383–387, 1978.
22. Knieriem, H-J., and Hueber, R. Quantitative morphologische untersuchugen an der aorta des menschen. *Beitr. Pathol. Anat. 140:* 280–297, 1970.
23. Leung, D. Y. M., Glagov, S., and Mathews, M. B. Elastin and collagen accumulation in rabbit ascending aorta and pulmonary trunk during postnatal growth: correlation of cellular synthetic response with medial tension. *Circ. Res. 41:* 316–323, 1977.
24. Manley, G. Changes in vascular mucopolysaccharides with age and blood pressure. *Br. J. Exp. Pathol. 66(2):* 125–134, 1964.
25. Martin, G. M., and Sprague, C. A. Symposium on *in vitro* studies related to atheroge-

nesis: life histories of hyperplastoid cell lines from aorta and skin. *Exp. Mol. Pathol. 18:* 125–141, 1973.
26. McKusick, V. *Heritable Disorders of Connective Tissue*, ed. 3. C. V. Mosby, St. Louis, 1966.
27. Mendez, J., and Tejada, C. Chemical composition of aortas from Guatemalans and North Americans. *Am. J. Clin. Pathol. 51:* 598–602, 1969.
28. Movat, H. Z., Moore, R. H., and Haust, M. D. The diffuse intimal thickening of the human aorta with aging. *Am. J. Pathol. 34:* 1023–1031, 1958.
29. Perdowitz, P., and Perell, A. Aneurysms complicated by pregnancy. I. Aneurysms of the aorta and its major branches. *Am. J. Obstet. Gynecol. 73:* 720–735, 1957.
30. Restrepo, C., Strong, J. P., Guzman, M. A., and Tejada, C. Geographic comparisons of diffuse intimal thickening of the aorta. *Atherosclerosis 32:* 177–193, 1979.
31. Roach, M. R. An experimental study of the production and time course of poststenotic dilatation in the femoral and carotid arteries of adult dogs. *Circ. Res. 13:* 537–551, 1963.
32. Sacks, A. H. The vasa vasorum as a link between hypertension and arteriosclerosis. *Angiology 26(5):* 385–390, 1975.
33. Sandberg, L. B., Soskel, N. T., and Leslie, J. G. Elastin structure, biosynthesis, and relation to disease states. *N. Engl. J. Med. 304:* 566–579, 1981.
34. Saruk, M., and Eisenstein, R. Aortic lesion in Marfan syndrome. *Arch. Pathol. Lab. Med. 101:* 74–77, 1977.
35. Schlatmann, T. J. M., and Becker, A. E. Histologic changes in the normal aging aorta: implications for dissecting aortic aneurysm. *Am. J. Cardiol. 39:* 13–20, 1977.
36. Schlatmann, T. J. M., and Becker, A. E. Pathogenesis of dissecting aneurysm of aorta. Comparative histopathologic study of significance of medial changes. *Am. J. Cardiol. 39:* 21–26, 1977.
37. Sirek, O. V., Sirek, A., and Fikar, K. The effect of sex hormones on glycosaminoglycan content of canine aorta and coronary arteries. *Atherosclerosis 27:* 227–233, 1977.
38. Stanley, J. C., and Fry, W. J. Pathogenesis and clinical significance of splenic artery aneurysms. *Surgery 76:* 898–901, 1974.
39. Sumner, D. S., Hokanson, E., and Strandness, D. E. Arterial walls before and after endarterectomy. *Arch. Surg. 99:* 606–611, 1969.
40. Suzuki, K., Hori, S., and Ooneda, G. Electron microscopic study on the medial defect at the apex of human cerebral arterial bifurcations. *Virchows Arch. (Pathol. Anat.) 382:* 151–161, 1979.
41. Thomas, W. A., Reiner, J. M., Florentin, R. A., and Scott, R. F. Population dynamics of arterial cells during atherogenesis. VIII. Separation of the roles of injury and growth stimulation in early aortic atherogenesis in swine originating in pre-existing intimal smooth muscle cell masses. *Exp. Mol. Pathol. 31:* 124–144, 1979.
42. Wilens, S. L., Malcolm, J. A., and Vazquez, J. M. Experimental infarction (medial necrosis) of the dog's aorta. *Am. J. Pathol. 47:* 695–711, 1965.
43. Wolinsky, H. Comparison of medial growth of human thoracic and abdominal aortas. *Circ. Res. 27:* 531–538, 1970.
44. Wolinsky, H. Response of the rat aortic media to hypertension: morphological and chemical studies. *Circ. Res. 26:* 507–522, 1970.
45. Wolinsky, H. Comparative effects of castration and antiandrogen treatment on the aortas of hypertensive and normotensive male rats. *Circ. Res. 33:* 183–189, 1973.
46. Wolinsky, H., and Glagov, S. Structural basis for the static mechanical properties of the aortic media. *Circ. Res. 14:* 400–413, 1964.
47. Wolinsky, H., and Glagov, S. A lamellar unit of aortic medial structure and function in mammals. *Circ. Res. 20:* 99–111, 1967.
48. Wolinsky, H., and Glagov, S. Nature of species differences in the medial distribution of aortic vasa vasorum in mammals. *Circ. Res. 20:* 409–421, 1967.
49. Wolinsky, H., and Glagov, S. Zonal differences in modelling of the mammalian aortic media during growth. *Fed. Proc. 26(2):* 357, 1967.
50. Wolinsky, H., and Glagov, S. Comparison of abdominal and thoracic aortic medial structure in mammals. Deviation of man from the usual pattern. *Circ. Res. 25:* 677–686, 1969.

CHAPTER 2

Physiology and Biomechanics of Aneurysms

PETER V. MOULDER, M.D.

Physiology and biomechanics have a mutual capability in precision of measurements and definitions in global descriptions of active processes, and in developing and describing systems—doing all of this in either micro- or macrocosms. Notably, the usual object of study is a normal situation. Sometimes even when the subject is normal, usually when it is distressed, and often when it is diseased or malfunctioning, these sciences require assumptions, restrictions, or limitations in definitions to such an extent that the descriptor is useless. Provincial differences in coding in various sciences often add to the confusion. Considerable limitation in the value of their contribution to the understanding and treatment of aneurysms would thus be predicted; however, useful information can be extracted from these resources which is of value in understanding aneurysms, and in selecting appropriate therapeutic systems.

INFRARENAL ABDOMINAL AORTA

The infrarenal abdominal aorta is a common site for development of arteriosclerotic aneurysms. An anatomic "fault," a startling species disparity in elastic lamination in the human infrarenal aorta, has been demonstrated by Wolinsky and Glagov (26). Is this sufficient cause for the infrarenal abdominal aorta to be a site of predilection for aneurysm? What abnormalities are present from the dynamic viewpoint?

Womersley (27) and others (8, 21) have shown that transmission of flowing blood through a junction is dependent upon the junctional cross-sectional area ratio (i.e., the ratio of the sum of the cross-sectional areas of the branch vessels to that of the vessel of origin). There is minimal reflection of the pressure pulse with a cross-sectional area ratio in the range of 1.15 to 1.26 for a two-vessel branch. This is referred to as "matched." In most species, the infrarenal aorta to the common iliac system is matched with the values greater than 1.15; however, humans are unmatched even at infancy with a value of 1.11—a value which continues to decrease, averaging about 0.75 at age 50 (20). In the presence of an ideal ratio, the increased cross-sectional area of the branch arteries results in a decrease in flow velocity, a decrease in tube Reynolds number (Re) (disturbance value), an increase in flow stability, and a minimization of pulsatile energy reflections. Therefore, the unmatching in the human aortoiliac system, which progresses over decades of life, undoubtedly contributes continuous detrimental effects on the hemodynamics of the infrarenal aorta, effects which are worsened in the presence of dilatation and aneurysm. A unique potential for disaster is presented when the obstructive/occlusive manifestations of arteriosclerotic disease can induce rapid, even sudden, decreases in the cross-sectional area ratio. In the experiments done by Newman and co-workers (16), studies were performed on the trifurcating canine terminal aorta, which has a cross-sectional area ratio of 1.23. Occlusion of the center or sural branch artery at this trifurcation reduces the ratio to 0.8, and produces a marked change in the character of the pulsatile pressure curves. Frequency and reflection phenomena demonstrate even more dramatic changes, which will be discussed below.

The distal portion of the infrarenal abdominal aorta has other unique characteristics as it forms the iliac arterial bifurcation. Measurements of elasticity and deformation indicate that it is the stiffest portion of the abdominal aorta (24). It is the primary site for receiving deleterious effects from distal obstructions, especially related to lateral pressure disturbances. It is also the important site for any dynamic disturbance which may be due to pulsatile reflections (10).

Attempts to measure elastic characteristics of the aneurysmal infrarenal abdominal aorta have produced little useful information, primarily due to the variability of the wall thickness. Applicable formulas are based on a homogenous viscoelastic wall and a constant wall thickness, both factors confounded by a variably thickened intima and overlying thrombus. There is also considerable variation in the degradation and thinning characteristics of the remaining elastic tissue, with no simple indication of the quantity or character of added collagen in the media and stimulated adventitia. Scattered data demonstrate obvious characteristics: an aneurysmal wall is weaker than a normal aorta, it is contained by the very hardness of the shell of vascular wall remnants with some support from the adventitia, and respite from dynamic factors is afforded by the thickened, fibrous intima and laminated thrombus.

LUMEN SHAPE AND ANEURYSMS

Tapering from beginning to end is a standard characteristic of the aorta. The relationships of velocity, flow, and diameter coincide with this taper. Attinger (1) demonstrated that geometrical tapering contributes to favorable transmission characteristics of the arterial tree by stabilizing the frequency-dependent factors of the input impedance. Appropriate taper is lost very early in the course of formation of an aneurysm and continues to be degraded with progressive enlargement of the aneurysm.

Divergence of blood flow, as occurs at the inlet of the aneurysm, leads to dynamic disturbances with a Bernoulli effect producing increased lateral pressure; retrograde vortices develop in the flow pattern and these are easily converted to turbulence (2, 4, 5). Suddenness of enlargement increases the disturbance and energy loss. Furthermore, these separation zones contribute to sites of sluggish flow where thrombosis can occur (18).

The human infrarenal abdominal aortic aneurysm is usually combined with other stigmata of atheromatous disease such as plaques, ulcers, and thromboses. These alterations produce a variety of obstructing lesions which contribute to the dynamic disturbances. The parabolic leading front of flow slows down before it meets an obstruction where it stops, thus producing points of stasis on the proximal as well as the distal side. Accelerations of flow occur on the surface and recirculating eddies occur beyond it, simulating the "wake" seen in the water behind a ship. In all of these situations, the critical Re at which turbulence can occur is lowered (i.e., disturbance and turbulence can occur at lower levels of velocity and/or in smaller-dimensioned vessel lumina).

FLOW CONCEPTS AND CLINICAL ANEURYSMAL DISEASE

Laminar flow represents flow as a set of parallel laminae, such that two entering branches to a single tube would produce two parallel sets of flow; thus, the equivalent term is streamline flow. Turbulent flow represents chaotic motion in the flow pattern. Disturbed flow represents a pattern between these two (20, 21).

The Reynolds number (Re) is the mathematical descriptor of flow disturbance. A Re is the ratio of inertial forces to frictional forces—the ratio of velocity × dimension × fluid density to viscosity. Think of a Re as velocity × dimension (usually diameter). Hydrodynamic studies in standard pipes indicate Re of 2,300 as the critical point where a disturbance in the wall will convert laminar to turbulent flow. The human, adult thoracic aortic blood flow has a Re of 1,200 to 2,000; large arteries have a Re of 110 to 850. Blunt points, divergence of walls, curved or sharp turns, and other factors lower this critical number. In pulsatile flow, a frequency or heart rate factor is added. Use of the Strouhal number or α indices brings frequency into the equation (11).

Goldstein (7) has developed a formulation of the effect of a projection in the lumen: if ϵ = height of projection, then $\epsilon/\text{radius} < 4/(\text{Re})^{1/2}$ must hold in the presence of a sharp-edged projection to maintain laminar flow. For example, a sharp-edge value of 1/5 would be tolerated in a vessel with a Re of 400. If a normal infrarenal abdominal aorta has flow characteristics associated at rest with Re of about 1,500, then an aneurysm with twice the diameter would double this number, and plaques would disturb any flow, and they would produce turbulence when over 2 mm in height.

Thus, it is unfortunate that calculation of actual Re's is not of value in discussing complex aneurysms. There may be some value in such measurements in evaluating berry aneurysms of the circle of Willis (3), or splenic artery aneurysms. Understanding the concept of critical levels of diameter-velocity relationship to turbulence and some of the factors which modify this, however, is of value to clinicians.

As blood is pulsated through the vascular tree, there are points where the flow is snubbed, dampened, and even blocked. From these sites, pulsatile reflections occur. The two major, normal reflection sites are the distal end of the aorta and the final small branches in the peripheral arterial bed. These reflections are generally dissipated or countered by other unique characteristics of the system (tethering, in particular) so that normal heart action is minimally disturbed. Many of the unique extra peaks on pulsatile pressure and flow waveforms are secondary to these reflections. As mentioned above, these reflections are exaggerated by abdominal aortic outlet abnormalities in the human.

Pulsatile flow is generally presented in a form representing an average of many different cross-sectional velocity patterns. Such is the pulsatile waveform obtained from an electromagnetic flowmeter. Observed throughout systole and diastole, however, the "neat" layers of laminar flow actually occur only at major points in systole. As systole is completed, there is stoppage and, eventually, even reversal of flow. Furthermore, these components are different across the cross-section of the vessel. The major point of motion is at the axis or center, whereas the velocity is much less and reversal of flow occurs earlier along the wall. Add this concept of cross-sectional uniqueness of flow characteristics to those flow differences occurring throughout systole and diastole, and all the aforementioned flow disturbances—the carefully conceived dynamics of flow—are lost in the complexity of flow of blood in an aneurysm.

FREQUENCY PHENOMENA AND ANEURYSMS

When a white light passes through a glass prism, a rainbow is produced. The rainbow represents the frequency-component colors composing white light. Many chemical analytic tools measure the magnitude of a transmitted or reflected signal—a frequency characteristic of the molecule or compound to be measured. Similarly, a continuously variable signal can be represented as a summation of sine waves of various frequencies. To look at these, a mathematical rather than glass prism is used. For pulsatile pressure and flow, which are almost periodic sine waves, the prism is a Fourier series which will dissect in rate-related or harmonic terms. This is used to define vascular impedance in pulsatile terms. The usual clinical measure of resistance is a non-pulsatile measurement, mean flow divided by mean pressure: $R = \overline{P}/\overline{F}$. To measure the oscillatory contribution to resistance, the Fourier series prism is applied to the pulsatile pressure divided by pulsatile flow. The measure or modulus at zero frequency is the same as the standard resistance measured from mean data. Production of a major obstruction of the abdominal aorta in an experimental animal produces minimal changes in the harmonic resistance values measured at the ascending aorta; therefore, the heart faces limited oscillatory resistive phenomena (23). Measurements of pressure and flow near the site of obstruction, however, demonstrate unique changes even with limited obstruction to flow. In addition to the form and size changes in the pulsatile pressures shown in the Newman and Bowden (15) experiments with occlusion of the sural artery of the dog, harmonic-related abnormalities were also demonstrated in the analysis of the pressure pulse which would modify the local impedance plot. Limited clinical use of impedance measurements has been striking in demonstrating resistive changes in the pulmonary artery (12), and shown to be of modest value from measurements in the ascending aortas (17). Whether the techniques will be of value with respect to evaluation of aneurysms is not clear, as sufficient data are not yet available. Impedance measurements represent a small area in the present context of frequency analysis, pattern analysis, and digital signal processing; therefore, more information in such analyses may be anticipated.

The last item of flow and frequency phenomena of consequence to aneurysmal dynamics is reflection (11, 25). When a pressure or flow pulse meets the iliac branching site it produces a reverberation, or reflected wave, of sufficient consequence to modify the true wave (referred to as incident wave) to produce the measured, transmitted wave. Similar major reflections occur from the distal, small vascular bed. Many minor reflections occur throughout the major branching vascular system and, of course, new reflections occur with major obstructions and distortions in diseased vessels. Reflected waves modify pulsatile waveforms and also change the modulus value of the low harmonics in impedance plots. A major reflection increases lateral pressure, and produces disconsonant flow effects on and near the aneurysmal wall. These are not measurable, so again we gain only from the knowledge, not from specific data.

INFORMATION FROM EXPERIMENTAL ANEURYSMS

Scherer's (19) studies of aneurysmal dynamics in glass models demonstrate the following: 1) Flow develops into a recirculating vortex within the aneurysm which is maintained until turbulence occurs. 2) The critical Re is high (2,000 to 3,000) in his models—estimates indicate the critical Re depends upon the dimensions of the aneurysm; and, as the aneurysmal lumen enlarges, this Re is soon passed (even in small aneurysms) with normal, quiescent-subject blood flows. 3) There are no abnormally high pressures as might be anticipated from boundary layer or other phenomena—that the pressures lie between those found above and below the aneurysm. 4) Estimates of shear stress indicate that it can be an order of magnitude higher than upstream or downstream before turbulence appears, and that it may be more important than turbulence in being responsible for deterioration of elastic laminae in the aneurysmal wall.

These studies with ink patterns in glass models cannot be used quantitatively; however, they point directly to the problems that the size of the aneurysm makes some difference (worse when large), but they also indicate that even small aneurysms are dramatic and destructive in their hydrodynamic properties. Jain (9) studied the latex aneurysm in plastic tube systems and his findings show deleterious effects from pulsatile pressure (especially from the peak of pressure), as well as from distal obstructions and occlusion. With double aneurysms, the proximal one is the more pulsatile and the one with greater *intrinsic* potential for rupture. The latter idea is striking as surgeons commonly see the smaller, proximal infrarenal aortic aneurysm rupture, no matter how great the disparity in size with respect to the second distal, larger aneurysm.

Ferguson (3), German and Black (6), and others (9, 19) have studied models of berry-like aneurysms. Valuable concepts from their studies are useful for understanding the different, systemic aneurysms, and the character of flow which produces stasis and clot formation. This is increasingly important in larger aneurysms, especially when the orifice is small in relation to the size of the aneurysm. This equates with the longevity of some huge lateral aneurysms with restricted orifices often seen even in the thoracic aorta. Small orifice size is common with false aneurysms and may contribute to their longevity.

Sumner *et al.* (22) studied 13 postmortem specimens of infrarenal aortic aneurysms, using careful segmental measurements and chemical analysis of collagen-elastin content. They found the aneurysms to be stiff but little different from that of control aortas, especially the normally stiff terminal aorta as mentioned above. Collagen and elastin content were much less than that of controls and these substances were concentrated in the outer shell. These data suggest that the compacted outer shell of the aortic aneurysm and a buffering layer of clot to impede shear stress are the major mechanisms of intrinsic control of rupture. We can infer the slimness of these controls.

This laboratory has used a frequency domain measurement technique, transfer function, akin to "black box" engineering measurements, for evaluation of left ventricular dynamics demonstrating an empiric value to this approach (13). Using a mathematical prism, the discrete Fourier transform, which extracts all-dimensional, even fractional, frequency content from the studied signal, power spectra and autocorrelations are obtained for each pressure and flow waveform. Specific interrelationships are then developed: cross-spectra, cross-correlations, transfer function, and coherence. Transfer function, which is a complex form of division of any two signals, has proved to be the most valuable tool (14). Analyses have been performed on three types of "aneurysms" in the thoracic aorta—a stiff Dacron sac on the side of a Dacron graft, a transplanted bicaval connected right atrium, and a rubber patch. Each type modifies the transfer function compared to the baseline state and the characteristics are different for each. Thus, these tools may prove helpful in distinguishing the stiff, clotted aneurysm with a near-normal central flow from the empty aneurysm with or without major wall pulsations. If subsequent data are supportive, there may also be useful information on size-pressure dynamic relations. The latter, if obtainable with echo-pulsed Doppler techniques, could be used to evaluate time changes and for evaluation of the probable deleterious effects of excessive activity and stress with their concomitant increases in blood flow velocity and pulsatility.

SUMMARY

In summary, studies from the dynamic sciences contribute to an understanding of the ubiquitous aneurysm and can aid in decisions concerning treatment; however, at present they offer little in actual measurements, the basic need for scientific decision.

1. Iliac arterial outlet mismatch, loss of tethering, increased reflections, wall divergence energetics, and wall stiffness add to the anatomic and biochemical characteristics which make the infrarenal abdominal aorta the major site for atherosclerotic aneurysmal formation.
2. Further outlet mismatch or increase in reflections, as commonly occurs with distal obstructive/occlusive disease, produces a greater dynamic disturbance and rupture potential at the proximal site of an aneurysm.
3. Local obstructions, distortions, and channel divergences are dynamically deleterious to aneurysms.
4. The importance of higher velocity and larger diameters, described in critical Re's, supports our recognition of the need for surgical intervention in aneurysms—especially when growing, large, pulsatile, and/or in a hypertensive patient.
5. The dynamics of unique, unruptured aneurysms, often cited as indicating lack of necessity of surgery, make more sense and such disclaimers can be contradicted with dynamic data as well as empiric case data.
6. The protection afforded by laminated intraluminal clots is clarified. It is also obvious that an inlet site with no clot and wide-angle divergence would nullify that protection, and that presence of a major luminal clot could obscure demonstration of such inlet divergence.
7. A proximal small aneurysm can rupture as readily as a large distal one.
8. Most of these and other points of interest acquired from dynamic studies strongly support the contention that we have no measure of aneurysmal rupture potential. An aneurysm of almost any size can be dangerous when considered from the viewpoint of the many potential dynamic phenomena that contribute to its rupture potential.

References

1. Attinger, E. O. (Ed.) *Pulsatile Blood Flow.* McGraw-Hill, New York, 1964.
2. Crowe, W. J., Jr., and Krovetz, J. Studies of arterial branching in models using flow birefringence. *Med. Biol. Engl. 10:* 415–426, 1972.
3. Ferguson, G. G. Turbulence in human intracranial saccular aneurysms. *J. Neurosurg. 33:* 485–497, 1970.
4. Forrester, J. H., and Young, D. F. Flow through a converging-diverging tube and its implications in occlusive vascular disease. I. Theoretical development. *J. Biomech. 3:* 297–305, 1970.
5. Forrester, J. H., and Young, D. F. Flow through a converging-diverging tube and its implications in occlusive vascular disease. II. Theoretical and experimental results and their implications. *J. Biomech. 3:* 307–316, 1970.

6. German, W. J., and Black, S. P. W. Intra-aneurysmal hemodynamics: turbulence. *Trans. Am. Neurol. Assoc. 79:* 163–165, 1954.
7. Goldstein, S. *Modern Developments in Fluid Dynamics*, vol. 2, p. 142. Clarendon Press, 1938.
8. Gosling, R. G., Newman, D. L., Bowden, N. L. R., and Twinn, K. W. The area ratio of normal aortic junctions. Aortic configuration and pulse wave reflection. *Br. J. Radiol. 44:* 850–853, 1971.
9. Jain, K. K. Mechanism of rupture of intracranial saccular aneurysms. *Surgery 54:* 347–350, 1963.
10. Kai-ming Tam, M., Melbin, J., and Knight, D. H. Hemodynamic phenomena in fusiform aneurysms. II. Pulsatile flow conditions. *IEEE Trans. Biomed. Eng. BME-24:* 24–28, 1977.
11. McDonald, D. A. *Blood Flow in Arteries*, ed. 2. Williams & Wilkins, Baltimore, 1974.
12. Milnor, W. R. Pulsatile blood flow. *N. Engl. J. Med. 287:* 27–34, 1972.
13. Moulder, P. V., Flauto, B., and Daicoff, G. R. Time series analysis for cardiovascular signals. In *Proceedings of the San Diego Biomedical Symposium*, vol. 16, pp. 487–492, Academic Press, New York, 1977.
14. Moulder, P. V., Flauto, B., Gallet, B., Galansky, S., and Alexander, J. A. Apperceptive signals demonstrating the dynamic disturbance of myocardial ischemia. *Surgery 85:* 71–81, 1979.
15. Newman, D. L., and Bowden, N. L. R. Effect of reflection from an unmatched junction on the abdominal aortic impedance. *Cardiovasc. Res. 7:* 827–833, 1973.
16. Newman, D. L., Gosling, R. G., Bowden, N. L. R., and King, D. H. Pressure amplitude increase on unmatching the aortic-iliac junction of the dog. *Cardiovasc. Res. 7:* 6–13, 1973.
17. Nichols, W. W., Conti, C. R., Walker, W. E., and Milnor, W. P. Input impedance of the systemic circulation in man. *Circ. Res. 40:* 451–458, 1977.
18. Roach, M. R. Blood flow and thrombosis, particularly in aneurysms. *Can. J. Surg. 23* (Supplement): 123–137, 1973.
19. Scherer, P. W. Flow in axisymmetrical glass model aneurysms. *J. Biomech. 6:* 695–700, 1973.
20. Stehbens, W. E. (Ed.) *Hemodynamics and the Blood Vessel Wall.* Charles C Thomas, Springfield, Ill., 1979.
21. Strandness, D. E., Jr., and Sumner, D. S. *Hemodynamics for Surgeons.* Grune & Stratton, New York, 1975.
22. Sumner, D. S., Hokanson, D. E., and Strandness, D. E., Jr. Stress-strain characteristics and collagen-elastin content of abdominal aortic aneurysms. *Surg. Gynecol. Obstet. 130:* 459–466, 1970.
23. Taylor, M. G. The input impedance of an assembly of randomly branching elastic tubes. *Biophys. J. 6:* 29–51, 1966.
24. Taylor, M. G. *The Optimum Elastic Properties of Arteries in Circulatory and Respiratory Mass Transport*, edited by G. E. W. Wolstenholme and J. Knight, pp. 136–147. Little, Brown, New York, 1969.
25. Wemple, R. R., and Mockros, L. F. Pressure and flow in the systemic arterial system. *J. Biomech. 5:* 629–641, 1972.
26. Wolinsky, H., and Glagov, S. Comparison of abdominal and thoracic aortic medial structure in mammals. *Circ. Res. 25:* 677–686, 1969.
27. Womersley, J. R. Oscillatory flow in arteries. II. The reflection of the pulse wave at junctions and rigid inserts in the arterial system. *Phys. Med. Biol. 2:* 313–323, 1958.

CHAPTER 3

Carotid and Subclavian Aneurysms

HUSHANG JAVID, M.D., PH.D.
GIACOMO A. DELARIA, M.S., M.D.

CAROTID ANEURYSMS

Aneurysms of the extracranial carotid arteries are rarely encountered by the vascular surgeon; nevertheless, they represent a significant diagnostic and management problem when found. Located in accessible regions of the neck, their presence is seldom difficult to define; however, carotid aneurysms must be differentiated from other commonly encountered cervical masses. Failure to make this differentiation has resulted in many early reports of catastrophe when a presumed abscess, subsequently determined to be an arterial aneurysm, was lanced (55).

Historical Perspective

A true incidence of carotid aneurysms has never been accurately determined. Large institutions with extensive carotid surgical experiences report few aneurysms. Raphael *et al.* (44), at the Mayo Clinic, found 6 cases during a 27-year period and Beall *et al.* (5), at Baylor, found 7 carotid aneurysms in a series of 2,300 aneurysms operated upon at their institution. More recent reviews from the Universities of Michigan and UCLA report an experience with 23 and 19 carotid artery aneurysms collected, respectively, over more than 15 years (8, 45). Series which limit themselves to true aneurysms are even smaller. Kaupp *et al.* (30) collected only 13 cases between two institutions' total experience with carotid artery aneurysms. Schechter (48, 49), in his large review of this subject, could find reports of only 853 cervical carotid aneurysms occurring in 820 patients over a period lasting 290 years and ending in 1977.

The natural history of carotid aneurysms is unclear. Winslow (65), in 1926, reported 35 patients left untreated with diagnosed carotid artery aneurysms. Of these patients, 71% died within one year of complications of their aneurysms; however, this is a very early experience with a heavy concentration of mycotic and traumatic aneurysms, both of which are more likely to grow rapidly and rupture. Recently, Busuttil *et al.* (8), in reviewing their experience, found 6 of 19 patients who were not surgically treated because of concern about distal control. Of these, one was lost to follow up and another experienced a single transient ischemic attack; the remaining four were neurologically unchanged. They argue that in the absence of neurologic symptoms these aneurysms are best left alone.

Pathophysiology

A carotid artery becomes aneurysmal in three ways with equal frequency: spontaneously, after infection, or following trauma. Spontaneous aneurysms are usually the result of atherosclerosis and are more common in males, occurring with equal frequency on the right and the left (36). Approximately 10% are bilateral (39). They can occur anywhere along the carotid tree, but usually involve the carotid bifurcation or the internal carotid artery. Only two cases of aneurysms limited to the external carotid artery have been described (29). Importantly, more than 25% of patients with atherosclerotic carotid aneurysms have evidence of aneurysms elsewhere in the arterial system (8, 36).

Congenital aneurysms do occur and are usually the result of medial disruption (20). Approximately four cases of carotid aneurysms associated with cystic medial necrosis are in the literature (20) and we have experienced one patient with medial necrosis and acute dissection producing an aneurysm. Occasionally, acute carotid dissection can present as a stroke and then produce an aneurysm (7). Carotid ectasia and "beading" is possible in patients with fibromuscular dysplasia, but a true aneurysm has not been described in this condition.

Mycotic carotid aneurysms are secondary to locally invasive sepsis or hematogenously spread infections. The former usually involve the high internal carotid artery and often present in the pharynx; the latter are located in the common carotid or at its bifurcation (48, 49). Pharyngeal abscess, mastoiditis, and cervical adenitis, especially tuberculosis, have all been associated with carotid aneurysms. Syphilis, in the past, was responsible for many aneurysms; but, recent experience documents no case of syphilis complicated by a cervical carotid aneurysm. Acute mycotic aneurysms have recently been added to the list of those complications of drug abuse. Three cases of heroin addicts who developed carotid artery infections and aneurysms following accidental carotid artery injection are described (31).

Traumatic carotid aneurysms represent the final, major category in this condition; most are the result of penetrating trauma. The majority of carotid artery injuries are lethal; however, delayed aneurysms following both high-velocity missile injuries and puncture wounds have been recorded (48, 49). The aneurysms usually involve the carotid bifurcation or internal carotid, as the common carotid rests deep and is protected from injury. However, the common carotid can be injured, particularly after stab wounds or fractures of the clavicle and first rib. One peculiar variety of carotid artery trauma is that associated with mandibular fracture. Force sufficient to crush the mandible can compress the internal carotid artery between the mandibular angle and the transverse process of the atlas (8). The artery is fractured and an aneurysm is produced. Other forms of blunt trauma, such as karate chops or neck-wrenching twists, have also resulted in carotid artery aneurysms, but these are rare (57).

Iatrogenic trauma can also be responsible for the development of carotid aneurysms, occurring following carotid angiography (particularly in those cases where direct puncture technique is utilized). Aneurysms can also develop following carotid endarterectomy. This particular complication of carotid surgery has almost disappeared since the introduction of braided polyester and monofilament sutures. Earlier cases were thought to result from suture-line disruptions associated with silk suture degeneration (36).

Clinical Presentation

Symptoms associated with carotid artery aneurysms result from either the mass or embolization of the material within the aneurysms. Many carotid aneurysms protrude into the pharynx and are, therefore, not noticed by the patient. This is particularly true for those internal carotid swellings high in the neck. Similarly, common carotid aneurysms can grow to a large size and remain ill-defined on physical examination. Aneurysms can often produce symptoms by traction, pressure, or irritation of adjacent normal structures. Pressure on the cervical sympathetic chain can produce Horner's syndrome, and vagus involvement can result in hoarseness. Symptoms of dysphagia have been caused by pressure on the glossopharyngeal nerve or the hypoglossal nerve. Earache occurs when the auriculotemporal nerve is compressed, and spinal accessory nerve pressure produces shoulder pain (48, 49).

Central symptomatology, characteristic of carotid aneurysms, does not differ from that constellation of problems associated with carotid artery disease. Sudden or complete aneurysmal occlusion by thrombosis can produce stroke. Partial occlusion is responsible for cerebral ischemic complaints such as lightheadedness, dizziness, or transient paresis. Emboli from the sac can produce profound stroke or transient ischemic attack, according to the size of the particle and its eventual location. Nine of 19 patients in the series of Rhodes *et al.* (45) had central neurologic complaints. Three had complete strokes, three had transient ischemic attacks, and three experienced amaurosis fugax. Twelve of 19 patients in the UCLA series (8) presented central symptoms, as did five of 34 patients in the report by McCollum *et al.* (36) from Baylor. Taber (61) discussed one patient with ball valve occlusion of a carotid aneurysm. Certain position changes produced carotid occlusion and symptoms of cerebral ischemia.

True carotid aneurysms increase in size with time, but rupture or bleeding is extremely uncommon (46). False aneurysms, particularly post-traumatic and mycotic types, do rupture spontaneously. Rapid growth and resultant inflammation around the enlarging vessel can make a differential diagnosis between an abscess and a rupturing aneurysm difficult. Aneurysms which increase rapidly in size require immediate diagnosis and surgical management. Ruptured cervical carotid aneurysms are difficult to control and the risk of major cerebral injury is high.

Cervical carotid aneurysms are not difficult to diagnose, except in the presence of marked inflammation or infection. In the absence of calcification or complete thrombosis, the aneurysms pulsate. Most aneurysms produce cervical systolic murmurs. Presence of a diastolic, continuous murmur indicates the rare complication of a carotid arteriovenous fistula rather than an aneurysm. An intraoral examination is imperative and visualization of a bulging pharynx or displacement of the uvula away from the aneurysm is typical. Bimanual examination will confirm the aneurysm's presence and location.

Diagnostic Evaluation

Noninvasive vascular diagnostic techniques have been infrequently applied to cervical aneurysms. Ultrasonic imaging would easily define most aneurysms and could be useful for long-term follow up. The advent of the computerized axial tomography (CAT) scan with contrast has provided surgeons with information concerning the lumen, amount of thrombus, and thickness of the walls and surrounding tissue. Evaluation of cerebral blood flow of oculoplethysmography is of value to exclude hemodynamically significant stenoses. This physiologic information is particularly useful in cases where carotid ligation is a therapeutic consideration. Supraorbital Doppler evaluation supplies similar information. Oculoplethysmography, in association with ipsilateral carotid compression, can provide important information about the competency of the circle of Willis. However, failure to document a reduction in ophthalmic artery pressure or supraorbital artery flow reversal does not guarantee the involved cerebral hemisphere will tolerate carotid occlusion. Additionally, in most cases the risk of cerebral embolism from carotid aneurysm manipulation is too high to warrant this diagnostic procedure.

X-ray is the keystone of diagnosis. Often, soft tissue films will outline an aneurysm, but diagnosis is confirmed by angiography. Angiograms must be four-vessel studies to completely define the arch, its branches, and status of the intracerebral circulation. Because atherosclerotic disease is responsible for more than 50% of all aneurysms, concomitant occlusive disease in the arch vessels must be diagnosed or excluded. The intracranial extension of an aneurysm, or the presence of multiple aneurysms, can be ascertained. Angiography is also important to define the type of aneurysm. Fusiform aneurysms are most typical of the atherosclerotic type, whereas saccular aneurysms are usually mycotic or posttraumatic. This information is important for both diagnosis and management, as saccular aneurysms are technically less difficult to manage. Finally, kinked or tortuous carotid arteries or cervical masses adherent to the carotid artery and masquerading as aneurysms, as well as carotid body tumors, can be differentiated best by contrast angiography.

Therapy

Operative management of the patient with a carotid artery aneurysm represents a major challenge. Not only does the surgeon have the responsibility of cerebral protection, but he must also deal with difficult anastomoses at the base of the skull and avoid injury to vital nerves which can be displaced from their usual location or buried in the wall of the pulsating mass. Both technical facility and complete familiarity with the various approaches to vascular reconstruction are essential.

The history of deliberate carotid aneurysm surgery begins with Sir Astley Cooper, as described in the review by Shipley *et al.* (55). Prior to his experience, carotid aneurysms had, for the most part, been diagnosed with lances. The early literature is replete with reports of explosive hemorrhage, carotid ligation, hemiplegia, and death. Cooper first ligated a common carotid aneurysm in 1805; this patient succumbed to complications of hemiplegia. Three years later, Cooper successfully performed the same operation and this patient survived 13 years without incident. Contemporary vascular surgical techniques were first applied to carotid artery surgery in 1956 by Dimtza (13). He resected an aneurysm and repaired the defect with an end-to-end anastomosis. Shea and Harrison (54) reported the same procedure in 1953. Subsequently, many authors have achieved successful control and repair of carotid artery aneurysms. There is little controversy regarding the indications and techniques in most cases; however, the various presentations of aneurysms require some discussion, particularly regarding techniques of repair.

The simplest form of aneurysm to repair is the saccular aneurysm—usually post-traumatic and false, but occasionally atherosclerotic. Although the aneurysm can be large, repair is less complex because the proximal and distal arteries are usually healthy. One case from our collection demonstrates a method for the management of a saccular aneurysm. Angiography (Fig. 3.1) defined a large, saccular aneurysm at the carotid bifurcation on the right. After careful dissection, the aneurysm was separated from adjacent structures and proximal and distal control were achieved (Fig. 3.2). The aneurysm was opened and a Javid shunt inserted to maintain cerebral perfusion (Fig. 3.3). Although carotid aneurysm surgery can be accomplished without shunting, these operations take longer than the usual carotid endarterectomy and satisfactory cerebral perfusion through shunting provides protection. Extra care is necessary during the insertion of the shunt. Aneurysms are filled with debris and a clean artery, above and below, must be assured to eliminate the possibility of cerebral embolization. Also, in the case of traumatic or mycotic aneurysms where vessel walls are fragile, direct visualization of the arterial lumen is required to avoid dissection and possible perfusion of a false channel. After control is obtained, most false and saccular aneurysms can be resected and repaired with a vein patch (Fig. 3.4). Usually autogenous saphenous vein is utilized for the patch, but standard graft materials can also be used.

Traumatic aneurysms can represent a difficult surgical challenge because of their size and the scar tissue between the aneurysm and the adjacent vital structures. Dissection for control can be difficult. A traumatic aneurysm taken from our earlier experience was the result of a missile wound. Typical of high-velocity injuries, the artery was trauma-

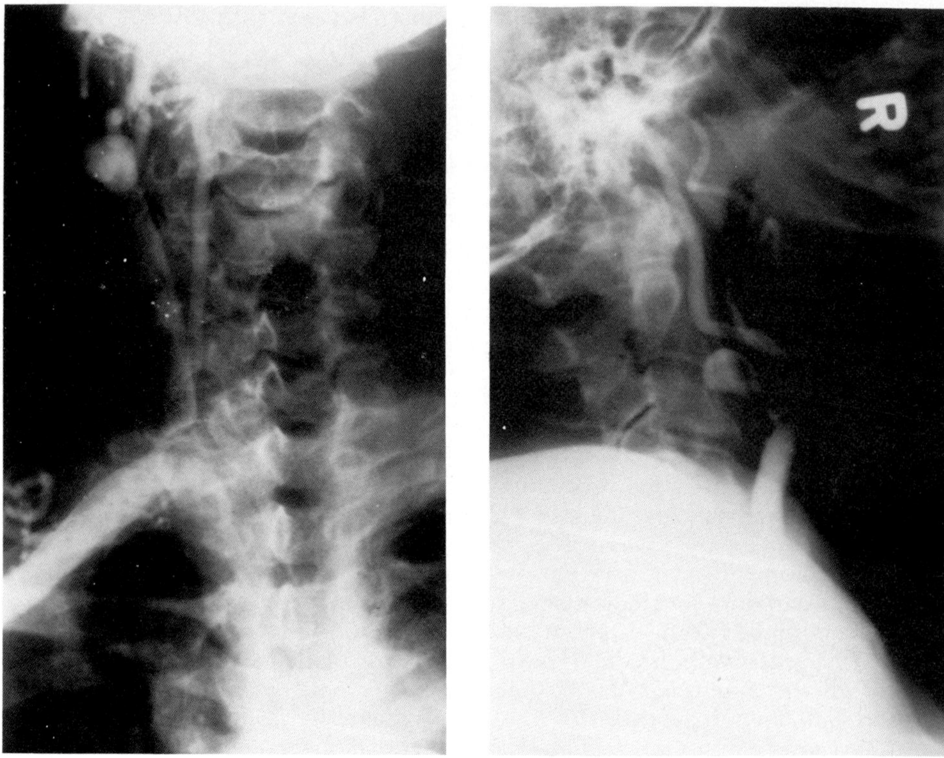

Figure 3.1. Arteriogram demonstrating large, saccular aneurysm arising at carotid bifurcation.

tized for a great distance. The aneurysm involved the common carotid, its bifurcation, and branches (Fig. 3.5). It could be easily seen and palpated and a plain X-ray of the neck showed a spherical mass (Fig. 3.6). The repair required resection of the bifurcation and internal carotid artery and continuity was restored by an arterial homograft (Fig. 3.7).

Carotid aneurysms involving the internal carotid and terminating high near the base of the skull require special techniques, making management difficult and controversial. In most cases, the aneurysm is small enough to resect and repair by end-to-end anastomosis. In another case from our experience, the aneurysm appeared high on carotid angiography (Fig. 3.8). Mobilization allowed exposure of the distal carotid and demonstration of the aneurysm (Fig. 3.9). By placing a shunt through a separate arteriotomy below and then through the aneurysm, it was possible to obtain control of the distal vessel and pull it down. The aneurysm was resected and end-to-end anastomotic repair of the internal carotid artery achieved over the shunt, which served both to maintain cerebral perfusion

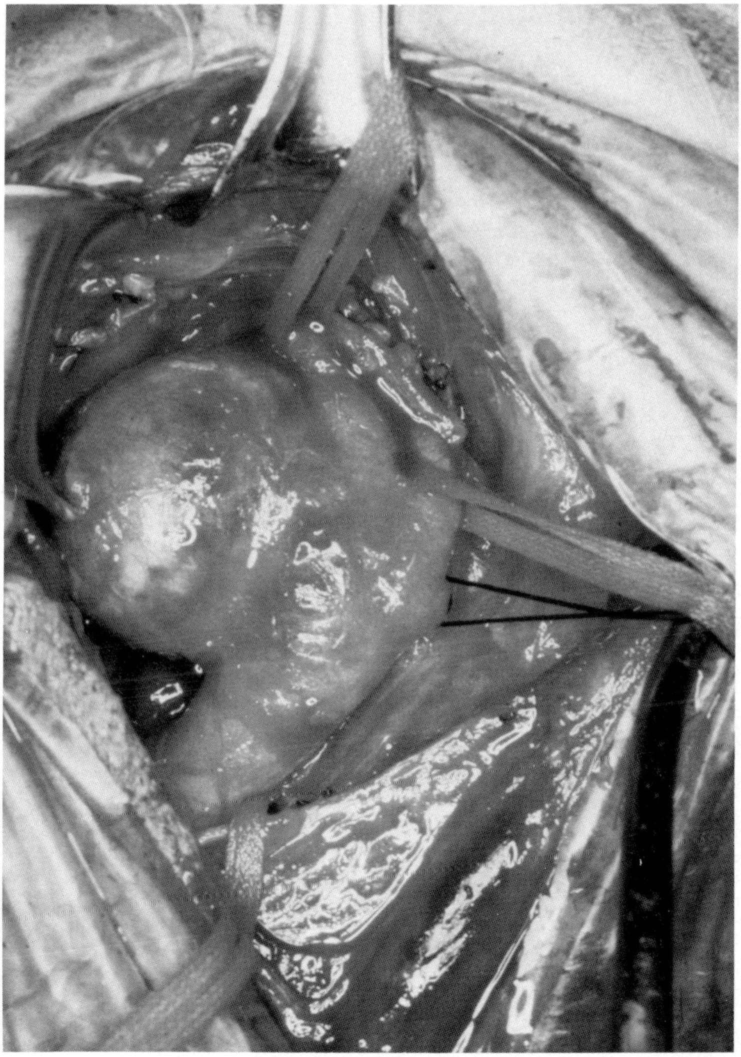

Figure 3.2. Saccular aneurysm at carotid bifurcation—tapes define normal-appearing common, internal, and external carotid arteries.

and stent the vessel (Fig. 3.10*A* to *D*). The shunt was easily removed and the low arteriotomy repaired.

Certain high carotid aneurysms cannot be managed in this fashion and the major technical problem becomes control of the distal carotid artery. Options for management include observation, ligation, direct repair, and extracranial carotid bypass.

Ligation is an effective treatment for high carotid aneurysms; however,

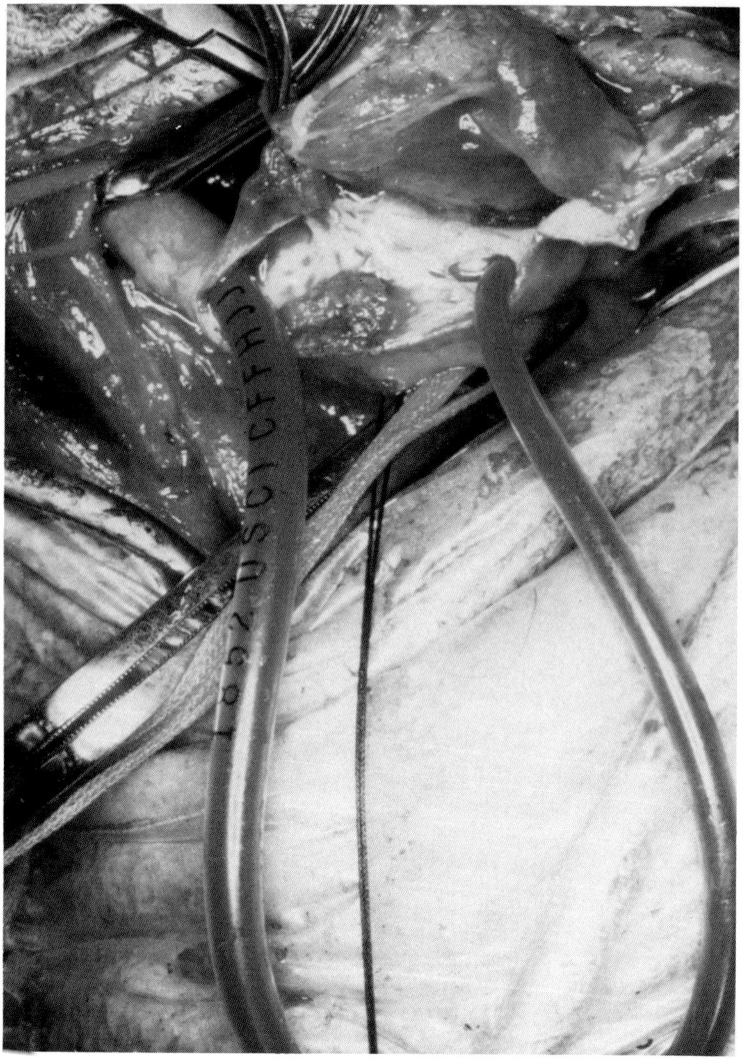

Figure 3.3. Cerebral perfusion maintained by an intraluminal shunt; aneurysmal sac partially excised.

the risk of major stroke is high and unpredictable. Most series quote a 30% risk of stroke following carotid ligation (21). If ligation of the aneurysm is to be undertaken, certain physiologic information is necessary to confirm its safety. Leech *et al.* (32) demonstrated that the brain will survive without injury in all cases where cerebral blood flow exceeds 40 ml per minute per 100 g of brain tissue. Flows less than 20 ml per minute per 100 g of brain tissue are always associated with significant brain damage. Between these two extremes, brain function is preserved

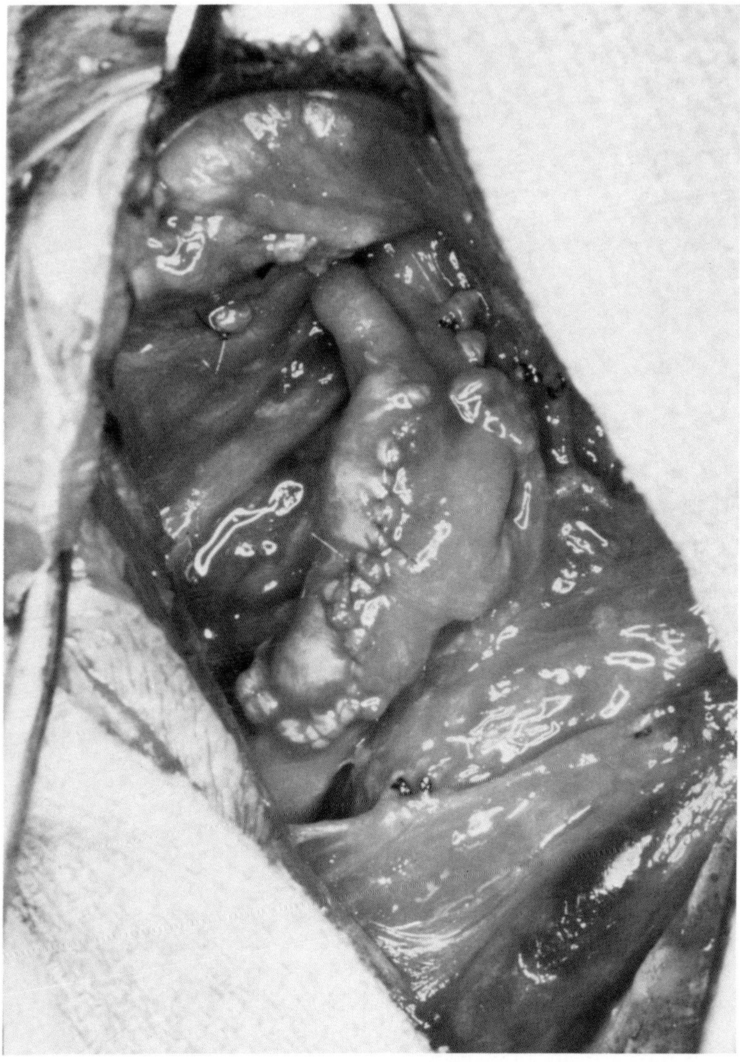

Figure 3.4. Defect in carotid artery repaired with vein patch.

if total cerebral blood flow is at least 75% of the pre-ligation value and the internal carotid stump pressure is greater than 60 mm Hg. Oller *et al.* (41) used oculoplethysmography as a guide to the safety of carotid ligation. They concluded, after studying four patients, that an ophthalmic artery pressure which remained above 80 mm Hg following ipsilateral temporary carotid occlusion indicated permanent occlusion was safe.

If carotid ligation is to be undertaken electively, it can be safely performed in the following manner. The patient should be operated on

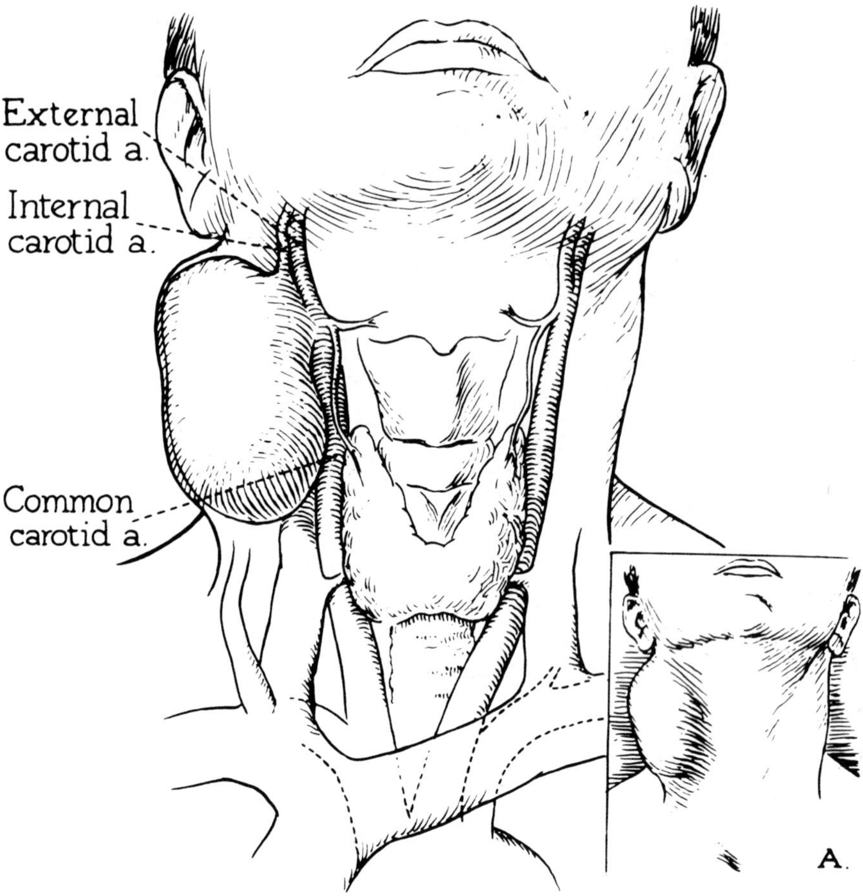

Figure 3.5. Large, traumatic, carotid aneurysm exhibiting a false sac involving common and internal carotid arteries; mass was easily seen and palpated (*inset*).

under local anesthesia. After clamp occlusion of the external and common carotid arteries, internal carotid stump pressure is measured. If this exceeds 60 mm Hg and the patient experiences no symptoms after five minutes of occlusion, permanent carotid occlusion is presumably safe. If not, the ligation attempt should be abandoned (21).

Other methods for dealing with the high carotid aneurysm involve technical maneuvers which permit control of the distal carotid artery until arterial continuity can be restored. Javid *et al.* (28), in a presentation on carotid body tumors, reported a 1957 case in which a dissecting sponge was used to occlude the lumen of the briskly bleeding distal internal carotid artery while a homograft was anastomosed to it. Hershey (22), in 1974, described the use of a tapered silastic catheter taken from a dialysis

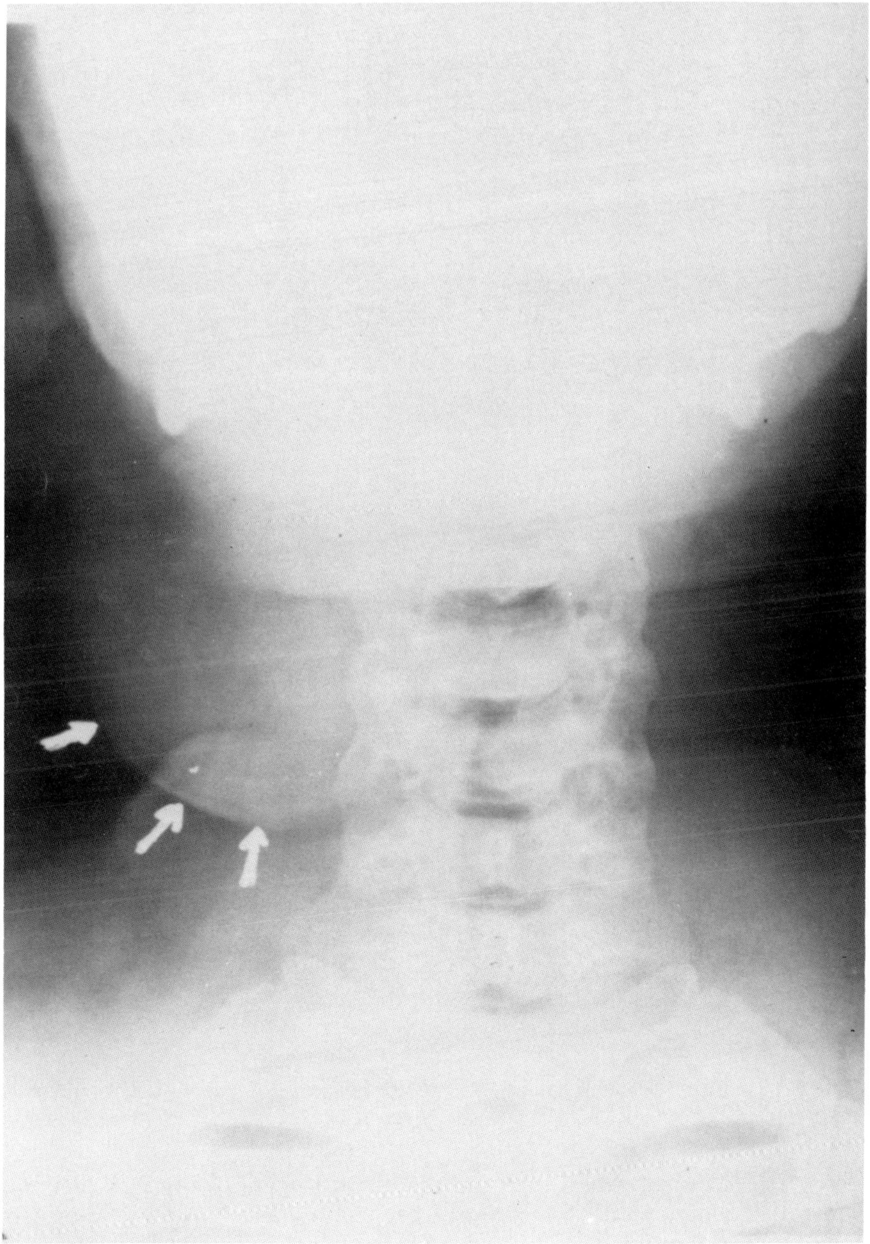

Figure 3.6. Large, carotid artery, false aneurysm appearing as a spherical mass, with uniform density on a plain X-ray of the neck.

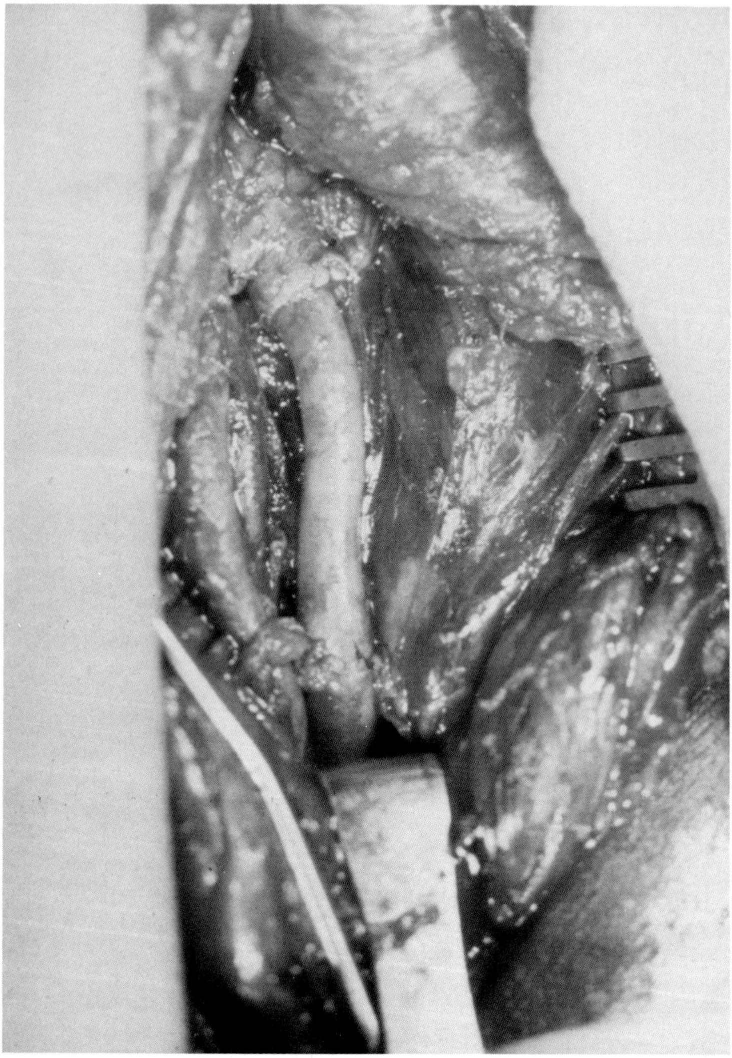

Figure 3.7. Arterial homograft used to restore vessel continuity after resection of aneurysm.

kit. With the tip pushed into the distal carotid, not only was bleeding controlled, but a route for cerebral perfusion was provided. This technique is recommended only for cases in which the aneurysm need not be excised, but can be controlled by endoaneurysmorrhaphy. Recent mention has been made of the application of modern neurosurgical extra-anatomic bypass techniques to the problem of the high carotid aneurysm. Theoretically, an aneurysm could be ligated and cerebral perfusion main-

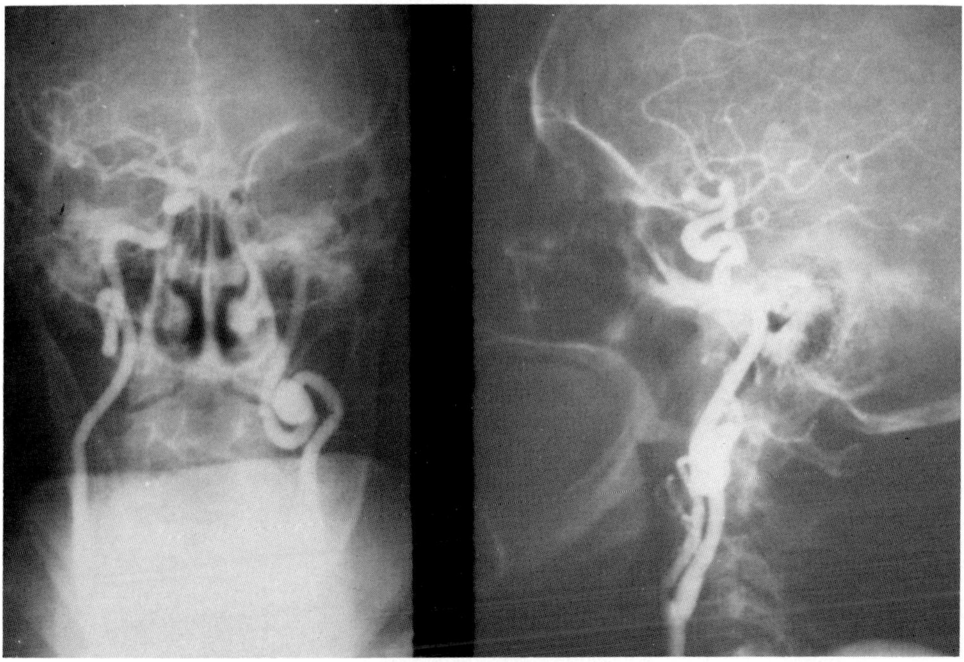

Figure 3.8. High, left internal carotid aneurysm demonstrated by contrast angiography.

tained through this technique. Although potentially effective, most aneurysms can be otherwise managed and only the exceptional case would require both ligation and extra-anatomic cerebral revascularization.

SUBCLAVIAN ANEURYSMS

Clinical manifestations, indications for surgical management, and surgical techniques in carotid and subclavian aneurysms differ sufficiently to justify division of this subject into two separate categories—carotid and subclavian aneurysms.

Aneurysms of the extracranial portion of the brachiocephalic system are uncommon, despite the frequent occurrence of atherosclerotic disease in the arteries of the neck. The etiology of subclavian aneurysms includes congenital origin, trauma, infection, dissection, atherosclerosis, and cystic medial necrosis. Luetic aneurysms, which were common in the past, have rarely been reported during the last few decades. Another cause of subclavian aneurysms is the cavitation effect of turbulent flow beyond a compressed area, for example, distal to a cervical rib.

Aneurysms of the subclavian artery are relatively rare in comparison to other peripheral aneurysms, and the exact incidence in the general population is unknown. Dent and associates (12) reviewed the location of atherosclerotic aneurysms in approximately 1,500 patients treated

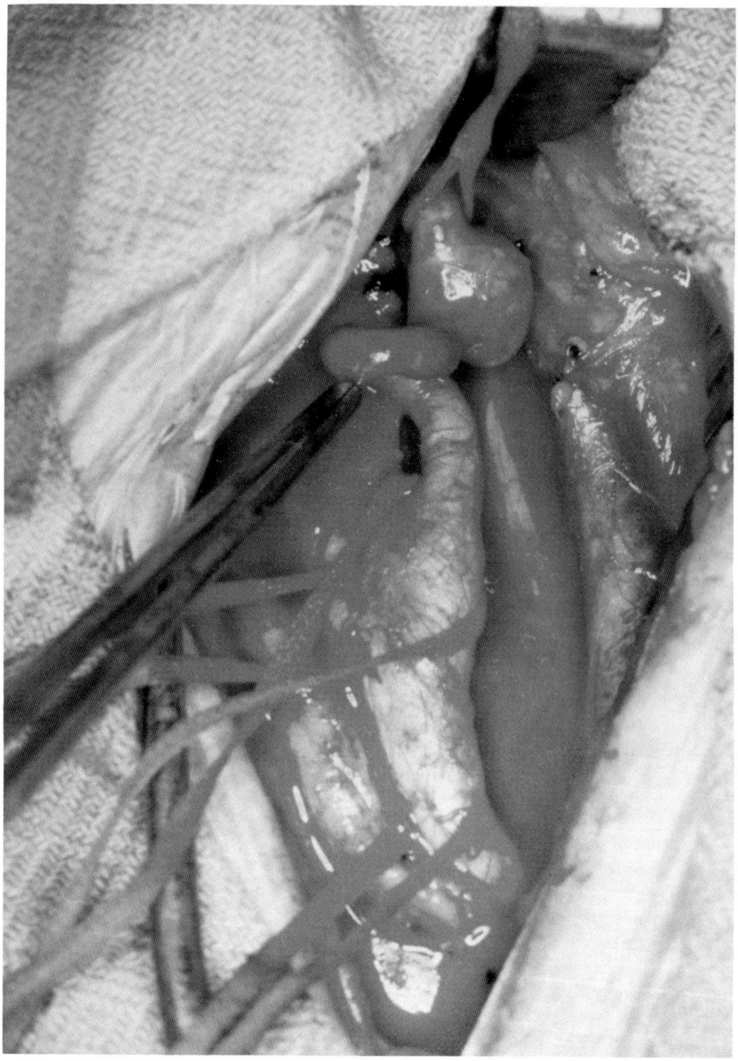

Figure 3.9. Careful dissection of a tortuous and elongated internal carotid artery, made possible by visualization of high-incidence carotid aneurysm.

during a ten-year period and reported only two subclavian aneurysms. Surgical intervention, as reported by Greenough (15), was first attempted in 1818 by Valentine Mott. His patient died of infection and hemorrhage on the 26th postoperative day. Steinberg (59) reported that Smyth of New Orleans obtained the first successful result in 1864 with proximal ligation. In the same article it is stated that Matas, also of New Orleans, introduced his innovative technique of endoaneurysmorrhaphy in 1888,

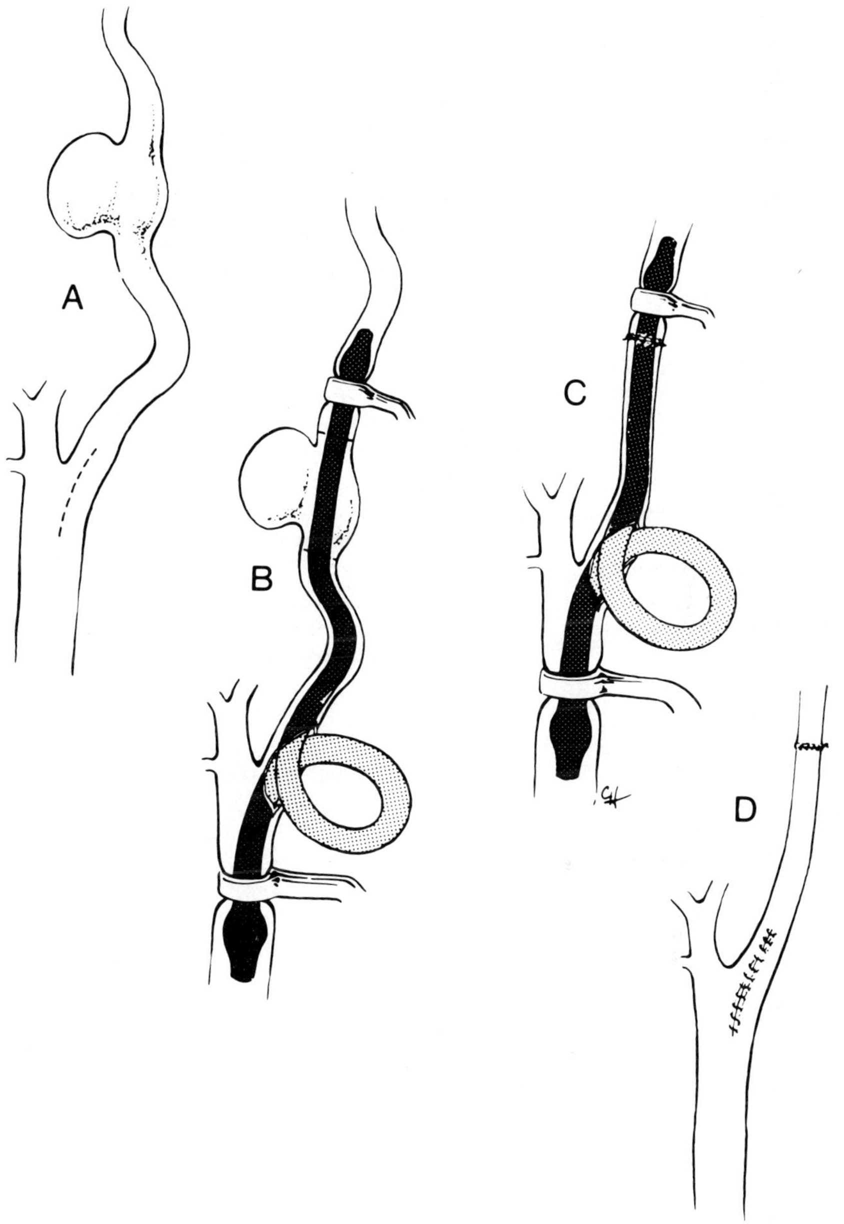

Figure 3.10. *A*, defined high internal carotid aneurysm and low carotid arteriotomy. *B*, intraluminal shunt advanced through the aneurysm to provide perfusion during resection. *C*, end-to-end anastomosis accomplished over the shunt after aneurysmectomy. *D*, repair completed and shunt removed.

when he first used this method of treatment in a subclavian aneurysm. Halsted (18), following some basic research that included proximal ligation and aluminum banding of the arteries in preparation for treatment of the subclavian aneurysm, reported success with excision of a subclavioaxillary aneurysm in 1892. At the turn of the century, the operative mortality rate for subclavian aneurysms was approximately 80% (6). The modern era of surgical management for this lesion began with Bahnson's report (2) of successful excision and graft replacement in 1953.

Atherosclerotic Aneurysms

PATHOPHYSIOLOGY

Aneurysms of the first portion of the subclavian artery are commonly caused by atherosclerosis. These lesions are often asymptomatic and are usually discovered in elderly individuals on routine chest X-ray—they appear as superior, anterior mediastinal masses, commonly mistaken for mediastinal or lung tumors. Useful roentgenographic signs are absence of a distinct border superiorly and presence of calcium deposits outlining the shadow (Fig. 3.11*A* to *C*). These lesions rarely extend into the supraclavicular region. A pulsating mass, particularly in the right medial portion of the supraclavicular area, does not necessarily represent a subclavian aneurysm. The aorta and arch branches may, with age, undergo dilatation and elongation due to chronic hypertension and generalized arteriosclerosis. In addition, kyphoscoliosis, which is commonly found in elderly individuals, results in displacement of the innominate subclavian junction into the right supraclavicular region. This has been reported by Honig *et al.* (26) in an angiographic study of hypertensive patients with atherosclerosis. In our experience, such lesions are benign and do not require surgical intervention. Angiography is indicated only if, in addition to the neck mass, there are also abnormal findings on chest X-ray, suggestive of aneurysmal dilatation of the innominate artery or the first portion of the subclavian artery. A tortuous subclavian artery may cast a shadow, which resembles a coin lesion, in the apex of the lung (Fig. 3.12). Rarely, tracheoesophageal symptoms or venous distention may result from external compression. The benign nature of this lesion has been emphasized by Thomas (63). It is important to be familiar with this lesion to avoid a potentially hazardous invasive diagnostic maneuver such as mediastinoscopy or needle biopsy. A diagnosis of a tortuous innominate subclavian junction should be established with absolute certainty before a decision is made to merely observe such a lesion. A true aneurysm of the first portion of the subclavian artery has the potential for rupture, thrombosis, or embolic manifestations in the upper extremity (64). Rupture of the subclavian artery can occur into the free pleural space, mediastinal tissue, or adjacent organs such as the esophagus or trachea. These lesions should be treated surgically whenever feasible.

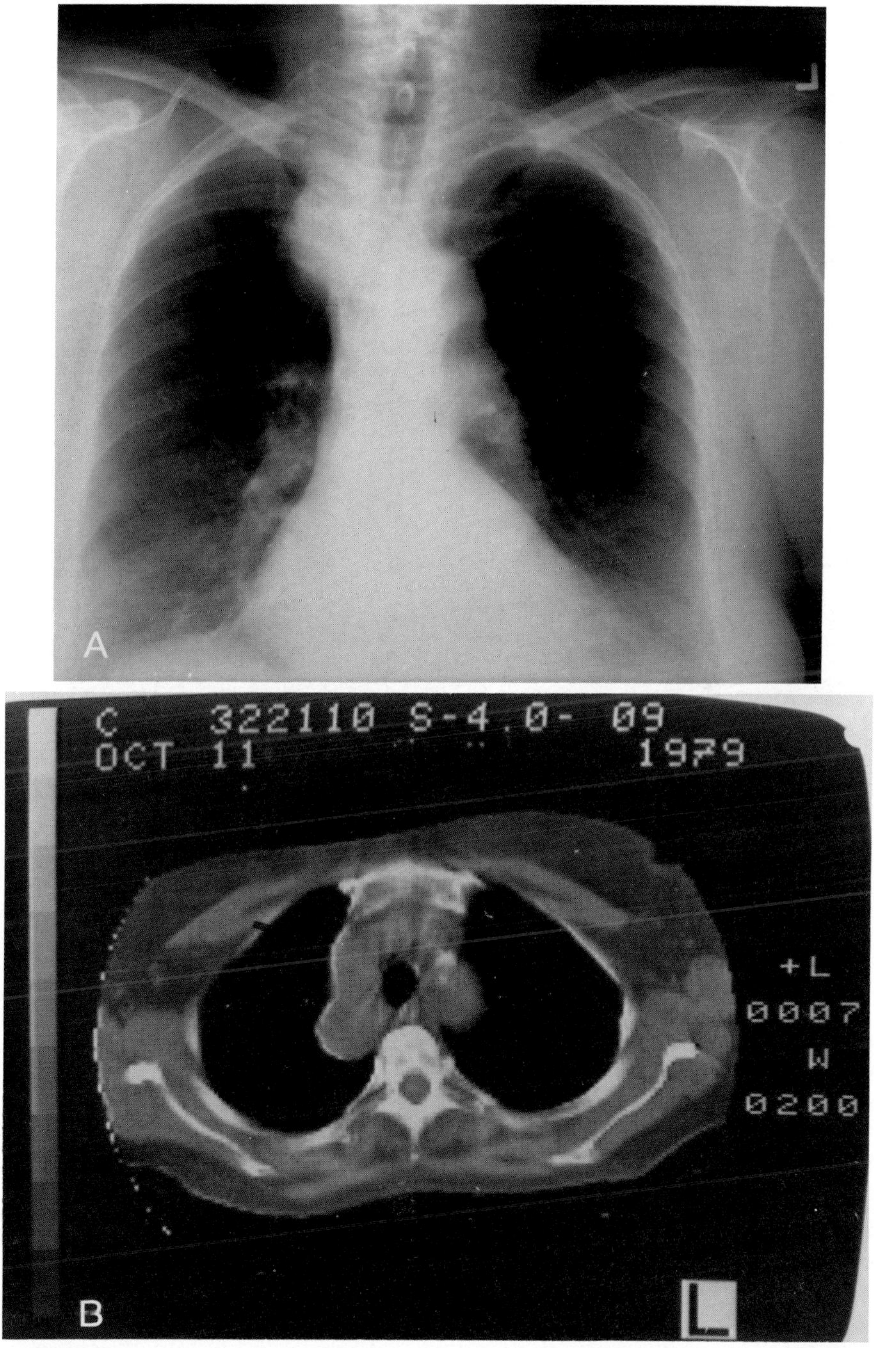

Figure 3.11. *A*, chest X-ray showing an anterior, superior mediastinal mass. *B*, CAT scan demonstrating clot-filled aneurysm of the subclavian artery. *C*, angiogram revealing aneurysm of the innominate and intrathoracic portion of the right subclavian artery.

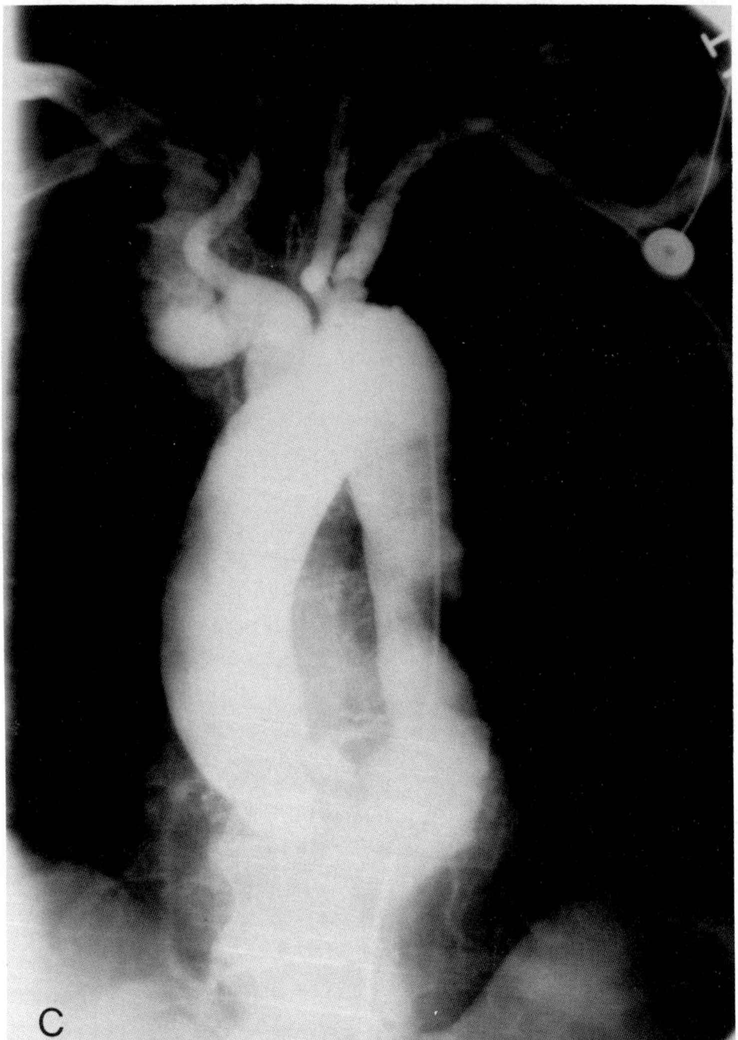

Figure 3.11 (*C*)

Diagnostic Evaluation

The diagnosis of a subclavian aneurysm and its relationship to the surrounding structures can best be evaluated with the use of short-exposure scanners and rapid injection of a bolus of intravenous contrast material (43). This method effectively visualizes the aneurysm and also demonstrates thrombus within the vessel. It is often impossible to accurately estimate the size of the aneurysm by angiography, since thrombus may fill much of the aneurysmal cavity. Noninvasive methods (e.g., ultrasonography and CAT scan) may be hampered by the clavicle or first rib. Nevertheless, they represent a safe step in the evaluation.

THERAPY

Surgical management of the aneurysm of the first portion of the subclavian artery requires optimal exposure, since repair often requires graft replacement. The right subclavian aneurysm can best be exposed through a median sternotomy incision with extension into the right supraclavicular region. The left subclavian aneurysm should be approached through a posterolateral thoracotomy through the left fourth intercostal space. If the aneurysm extends into the second portion of the subclavian artery, better exposure can be obtained through an anterolateral fourth intercostal space incision to permit supraclavicular control, if necessary. Resection of the clavicle has not been necessary in elective cases managed at our institution.

Aberrant Subclavian Artery

PATHOPHYSIOLOGY

Aneurysmal dilatation of the origin of an aberrant right subclavian artery from the descending thoracic aorta is termed Kommerell's diverticulum. Embryologically, this is a persistent distal end of the right aortic arch. An aberrant right subclavian artery, arising from the posterior aspect of the descending arch, is the most common anomaly of the aortic arch. The artery passes behind the esophagus in front of the spine and then assumes a normal position as it enters the thoracic outlet tract. Aberrant subclavian artery occurs in approximately 1% of the population (11). Although the anomalous origin of the right subclavian artery as a cause of dysphagia in children is well known (47), the majority of elderly individuals with this anomaly are asymptomatic. In 1794, Bayford (4) described in detail the case of a 62-year-old woman who had suffered dysphagia of increasing severity for 20 years. She died with extreme emaciation, as a result of esophageal obstruction due to an anomalous right subclavian artery. Bayford used the phrase "dysphagia lusoria" in this case to describe the difficulty in swallowing because of a freak occurrence of nature.

Stauffer and Pote (58) described such a lesion in a paper presented in 1946 in which the diagnosis was determined radiologically. Shannon (53), in 1961, recognized this anomaly during an operation. The patient expired three months postoperatively, though the cause of death was not stated. Lynn (34) presented a case with an esophagoaortic fistula associated with Kommerell's diverticulum; the patient expired after emergency surgery. Campbell (9), in 1971, reported successful operative management of this lesion with the interposition of a segment of Dacron graft. In 1980, McIntyre and Lynn (38) reported satisfactory results with proximal and distal ligation of the aberrant subclavian aneurysm. Their patient denied dysphagia, cough, or dyspnea prior to surgery. The diagnosis was

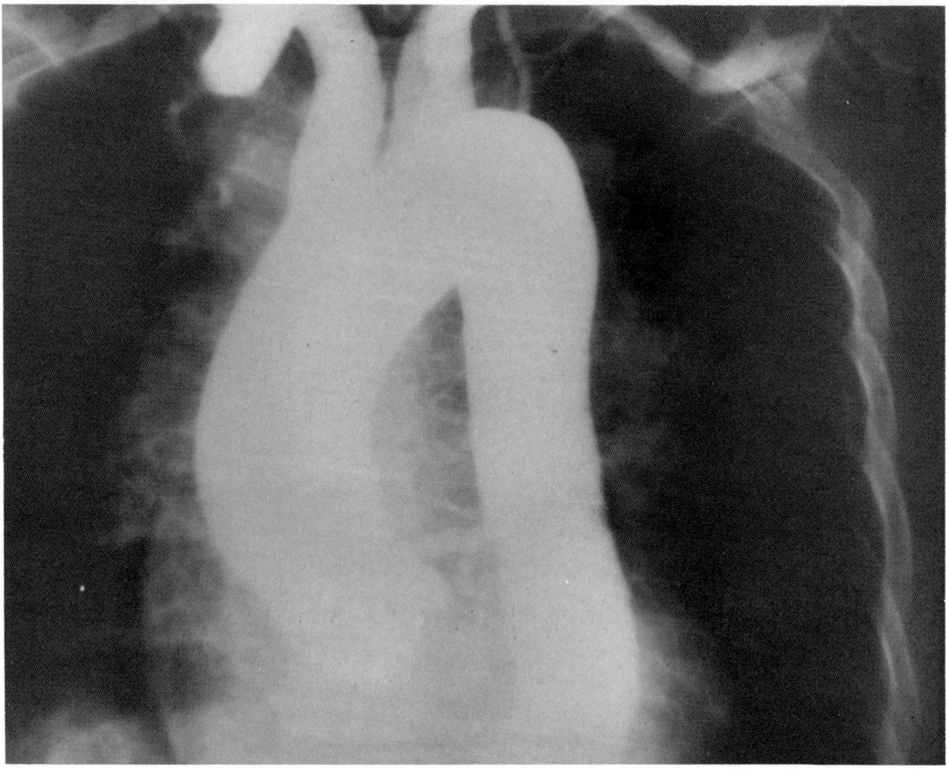

Figure 3.12. Angiography revealing the coin-shaped lesion representing a loop of subclavian artery.

confirmed with a CAT scan and an arteriogram was not obtained. The nature of the pulsatile mass was confirmed through a right thoracotomy incision. After proximal and distal ligation, the right radial pulse was obliterated postoperatively, but there was no color change in the hand. The patient was followed for approximately 18 months, with no claudication or symptoms referable to his cerebral circulation.

DIAGNOSTIC EVALUATION

The diagnosis of aberrant subclavian artery can be readily made by an esophagram and angiogram. The lesion typically compresses the esophagus from behind, presenting a pathognomonic sign (Fig. 3.13).

THERAPY

Gross and Ware (16), in 1946, successfully divided the anomalous subclavian artery through a left thoracotomy incision in a child with esophageal obstruction. Division of the anomalous subclavian artery was also advocated in adults by Lichter (33) in 1963. Although ligation of the

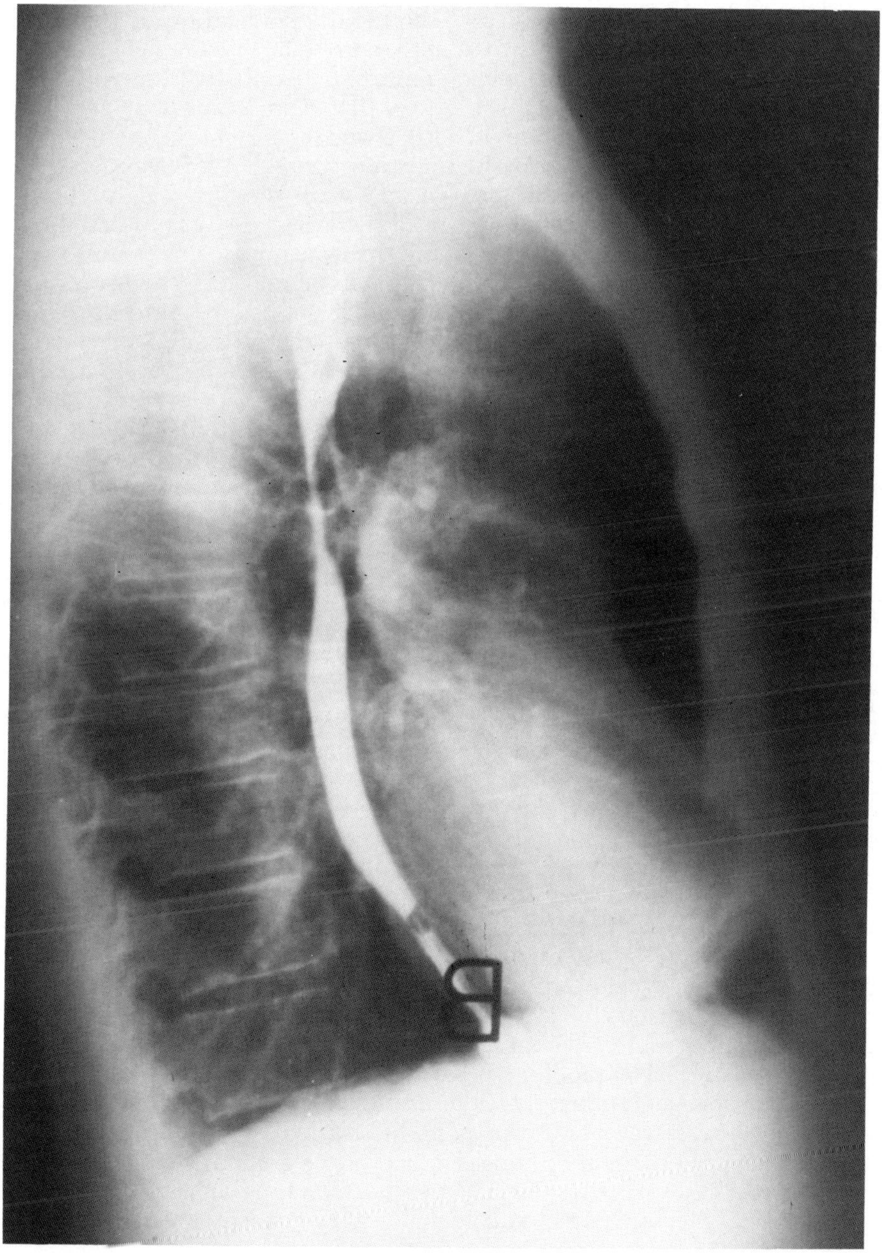

Figure 3.13. Compression of the esophagus from behind by an aberrant right subclavian artery.

subclavian artery is commonly well tolerated, claudication of the arm, significant ischemic changes in the upper extremity, and the vertebral subclavian steal syndrome have been reported (17). Reattachment of the distal end of the subclavian artery to the right carotid artery was accomplished in 1969 by Siderys (56) through a right neck incision, followed by removal of the proximal portion through a left thoracotomy incision. Bailey *et al.* (3) described an operation through a right thoracotomy to preserve the circulation to the right arm. They transected the anomalous right subclavian artery behind the esophagus as far into the left chest as possible, and reimplanted the distal end into the ascending aorta, posterior to the vena cava. A similar procedure, interposing a segment of 10-mm Dacron graft between the cut end of the subclavian artery and the ascending aorta, was accomplished through a left thoracotomy approach by Pifarre and associates (42).

Although the tendency for dilatation of an aberrant right subclavian artery has been commented on in the literature (60), true aneurysmal dilatation of this common congenital anomaly has been extremely rare. McCallen and Schaff (35) reported the first such aneurysm in 1956. The diagnosis was confirmed during thoracotomy but resection was not attempted. Gomes *et al.* (14), in 1968, reported a similar lesion which was successfully treated with proximal and distal ligation. In 1970, Hunter *et al.* (27) reported three patients with symptomatic anomalous right subclavian artery aneurysms. Errors made in the preoperative diagnosis of the first case seen in 1961, an improper surgical approach through a median sternotomy incision, and the fragile aneurysmal nature of the descending aorta resulted in a difficult surgical procedure. The patient expired during the postoperative period. Two other patients were properly diagnosed by angiography and treated successfully through a left thoracotomy incision. These patients required resection and graft replacement of the descending arch for management of large aneurysms of the aberrant subclavian artery (60). Retrograde flow from the subclavian artery was controlled in each of these two patients by tamponading the orifice with a balloon catheter. Distal closure of the subclavian artery was accomplished by suturing the vessel through the aneurysmal sac. Schmidt *et al.* (51), in February of 1980, reported managing a large aneurysm of the proximal portion of the anomalous right subclavian artery by proximal and distal ligation. The proximal end was repaired through a transaortic approach after proximal and distal cross-clamping. The patient's postoperative course was complicated by a profound neurologic deficit, including cortical blindness; however, he gradually recovered to a near-normal state. During the past year, a fourth patient with an aneurysm of the aberrant right subclavian artery presented as a vascular lesion simulating neoplasm (52).

Most of the patients reported in the literature have been managed with subclavian ligation. None of the surviving patients have noted ischemic symptoms of the brain or have experienced claudication of the upper extremity. A review of past experience shows these lesions to have an ominous prognosis. Appropriate surgical care requires an accurate preoperative diagnosis, good exposure through a left fourth intercostal space posterolateral thoracotomy, and readiness for possible vessel grafting. Control of the subclavian artery distal to the aneurysm may be impossible until the aneurysmal sac is opened. Control of backflow may be accomplished by intraluminal occlusion with a balloon-tipped catheter (27, 63).

False Aneurysms Due to Compression and Trauma

ETIOLOGY AND SYMPTOMS

Deceleration injuries may disrupt the innominate junction from the aortic arch, producing a false aneurysm with involvement of the superior mediastinum, as well as the supraclavicular region (Fig. 3.14*A* and *B*). Other causes of aneurysmal dilatation of the first portion of the subclavian artery include coarctation of the aorta, dissection, and cystic medial necrosis.

Aneurysms of the extrathoracic portion of the subclavian artery are caused mainly by external compression and trauma. Mechanical compression of the subclavian artery by the structures of the thoracic outlet (such as the first rib, scalenus anticus muscle, anomalous first rib, elongated transverse process, exostosis, and healing fracture) results in turbulence of flow leading to poststenotic dilatation and eventual aneurysmal formation (61).

In 1927, Adson and Coffey (1) focused attention on the possibility of muscle compression of the subclavian artery. The proposal of an active participation of the scalenus anticus muscle in causing the symptoms was presented by Ochsner *et al.* (40) in 1935. Poststenotic dilatation caused by scalenus anticus muscle compression has rarely been reported.

Mural thrombi form at the site of intimal damage. Frequent distal embolization and eventual thrombosis represent the serious complications of this lesion. Early diagnosis is extremely important because upper extremity symptoms (e.g., pain, numbness, and paresthesia) are often ignored or thought to be neurologic in origin. Peripheral artery occlusion, due to embolization, may result in gangrene of the fingertips and loss of digits.

DIAGNOSTIC EVALUATION

Early diagnosis requires a thorough physical examination of the neck to detect aneurysmal dilatation or vascular compression. Auscultation of the supraclavicular region with the arm in various positions is most informative. It should, however, be recognized that pulse and blood pressure changes and bruits in the neck may be present in a normal individual with the arm in extreme abduction. Positional angiography is often helpful. Even mild poststenotic dilatation in a symptomatic patient deserves attention. Mural thrombi may not be evident on roentgenographic evaluation, but will usually be found during surgery. As originally observed by Halsted (19), stenosis of any vessel leads to the phenomenon of poststenotic dilatation. Holman (24, 25) demonstrated that "structural

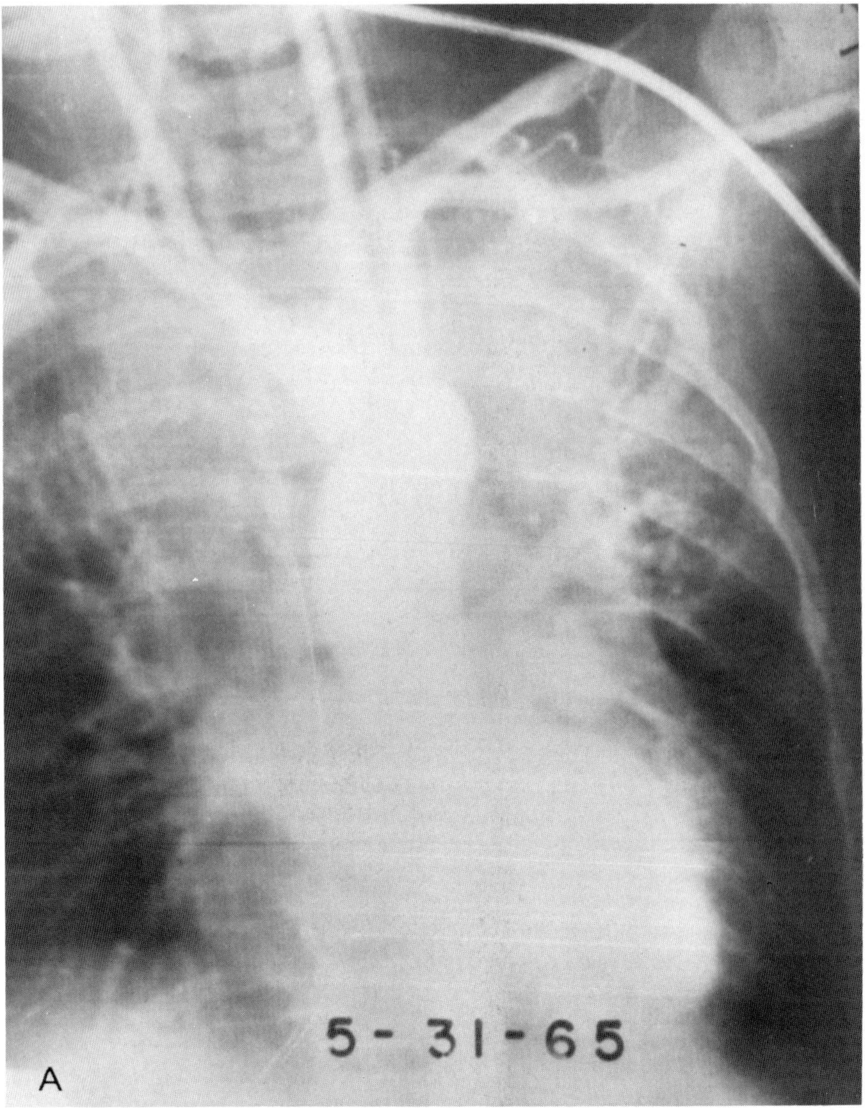

Figure 3.14. *A*, avulsed innominate artery producing widened mediastinum, as well as a pulsating supraclavicular mass. B, postoperative angiogram showing an aortosubclavian bypass around the mediastinal mass.

fatigue" will develop in arterial segments distal to a stricture. As the flow passes through the stenotic area, it enters an area of lower pressure. This transformation of high kinetic energy to high lateral energy results in turbulence of flow and cavitation effect. As the process continues, struc-

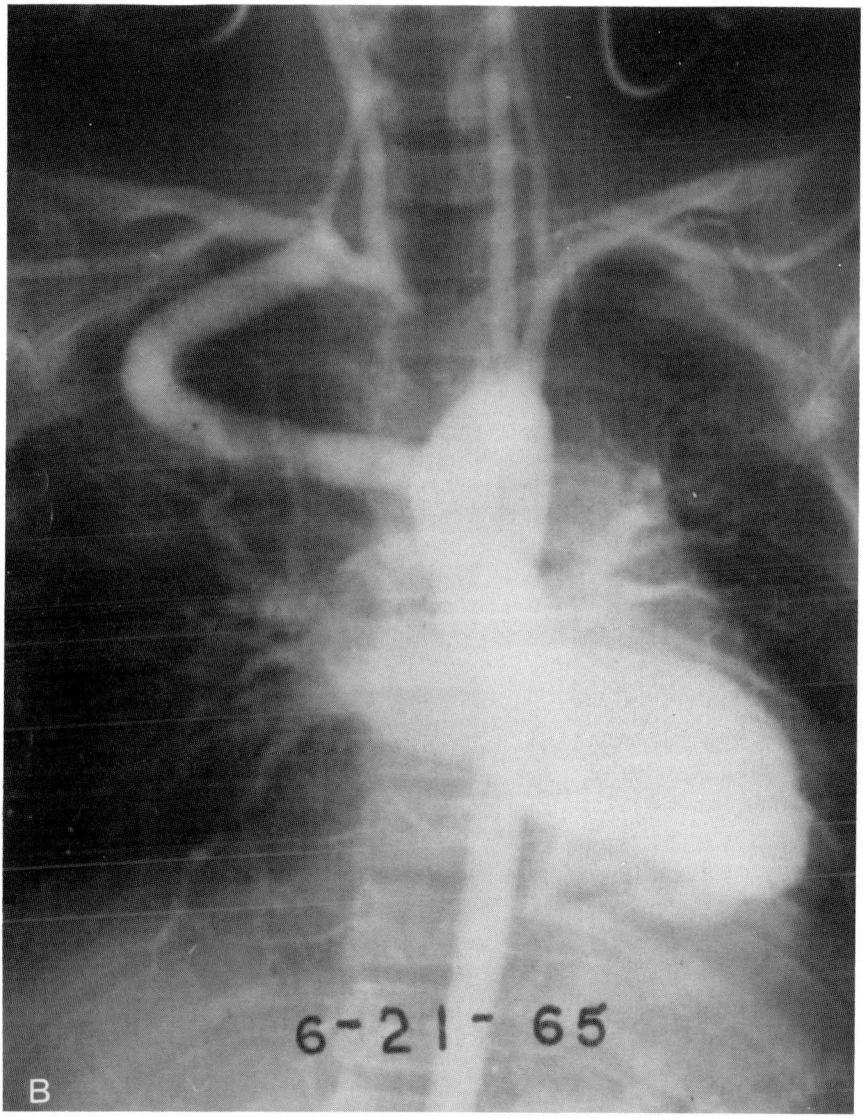

Figure 3.14 (*B*)

tural failure of the elastic tissue in the arterial wall occurs with development of a typical arteriosclerotic aneurysm containing laminated clots (see Chapter 2). Although rupture of these aneurysms is rare, thrombosis and embolization are common complications. Thrombosis of the subclavian artery may be severely disabling. In a series of 31 patients reported by Schein and associates (50), the gravity of the thrombosis was illustrated by the fact that 11 patients lost portions of their fingers, two required major upper extremity amputations, and three suffered hemiplegia as a result of the extension of the thrombotic process into the common carotid artery.

THERAPY

A false aneurysm caused by a penetrating or blunt trauma demands prompt and wide exposure, thus often necessitating removal of the medial portion of the clavicle. The operation should relieve compression of the artery and remove the emboli. Excision of the involved segment and graft replacement is often necessary. Hilton (23), in 1879, at Guys Hospital in London, is credited as the first to describe subclavian artery compression caused by exostosis of the first rib. Coote (10), in 1861, performed the first excision of a cervical rib to relieve compression of the subclavian artery.

CASE REPORTS

Case Report I

A 63-year-old white female was admitted to Presbyterian-St. Luke's Hospital because of pain and numbness of the right hand and forearm of 18 months' duration. She also noted intermittent claudication and blanching followed by cyanosis. Examination revealed atrophy of the muscles of the forearm and hand, cyanosis of the fingertips, absence of arm pulses, and a supraclavicular pulsatile mass. Angiography (Fig. 3.15*A* and *B*) showed aneurysmal dilatation of the subclavian artery resulting from compression by the cervical rib. The brachial artery beyond the aneurysm was totally occluded. Resection of the aneurysm, removal of the cervical rib, and distal thrombectomy were accomplished. Pulses were restored down to the elbow level, but not to the wrist. Arteriogram, after three months, demonstrated patency of the brachial artery; a few months later, however, the vessel occluded again and a dorsal sympathectomy was necessary.

Case Report II

A 35-year-old white male presented with pain and numbness of the right hand and claudication of the right arm of one year's duration. Gradual deterioration caused total disability and he was unable to pursue his occupation as a garbage collector. Examination showed a pulseless, cold, somewhat cyanotic right hand. No pulses were palpable in the right upper extremity, but there was a pulseless mass in the right supraclavicular region. There was also a pulsatile aneurysmal dilatation of the cervical portion of the *left* subclavian artery with a thrill and loud bruit. Angiography demonstrated complete occlusion of the right subclavian artery with late filling of the brachial artery (Fig. 3.16*A* and *B*). At surgery, the subclavian artery was found to be flattened by a markedly hypertrophied scalenus anticus muscle (Fig. 3.17). Poststenotic dilatation beyond the edge of the muscle and lack of other compressive structures confirmed the diagnosis of scalenus anticus syndrome. The thrombosed

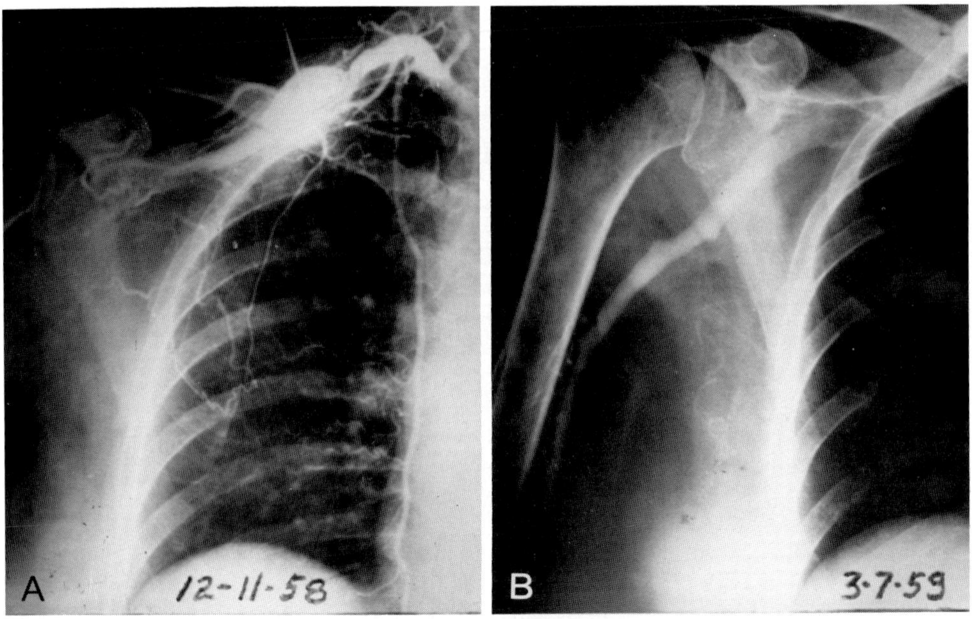

Figure 3.15. *A*, preoperative angiogram showing subclavian aneurysm with distal thrombosis B, postoperative angiogram three months later showing patency of the channel down to the elbow level.

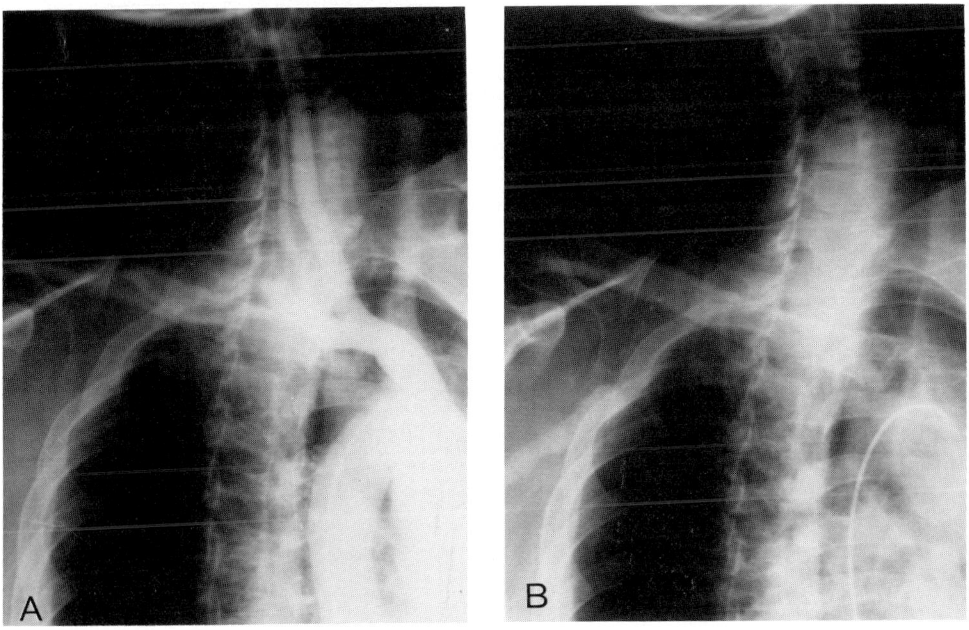

Figure 3.16. *A*, complete occlusion of the right subclavian artery. *B*, late filling of the brachial artery.

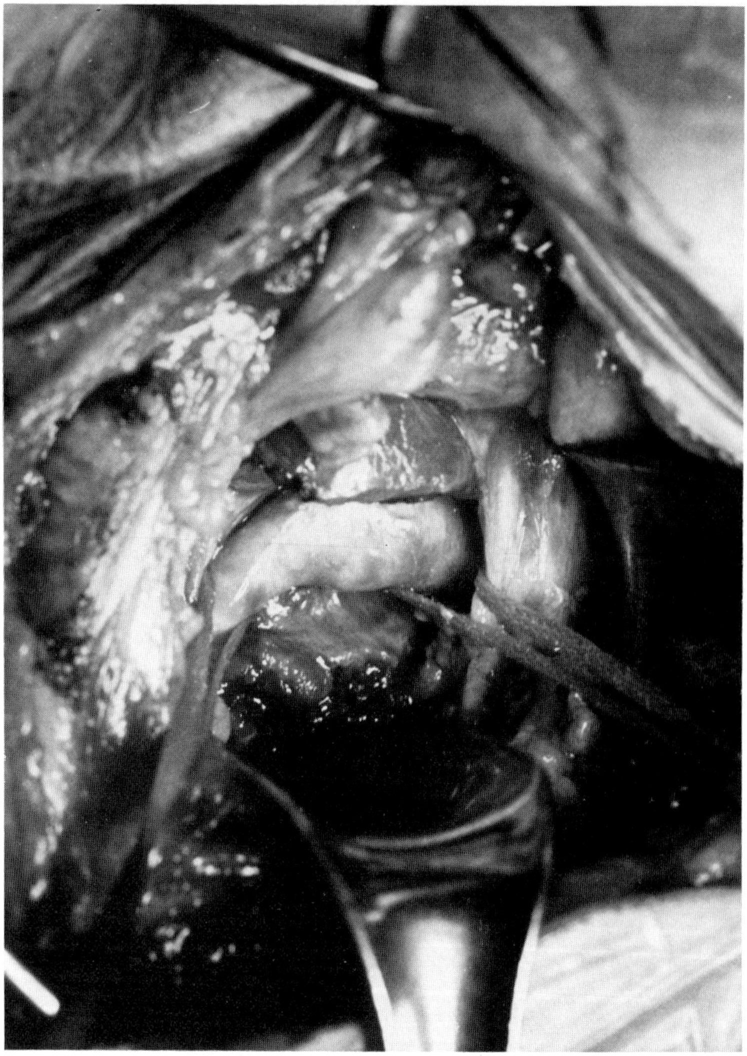

Figure 3.17. Division of hypertrophied scalenus anticus muscle exposed, with flattened subclavian artery immediately underneath the muscle.

segment was excised (Fig. 3.18) and a 10-mm Dacron graft was used to bridge this defect. The two anastomoses were accomplished through separate incisions above and below the clavicle. It was not necessary to remove the clavicle in this patient. Return of the peripheral pulses and the elimination of symptoms encouraged us to repeat a similar procedure on the opposite side a few months later.

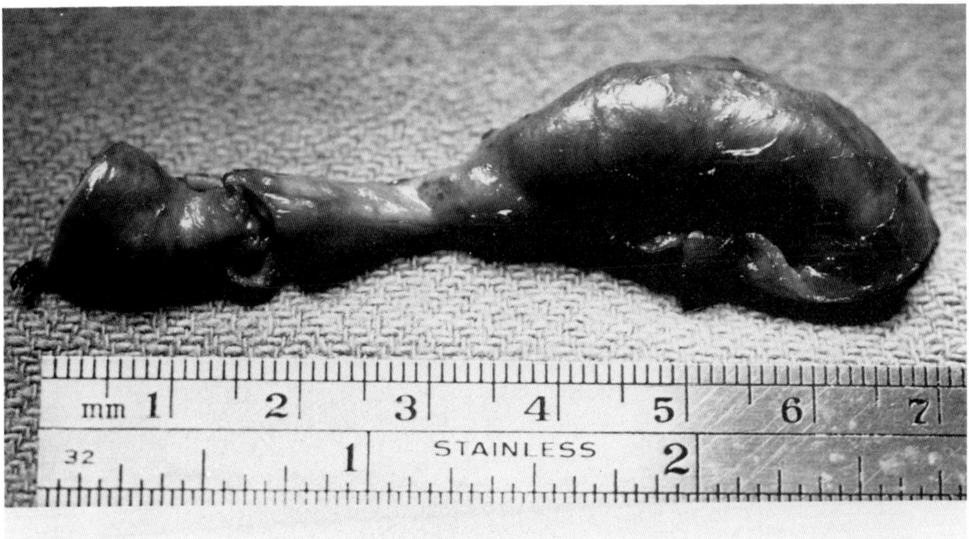

Figure 3.18. Thrombosed subclavian artery with compressed area and aneurysmal poststenotic segment well demonstrated.

COMMENT

According to the study of Telford and Mattershead (62), the thickness of the scalenus anticus muscle varies from 0.4 to 2.5 cm in normal individuals. The word hypertrophy should therefore be used with caution, as it pertains to an abnormal state. This is the only patient in our institution with poststenotic dilatation of the subclavian artery caused by hypertrophy of the scalenus anticus muscle. The occupation of the patient as a garbage collector may have contributed to the abnormal size of this particular muscle.

Case Report III

A 58-year-old white male presented with a left neck pulsatile mass and left arm numbness and pain of many years' duration. While serving in the army in 1940, he had operative transection of the left scalenus anticus muscle with relief of symptoms. He did well until March 1981, when he developed sudden left arm numbness and weakness which lasted for several hours. In addition, he noted left hand numbness on turning his head to the left side. Examination revealed a supraclavicular bony prominence representing a large cervical rib; palpation revealed a pulsating mass and a thrill; auscultation revealed a loud bruit; and angiography demonstrated poststenotic dilatation beyond a large cervical rib (Fig. 3.19). Resection of the rib resulted in improvement of symptoms.

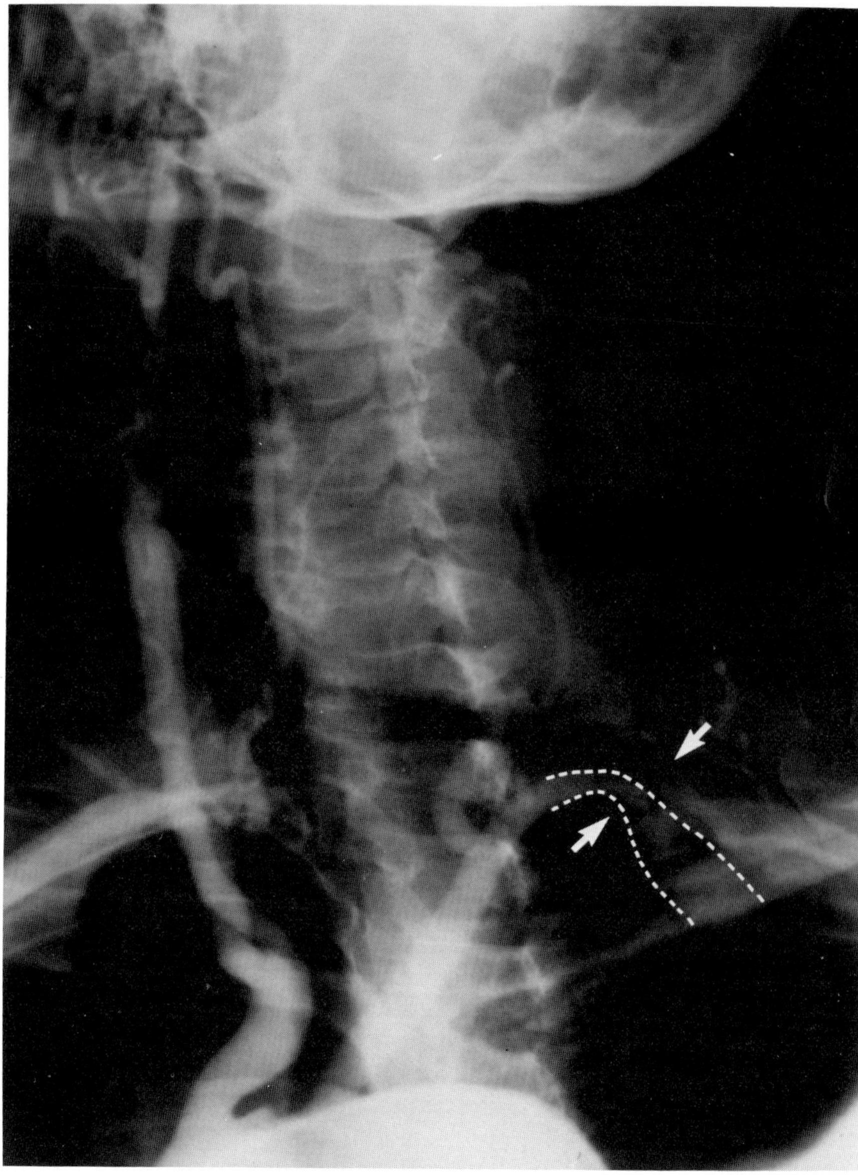

Figure 3.19. Angiogram revealing area of subclavian compression by a cervical rib and poststenotic dilatation of the vessel.

COMMENT

Another site of compression in the thoracic outlet is the costoclavicular space. McGovern and Velensky (37), in a study of 108 presumably normal soldiers, reported that the attention position test resulted in alteration of the radial pulse in three individuals. Of these soldiers, two had symptoms of costoclavicular compression, diminution of the pulse below the clavicle, presence of a bruit during the attention position, and development of engorged arm veins, all of which are diagnostically significant. Figure 3.20 clearly demonstrates the exact site of compression and the tendency for poststenotic dilatation.

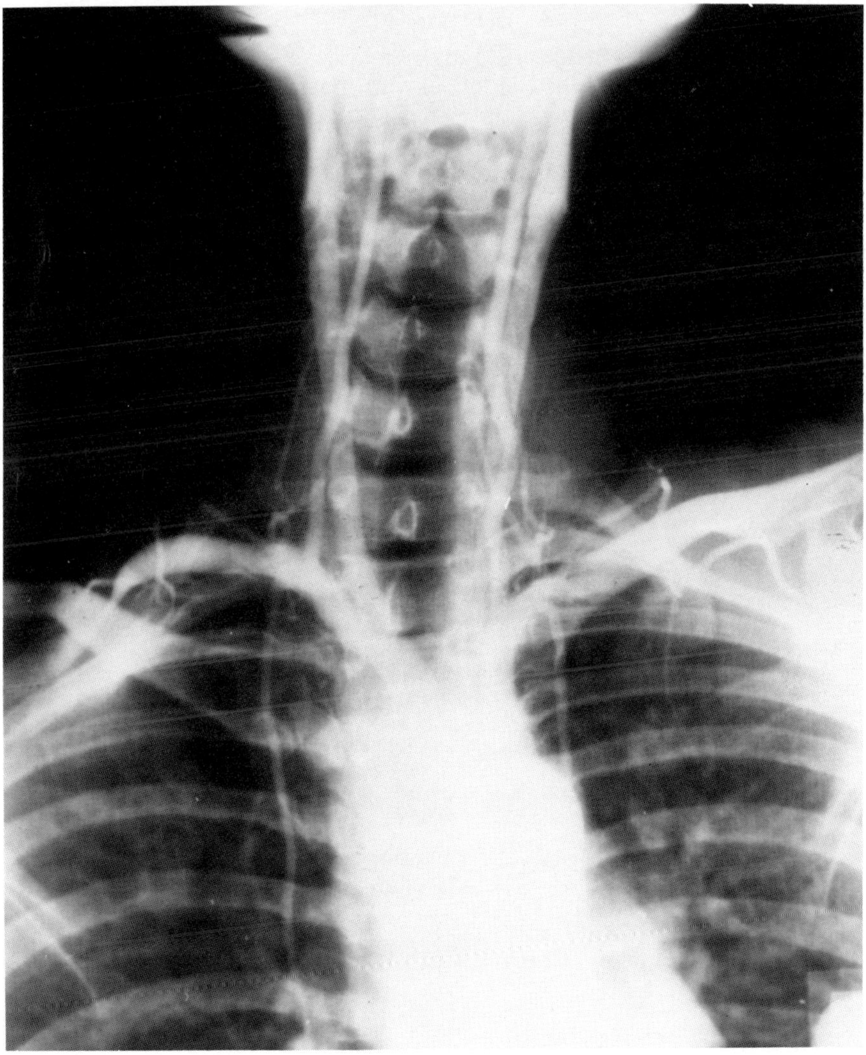

Figure 3.20. Angiogram showing area of compression and poststenotic dilatation in costoclavicular syndrome.

UNUSUAL PRESENTATIONS

Mycotic aneurysms in the subclavian artery are extremely rare. In our experience, two such cases have been seen in the last three decades. Both of these patients had aneurysms in the axillary region which were caused by subacute bacterial endocarditis. After a prolonged course of antibiotics, resection and vein graft replacement resulted in restoration of flow and excellent long-term results (see Chapter 8).

SUMMARY

Aneurysms of the extracranial carotid and subclavian arteries represent a unique challenge in diagnosis and management. In most cases, direct operative management is the preferred treatment. With proper case selection, careful preoperative evaluation, and meticulous surgical technique, aneurysmal resection can be performed with minimal risk. Most aneurysms are filled with debris, necessitating gentle manipulation during dissection. Close proximity of these lesions to vital cranial nerves demands precise knowledge of the anatomy and careful separation of these important structures from the wall of the aneurysm. Intraluminal shunting, when feasible, is recommended for dealing with aneurysms of the carotid system.

Occasionally, aneurysms should be left alone if the risk of surgical intervention is deemed greater than the potential for rupture or thrombosis. Small, asymptomatic aneurysms may be observed. No single approach is always effective, and careful planning is necessary to provide a satisfactory outcome.

References

1. Adson, A. W., and Coffey, J. R. Cervical rib. A method of anterior approach for relief of symptoms by division of the scalenus anticus. *Ann. Surg. 85:* 839–857, 1927.
2. Bahnson, H. T. Definitive treatment of saccular aneurysms of the aorta with excision of sac and aortic suture. *Surg. Gynecol. Obstet. 96:* 383–402, 1953.
3. Bailey, C. P., Hirose, T., and Alba, J. Re-establishment of the continuity of the anomalous right subclavian artery after operation for dysphagia lusoria. *Angiology 16:* 509–513, 1965.
4. Bayford, D. Singular case of obstructed deglutition. *Memoirs of the Medical Society of London*, ed. 2. American College of Surgeons, vol. 2, pp. 275–286, 1794.
5. Beall, A. C., Jr., Crawford, E. S., Cooley, D. A., and DeBakey, M. E. Extracranial aneurysms of the carotid artery: report of seven cases. *Postgrad. Med. 32:* 93–102, 1962.
6. Bjork, V. O. Aneurysm and occlusion of the right subclavian artery. *Acta Chir. Scand. (Supplement) 356:* 103–109, 1965.
7. Burklund, C. W. Spontaneous dissecting aneurysm of the cervical carotid artery. A report of surgical treatment in two patients. *Johns Hopkins Med. J. 126:* 154–159, 1970.
8. Busuttil, R. W., Davidson, R. K., Foley, K. T., Linesay, J. T., and Barker, W. F. Selective management of extracranial carotid arterial aneurysms. *Am. J. Surg. 140:* 85–91, 1980.
9. Campbell, C. F. Repair of an aneurysm of an aberrant retroesophageal right subclavian artery arising from Kommerell's diverticulum. *J. Thorac. Cardiovasc. Surg. 62:* 330–334, 1971.
10. Coote, H. Pressure on the axillary vessels and nerve by an exostosis from a cervical rib—interference with the circulation of the arm—removal of the rib in exostosis recovery. *Med. Times Gaz. 2:* 108, 1861.

11. Daseler, E. H., and Anson, B. J. Surgical anatomy of the subclavian artery and its branches. *Surg. Gynecol. Obstet. 108:* 149–174, February 1959.
12. Dent, T. L., Lindenauer, S. M., Ernst, C. B., and Fry, W. J. Multiple arteriosclerotic arterial aneurysms. *Arch. Surg. 105:* 388–394, 1972.
13. Dimtza, A. Aneurysm of the carotid arteries. Report of two cases. *Angiology 7:* 218–227, 1956.
14. Gomes, M. M. R., Bernatz, P. E., and Forth, R. J. Arteriosclerotic aneurysm of an aberrant right subclavian artery. *Dis. Chest 54:* 549–552, 1968.
15. Greenough, J. Operations on the innominate artery: report of a successful ligation. *Arch. Surg. 19:* 1484–1544, 1929.
16. Gross, R. E., and Ware, P. F. The surgical significance of aortic arch anomalies. *Surg. Gynecol. Obstet. 83:* 435, 1946.
17. Hallman, G. L., and Cooley, D. A. Congenital aortic vascular ring. Surgical considerations. *Arch. Surg. 88:* 666–675, 1964.
18. Halsted, W. S. Ligation of the first portion of the left subclavian artery and excision of a subclavio-axillary aneurysm. *Johns Hopkins Hosp. Rep. 3:* 93–97, 1892.
19. Halsted, W. S. An experimental study of circumscribed dilation of an artery immediately distal to a partially occluding band, and its bearing on the dilation of the subclavian artery observed in some cases of cervical rib. *J. Exp. Med. 24:* 271–286, 1916.
20. Hammon, J. W., Jr., Silver, D., and Young, W. G., Jr. Congenital aneurysm of the extracranial carotid arteries. *Ann. Surg. 176:* 777–781, 1972.
21. Haywood, I. R., and Ellis, H. Extra-cranial aneurysm of the internal carotid artery treated by proximal ligation. *Postgrad. Med. J. 55:* 30–35, 1979.
22. Hershey, F. B. Operation following aneurysm of the internal carotid artery high in the neck: a new and an old technique. *Angiology 25:* 24–30, 1974.
23. Hilton, J. *On Rest and Pain*, ed. 2, pp. 113–116. William Wood & Company, New York, 1879.
24. Holman, E. On circumscribed dilatation of an artery immediately distal to a partially occluding band: poststenotic dilatation. *Surgery 36:* 3–24, 1954.
25. Holman, E. The development of arterial aneurysms. *Surg. Gynecol. Obstet. 100:* 599–611, 1955.
26. Honig, E. I., Dubilier, W., and Steinberg, I. Significance of the buckled innominate artery. *Ann. Intern. Med. 39:* 74–80, 1953.
27. Hunter, J. A., Dye, W. S., Javid, H., Najafi, H., and Julian, O. C. Arteriosclerotic aneurysm of anomalous right subclavian artery. *J. Thorac. Cardiovasc. Surg. 59:* 754–758, 1970.
28. Javid, H., Dye, W. S., Hunter, J. A., Najafi, H., and Julian, O. C. Surgical management of carotid body tumor. *Arch. Surg. 95:* 771–779, 1967.
29. Johnson, J. N., Helsby, C. R., and Stell, P. M. Aneurysm of the external carotid artery. *J. Cardiovasc. Surg. 21:* 105–107, 1980.
30. Kaupp, H. A., Haid, S. P., Jurayj, M. N., Bergan, J. J., and Trippel, O. H. Aneurysms of the extracranial carotid artery. *Surgery 72:* 946–952, 1972.
31. Ledgerwood, A. M., and Lucas, C. E. Mycotic aneurysm of the carotid artery. *Arch. Surg. 109:* 496–498, 1975.
32. Leech, P. J., Miller, J. D., Fitch, W., and Barker, J. Cerebral blood flow, internal carotid artery pressure and the EEG as a guide to the safety of carotid artery ligation. *J. Neurol. Neurosurg. Psychiat. 37:* 854–862, 1974.
33. Lichter, I. The treatment of dysphagia lusoria in the adult. *Br. J. Surg.* 50: 793–796, 1963.
34. Lynn, R. B. Kommerell's diverticulum with esophago-arterial fistula. *Can. J. Surg. 12:* 331–333, 1969.
35. McCallen, A. M., and Schaff, B. Aneurysms of anomalous right subclavian artery. *Radiology 66:* 561–563, 1956.
36. McCollum, C. H., Wheeler, W. G., Noon, G. P., and DeBakey, M. E. Aneurysms of the extracranial carotid artery. Twenty-one years' experience. *Am. J. Surg. 137:* 196–200, 1979.
37. McGovern, J. M., and Velensky, M. Costoclavicular compression. Relation to the scalenus anticus and thoracic outlet syndrome. *Arch. Surg. 59:* 62–73, 1949.

38. McIntyre, M. D., and Lynn, R. B. Kommerell's diverticulum. *Can. J. Surg. 23:* 356, 1980.
39. Nesbit, R. R., Neistadt, A., and May, A. G. Bilateral internal carotid artery aneurysms. *Arch. Surg. 114:* 293–295, 1979.
40. Ochsner, A., Gage, M., and DeBakey, M. Scalenus anticus (Naffziger) syndrome. *Am. J. Surg. 28:* 669–695, 1935.
41. Oller, D. W., Gee, W., and Kingsley, J. R. Treatment for high extracranial internal carotid aneurysms. *Am. Surg. 42:* 311–315, 1976.
42. Pifarre, R., Dieter, R. A., and Niedballa, R. G. Definitive surgical treatment of the aberrant retroesophageal right subclavian artery in the adult. *J. Thorac. Cardiovasc.*
43. Pond, G. D., and Hillman, B. Evaluation of aneurysms by computed tomography. *Surgery 89:* 216–223, 1981.
44. Raphael, H. A., Bernatz, P. E., Spittel, J. A., Jr., and Ellis, F. H., Jr. Cervical carotid aneurysm: treatment by excision and restoration of arterial continuity. *Am. J. Surg. 105:* 771–778, 1963.
45. Rhodes, E. L., Stanley, J. C., Hoffman, G. L., Cronenwett, J. L., and Fry, W. L. Aneurysms of the extracranial carotid arteries. *Arch. Surg. 111:* 339–343, 1976.
46. Rittenhouse, E. A., Radke, H. M., and Sumner, D. S. Carotid artery aneurysm. Review of the literature and report of a case with rupture into the oropharynx. *Arch. Surg. 105:* 786–789, 1972.
47. Rodgers, B. M., Talbert, J. L., and Hollenbeck, J. I. Aneurysm of anomalous subclavian artery: an unusual cause of dysphagia lusoria in childhood. *Ann. Surg. 187:* 158–160, 1978.
48. Schechter, D. C. Cervical carotid aneurysms. Part I. *N.Y. State J. Med. 79(1):* 892–901, 1979.
49. Schechter, D. C. Cervical carotid aneurysms. Part II. *N.Y. State J. Med. 79(1):* 1042–1048, 1979.
50. Schein, C. J., Haimovici, H., and Young, H. Arterial thrombosis associated with cervical ribs: surgical considerations. Report of a case and review of the literature. *Surgery 40:* 428–443, 1956.
51. Schmidt, F. E., Hewitt, R. L., and Flores, A. A., Jr. Aneurysm of anomalous right subclavian artery. *South. Med. J. 73:* 255–256, 1980.
52. Shahian, D. M., Javid, H., Faber, L. P., Kittle, C. F., and Matthew, G. R. Lesions of the thoracic aorta and its arch branches simulating neoplasm. *J. Thorac. Cardiovasc. Surg. 81:* 251–263, 1981.
53. Shannon, J. M. Aberrant right subclavian artery with Kommerell's diverticulum. Report of a case. *J. Thorac. Cardiovasc. Surg. 41:* 408–411, 1961.
54. Shea, P. C., and Harrison, J. H. Anastomosis of common and internal carotid arteries following resection of the defective portion. Report of a case. *Surgery 34:* 895–901, 1953.
55. Shipley, A. M., Winslow, N., and Walker, W. W. Aneurysm in the cervical portion of the internal carotid artery: an analytical study of the cases recorded in the literature between August 1, 1925 and July 31, 1936. Report of two new cases. *Ann. Surg. 105:* 673–699, 1937.
56. Siderys, H. A new operation for symptomatic aberrant right subclavian artery in the adult (dysphagia lusoria). *J. Thorac. Cardiovasc. Surg. 57:* 269–272, 1969.
57. Solheim, K. Common carotid artery aneurysm after blunt trauma. *J. Trauma 19:* 707–709, 1979.
58. Stauffer, H. M., and Pote, H. H. Anomalous right subclavian artery originating on the left as the last branch of the aortic arch. Report of a probable case diagnosed roentgenologically. *Am. J. Roentgenol. Rad. Ther. Nucl. Med. 56:* 13–17, 1946.
59. Steinberg, I. A true and a false arteriosclerotic aneurysm of the subclavian artery. *Am. J. Roentgenol. Rad. Ther. Nucl. Med. 78:* 1007–1012, 1957.
60. Steinberg, I. Poststenotic dilatation (aneurysm) of the subclavian artery associated with cervical rib. Report of two cases. *Am. J. Roentgenol. Rad. Ther. Nucl. Med. 92:* 1328–1330, 1964.

61. Taber, R. E. Surgical management of carotid artery aneurysm with ball valve thrombus. *J. Cardiovasc. Surg. 20:* 477–480, 1979.
62. Telford, E. D., and Mattershead, S. Pressure at cervicobrachial junction. *J. Bone Joint Surg. 30B:* 249–265, 1948.
63. Thomas, V. T. Control of bleeding in complicated peripheral vascular lesions. *Surg. Gynecol. Obstet. 132:* 1015–1018, 1971.
64. Thomas, V. T. Intrathoracic aneurysms of the innominate and subclavian arteries. *J. Thorac. Cardiovasc. Surg. 63:* 461–471, 1972.
65. Winslow, N. Extracranial aneurysm of the internal carotid artery: history and analysis of the cases registered up to August 1, 1925. *Arch. Surg. 13:* 689–729, 1926.

CHAPTER 4

Surgical Treatment of Thoracic and Thoracoabdominal Aortic Aneurysms

E. STANLEY CRAWFORD, M.D.
DONALD M. SNYDER, M.D.

Operations for aneurysms of the thoracic aorta have been increasingly successful in recent years. Improved surgical technique has extended treatment, regardless of type, location, and magnitude of disease, resulting in a substantial decrease in operative mortality and an increase in long-term survival. Refinements in anesthesia and monitoring techniques have also contributed to the success of operative treatment. All aneurysms of the aorta are now surgically accessible, and this chapter emphasizes the current concepts of disease and principles of treatment of thoracic aortic aneurysms.

For the purpose of simplifying this discussion, operative treatment will be described according to segment of aortic involvement, starting with the most proximal lesions. The thoracic aorta extends from the aortic annulus to the diaphragmatic hiatus and is divided into ascending, arch, and descending segments. The ascending aorta is bounded proximally by the aortic annulus and extends distally to the orifice of the innominate artery. The aortic arch is defined as that segment of aorta from which the brachiocephalic vessels arise and is bounded proximally by the origin of the innominate artery and distally by the origin of the left subclavian artery. The descending thoracic aorta starts just distal to the left subclavian artery and extends to the diaphragm. The thoracoabdominal segment includes the descending thoracic and abdominal aorta.

ETIOLOGY

Multiple etiologic agents account for aneurysmal disease in the thoracic aorta. Arteriosclerosis, a degenerative process affecting both the intima and media, may affect any segment and cause aneurysms. Males are affected more frequently than females, generally in the sixth and seventh decades of life but occasionally earlier. Disruption of the fibroelastic elements of the media with destruction of tissue integrity and calcification results in dilatation, elongation, and tortuosity of the aorta which, in its severest form, is aneurysmal transformation. The entire circumference of the aorta is usually involved, resulting in fusiform aneurysms; however, if there is only partial wall involvement, the aneurysm may be saccular in nature.

The common medial diseases that cause aneurysms are cystic medial necrosis and myxomatous degeneration. Both tend to involve the ascending aorta and aortic annulus and cause aortic insufficiency, but may involve any part or all of the aorta. The former tends to occur in middle and old age and the latter may occur at any age and be genetically linked and manifested as Marfan's syndrome with characteristic ocular, musculoskeletal, and cardiovascular complications. The latter form of the disease occurs early in life and causes death in 50% of cases by the age of 32 years. The media in other cases may be weakened or destroyed by arteritis (i.e., nonspecific or giant cells) of unknown etiology and cause aneurysms. These diseases occur at any age and the ages of our cases have varied from 19 to 63 years (1, 3, 5, 8).

Dissection in the aortic wall may also lead to aneurysmal formation. Unless due to an acute traumatic event, most dissections are initiated by medial degeneration in the aortic wall which result in decreased cohesiveness of the layers. Repeated aortic pulsations with each cardiac cycle create flexion stresses that result in an intimal tear, occurring most commonly in the ascending or descending thoracic aorta. The hydrodynamic pressures of the bloodstream exert pressure through the intimal tear, leading to dissection of the aortic layers which may progress proximally, distally, or in both directions simultaneously. The dissecting hematoma may then spontaneously rupture back into the true aortic lumen terminating the event, or rupture into the pericardium or pleural cavity, leading to early death in most cases. Once the dissection has stabilized, the resulting false lumen may continue to undergo dilatation, forming a fusiform aneurysm. This disorder usually occurs in the sixth to seventh decades of life and earlier in patients with myxomatous degeneration and more commonly affects males. Eighty-five percent of patients have hypertension on admission or a history of hypertension (1, 3, 5, 8).

Microbial infections may result in mycotic aneurysms which are predominantly saccular in nature. Syphilitic aneurysms, although now rare, usually affect the ascending and aortic arch. Occasionally, fusiform aneurysms may occur with diffuse syphilitic aortitis. Pyogenic bacteria, usually in association with acute or chronic endocarditis, may produce saccular aneurysms occurring in the aortic arch and the abdominal aorta behind the mesenteric vessels (1, 3) (see Chapter 8).

Traumatic aneurysms usually result from acute deceleration injuries which lead to disruption of the aortic intima and media. The most common site of such injuries is just distal to the left subclavian artery where the aorta is most fixed. The transverse tear (usually posterior) that ensues may occasionally be contained by the surrounding adventitia, resulting in a pulsating hematoma. If rupture does not occur within several weeks, fibrosis stabilizes the lesion, resulting in a chronic traumatic aneurysm. Such lesions usually undergo calcification and may remain stable and asymptomatic for years.

False aneurysms may occur following previous aortic operations and are usually due to deterioration of suture material including silk, polyethylene, and nylon. Infection, tension, or progression of the underlying disease at the anastomosis may also result in false aneurysmal formation. This type of aneurysm may be either fusiform or saccular and, fortunately, does not occur in the chest as often as in peripheral locations (1, 3).

CLINICAL MANIFESTATIONS

Symptoms and signs of thoracic aortic aneurysms are usually due to expansion or dissection of the aortic wall, compression, obstruction, or erosion of the adjacent structures, or frank rupture. Pain is the most common symptom and may be acute in onset, as with dissection or rupture, or may develop gradually as the aneurysm expands. The discomfort is usually in the region of aortic involvement, but may radiate to the neck, back, shoulders, or abdomen. In all cases, progression in the intensity of pain suggests impending rupture and demands expedient treatment.

Although aneurysms at any level may remain asymptomatic for long periods of time, symptoms (when they do occur) may be very similar in each region. Aneurysms of the ascending aorta or aortic arch may both produce fulminant heart failure by induction of aortic insufficiency, or secondary to creation of high-flow shunts by erosion into the heart, pulmonary arteries, or great veins. Compression of the superior vena cava or innominate veins may produce venous distention of the neck and upper extremities. Compression of the trachea or bronchus may lead to wheezing, cough, or pneumonitis distal to the area of obstruction, whereas erosion into the airway or pulmonary parenchyma can produce hemoptysis. Pericardial tamponade may also result from rupture of the aneurysm into the pericardium (1, 3, 5).

In addition to pain and airway compression or erosion, aneurysms of the descending thoracic aorta or thoracoabdominal segment may also present with symptoms more unique to these areas. Obstruction of, or erosion into, the esophagus, although rare, may occasionally produce dysphagia or hematemesis. Compression of the vagus or recurrent laryngeal nerve may occasionally produce hoarseness. Neurologic deficits secondary to spinal cord ischemia may develop, but are most often associated with acute dissection. With thoracoabdominal involvement, duodenal and inferior vena cava fistulas may occur as with any aneurysm involving the aortic segment (1, 3, 5, 7, 8, 11).

Acute dissecting aneurysms of the aorta may present with protean manifestations, since any or all of the aorta may be involved. Pain described as sharp, tearing, or knifelike in quality (usually severe, steady, or intermittent) may be located in the back, epigastrium, or both, although nausea, vomiting, and abdominal tenderness are rare. With ascending aortic involvement, which is most commonly seen, acute aortic insufficiency may be precipitated, and rupture into the pericardium may occur and produce tamponade. Dissection may produce myocardial insufficiency by causing obstruction of the orifices, or by direct extension into the coronary arteries. With involvement of the aortic arch, any or all of the brachiocephalic vessels may be compromised, leading to ischemia of the upper extremities or to hemiplegia. Acute dissection in the descending thoracic aorta may produce spinal cord ischemia which results in paraplegia (as previously described). As the dissecting process enters the abdominal aorta, it may either terminate by re-entering the true lumen or proceed into the common femoral arteries, producing ischemia of the lower extremities. The blood supply to the visceral vessels can be severely compromised, producing intestinal and renal ischemia that may result in oliguric or anuric renal failure. If the dissection enters a chronic state, the wall of the false lumen may undergo fusiform aneurysmal dilatation and, depending upon the segment involved, produce symptoms by compression, obstruction, or erosion (as previously described).

Regardless of the location of the aneurysm, frank rupture into the mediastinum, pleura, or peritoneal cavity represents the most devastating manifestation of these lesions. In a review of 176 patients with a diagnosis of thoracic aortic aneurysm, rupture of the aneurysm was the leading cause of death in 135 patients who were not surgically treated. Of this group, death by rupture occurred in 77% of the patients with dissecting aneurysms and 44% with arteriosclerotic aneurysms. In these two groups, symptoms prior to rupture occurred in 78 and 42% of patients, respectively (1, 3, 5, 7, 8, 11).

DIAGNOSIS

Although in some cases the diagnosis can be made from the history and physical examination, most cases require thorough radiologic investigation. Aneurysms of the thoracic aorta may be suspected in the presence of mediastinal widening or masses contiguous with the aortic shadow on plain chest roentgenograms. In the presence of syphilitic or arteriosclerotic aneurysms, calcification in the wall of the aneurysm may be readily seen. Involvement of the ascending aorta and proximal aortic arch usually presents radiologically in the upper right and middle mediastinum, while involvement of the distal arch and descending thoracic aorta presents to the left of the midline. An acute dissecting aortic aneurysm should be suspected on the plain film in the presence of a change in aortic shadow on successive films, evidence of aortic wall thickening by displacement of intimal calcification, or widening of the mediastinum with concomitant pleural effusion (1, 3, 5).

For precise diagnosis of disease, its extent, and location, contrast aortography under high-pressure injection is required. Anteroposterior, oblique, and lateral views should be obtained, with views of any potentially involved branch vessels for accurate delineation. With most aneurysms, aortography will usually demonstrate a dilated arterial lumen, but occasionally the lumen may appear normal because of the presence of laminated clot. In such cases, the presence of calcification in the aortic wall beyond the contrast-filled lumen may allow for the determination of whether or not an aneurysm actually exists. Unsuspected concomitant occlusive disease of the branch vessels may also be visualized, allowing for a precise approach to treatment. In the presence of either an intimal tear and a false channel or compression of the true aortic lumen by the dissecting hematoma, a definitive diagnosis of a dissecting aortic aneurysm may be made. Ultrasonography, a valuable tool in the diagnosis of abdominal aortic aneurysms, is minimally effective in the diagnosis of thoracic aneurysms due to interference caused by the air-filled lungs. Computerized axial tomography (CAT) scan, however, provides an excellent method of study, especially in patients with dissection, clot-filled aneurysms, and postoperative perigraft complications. It has been suggested this form of noninvasive investigation may offer a valuable advantage over invasive angiography in elderly patients with localized lesions by obviating the potential development of renal impairment caused by angiographic contrast medium (1, 3, 5, 13).

OPERATIVE SELECTION AND PREOPERATIVE ASSESSMENT

All patients with asymptomatic aneurysms of the thoracic aorta should have elective operative treatment of these lesions unless other underlying medical conditions contraindicate operation. However, all patients who present with symptomatic aneurysms should be submitted to emergent operation, regardless of severity of concurrent medical problems, because of the dismal results associated with rupture. Indications for operation in patients with acute and chronic dissection are covered in the "Treatment" section.

Associated diseases should be thoroughly assessed before operation and appropriate treatments administered to minimize operative risks. Hypertension should be controlled by the administration of rapid-acting vasodilators and pulmonary insufficiency improved, as much as possible, by available techniques. Digitalization should be instituted preoperatively in all patients and carried through the postoperative period. A broad-spectrum antibiotic should be started at least one to two hours prior to operation and continued into the postoperative period to assure adequate tissue levels. Adequate hydration and correction of electrolyte imbalance should be secured prior to the undertaking of operation.

As previously described, all patients should undergo thorough radiologic investigation; and, if their condition permits, an assessment of the extent of the disease, presence of other unsuspected aneurysms, and presence of associated occlusive diseases should be determined. Similarly, patients with evidence of coronary insufficiency should have selective coronary angiography so that appropriate treatment can be designed. Naturally, in patients with symptomatic myocardial or cerebrovascular disease, appropriate staging of operation is needed to minimize the patient's operative risks. In such cases, patients with unstable, nocturnal, or preinfarction angina and evidence of transient ischemic attacks should first undergo coronary artery bypass and/or carotid endarterectomy, with replacement of the aneurysm done as soon as is clinically feasible (usually in four to six weeks). All may be accomplished at one operation if the aneurysm involves only the ascending or arch aorta (1–3, 7, 9, 10, 12).

Special consideration must also be given to patients with multiple aneurysms. Patients with concurrent aneurysms of the ascending or arch aorta and descending or thoracoabdominal segment should have the symptomatic lesion treated first. However, if all the lesions are asymptomatic, the proximal aneurysm is usually replaced first in order to prevent its possible rupture during aortic cross-clamping for repair of the more distal lesion. Similarly, it is not uncommon to encounter patients who have concomitant descending thoracic and infrarenal abdominal aortic aneurysms. A decision must be made as to which aneurysm should receive treatment priority, or whether both lesions should be corrected at the same operation. Rupture of thoracic aortic aneurysms has occurred in the postoperative period following successful graft replacement of infrarenal aortic aneurysms; and, likewise, rupture of abdominal aortic aneurysms has occurred in the postoperative period following successful correction of thoracic aortic aneurysms. Because of this potential threat, both aneurysms should ideally be replaced at the same operation, but this is not always feasible. Priority should be given to the symptomatic lesion or to the descending thoracic aneurysm if both lesions are asymptomatic, with the other lesion being corrected if the patient's condition warrants. We believe the advantage of this approach is that complications occurring in the postoperative period from abdominal aortic aneurysms are easier to detect than those occurring in the thorax. In our experience, eight patients have had successful replacement of both aneurysms at one operation (1, 3, 5, 6, 9, 13).

SPECIAL CONSIDERATIONS

Improved results in thoracic aneurysm operations are secondary to advances in surgical technique, anesthesia, monitoring, and application of component therapy for the normalization of coagulation. Aneurysms are no longer excised, rather, they are incised longitudinally with cautery after proximal and distal control. Clot is removed from the aneurysm and bleeding points not to be revascularized are suture-ligated from within. Back bleeding from any intercostal, lumbar, visceral, or major arterial branch to be revascularized is controlled with Fogarty catheters of appropriate size. The graft is sutured from within the aneurysm to the proximal aorta. Serially, side holes are appropriately made on the graft and the arterial branches to be revascularized are again reattached from within. Finally, the distal anastomosis is performed in a similar fashion, but distal and proximal flushes are performed prior to completion of the graft. Before declamping, the patient's head is lowered to prevent any residual air in the graft system from embolizing into the brain. The aneurysmal wall is used to the advantage of the surgeon as a hemostatic blanket around the graft; it is sutured around the graft material and forms a watertight wrap to prevent annoying bleeding from the graft and/or suture sites. Using the inclusion technique, minimal preliminary dissection is required and the operative field is dry at the completion of the procedure. Although no shunts or heparin are used for treatment of aneurysms not requiring extracorporeal bypass, we have not encountered difficulty with arterial thrombosis and/or embolization. These large, long aneurysms can be associated with massive blood loss which needs to be replaced. This blood loss makes the patient mildly hypocoagulable and adding heparin would only increase the bleeding. Recently, in an attempt to preserve the patient's own blood, we have used a cell saver for autologous transfusion of red blood cells and have saved up to ten units of the patient's own blood for any one operation. We routinely use component replacement therapy, including fresh frozen plasma, platelets, and cryoprecipitate, to render the patients normo-coagulable at the end of the procedure (4–9).

During the past four years, the same anesthetic protocol has been employed exclusively with very gratifying results. Non-cardiac depressant agents (Sublimaze and Valium) are used to induce anesthesia and muscle relaxation is obtained with pancuronium bromide. Cardiocompression and lung injury during operative manipulation are avoided by insertion of a Carlen's double-lumen endobronchial tube, which allows collapsing of the left lung on command. Multiple percutaneous lines are inserted that include bilateral radial artery catheters for blood pressure recording, a subclavian catheter singular for central venous pressure monitoring and the administration of drugs, a right pulmonary artery thermodilution Swan-Ganz catheter for monitoring the pulmonary artery and pulmonary capillary wedge pressure and cardiac output, and four peripheral intravenous catheters for rapid volume replacement. Blood gases, chemistry, and acid-base balance are monitored every 30 minutes and appropriate adjustments are made. Mannitol (25 g) is administered at the induction of anesthesia and the urinary output continuously monitored.

Abnormalities detected by the various monitoring modalities are treated before or at the time of occurrence. Normal blood volume and good cardiac output are assured before induction of anesthesia by proper administration of intravenous fluids, if necessary. Proximal blood pressure, cardiac hemodynamics, and peripheral resistance are maintained at desirable levels during the period of aortic clamping by the administration of nitroprusside solution and appropriate replacement of blood and fluid losses. Ventricular arrhythmias are treated with lidocaine (Xylocaine) and/or propranolol hydrochloride (Inderal). Declamping hypotension is avoided and the desired cardiac hemodynamics are obtained first by discontinuing the nitroprusside, then by rapidly administering blood elements and electrolyte solution for restoration of losses as the proximal aortic clamp is slowly removed. Bicarbonate solution is administered routinely by drip to prevent or treat post-clamping acidosis (4–9).

TREATMENT

Ascending Aortic Aneurysms

Operative treatment of aneurysms in unselected patients involving the ascending aorta has resulted in survival rates as high as 92%. Operative approach is through the median sternotomy incision using cardiopulmonary bypass. Prior to the exposure of the aneurysm, partial cardiopulmonary bypass is secured through the femoral approach to augment cardiopulmonary function and aid in the autotransfusion of blood during exposure. Occasionally, the aneurysm may be large enough to preclude double cannulation of the right atrium for venous return and, with partial bypass previously obtained through the groin, only the superior vena cava remains to be cannulated through the limited exposure available. Saccular aneurysms may occasionally be treated by excision and lateral aortorrhaphy, but more frequently require closure by Dacron patch tube grafts.

Following exposure of the aneurysm and establishment of cardiopulmonary bypass, the ascending aorta is cross-clamped as close to the innominate artery as possible. The aneurysm is incised longitudinally and the cut edges of the aneurysmal sac retracted with stay sutures. The annulovalvular apparatus and coronary ostia are then inspected. If there is no evidence of involvement of these structures and all pathology appears to be in a supracoronary location, which is most often the case with arteriosclerotic aneurysms, the aneurysmal segment is simply replaced by an appropriately sized, woven Dacron tube graft using the previously described inclusion technique. Continuous suture of 3-0 polypropylene is used to complete the anastomosis to the uninvolved segments of aorta. Prior to completion of the distal anastomosis, blood is allowed to enter the heart and graft to evacuate air and the anastomosis carried to completion. The distal aortic clamp is then removed and cardiac function restored on partial bypass. The aneurysmal sac is securely closed over the graft providing complete hemostasis; cardiopulmonary bypass is discontinued. Coagulation is restored by previously described techniques and the wound is closed (1–3).

The above technique is modified in the presence of annulovalvular involvement. Following opening of the aneurysm, if valvular insufficiency or sinus dilatation are noted, the aortic valve should be either resuspended or replaced, depending upon etiology. Resuspension may occasionally be employed in those patients with dissection in whom the tough inner layer of aorta remains, from which the valve may be securely resuspended; however, when the proximal aortic intima has been fragmented or destroyed, the aortic valve is removed and replaced by a prosthetic valve (Figs. 4.1 and 4.2). The proximal segment of ascending aorta is then replaced (as previously described) with one modification in the case of dissection. Prior to performing the proximal and distal anastomoses, the edges of the aorta are first coapted between strips of Dacron felt using

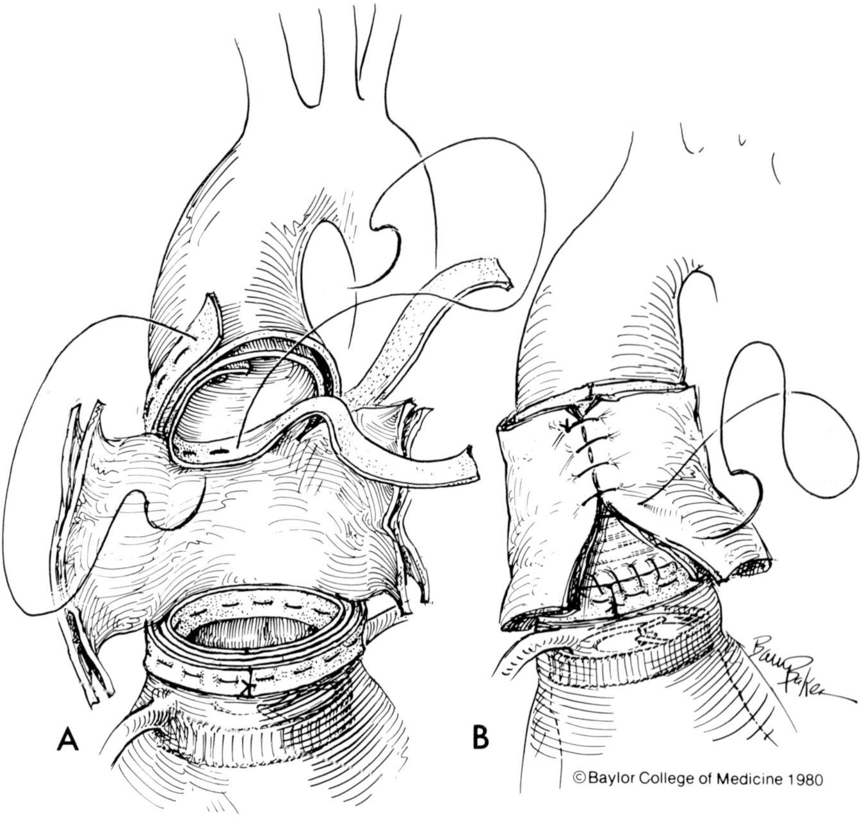

Figure 4.1. Technique of a separate valve-graft replacement in patients with types I and II dissection associated with aortic insufficiency. *A*, aortic valve replaced with a prosthetic valve and the aortic wall reconstituted proximally and distally using Dacron felt. *B*, proximal ascending aorta replaced with Dacron graft and the aortic wall sutured around the graft.

interrupted mattress sutures to obliterate the false lumen. This technique holds the friable inner layer in place and offers a more secure sewing surface for the proximal and distal anastomoses. Care should be exercised in inserting the Dacron strips to avoid narrowing of the aortic lumen (14).

The technique of prosthetic valve replacement and supracoronary grafting does not eliminate the potential for aneurysmal dilatation of the sinuses of Valsalva which has occurred in 16% of patients reported in one series who were followed for a mean of 72 months. Re-operation in this group resulted in an operative mortality of 60%. Paravalvular leakage and suture line bleeding in the early postoperative period was also observed in 10 to 20% of cases. As a result of these problems, most surgeons now agree that the composite graft-valve technique should be employed in all patients with annular dilatation, or in those in whom the

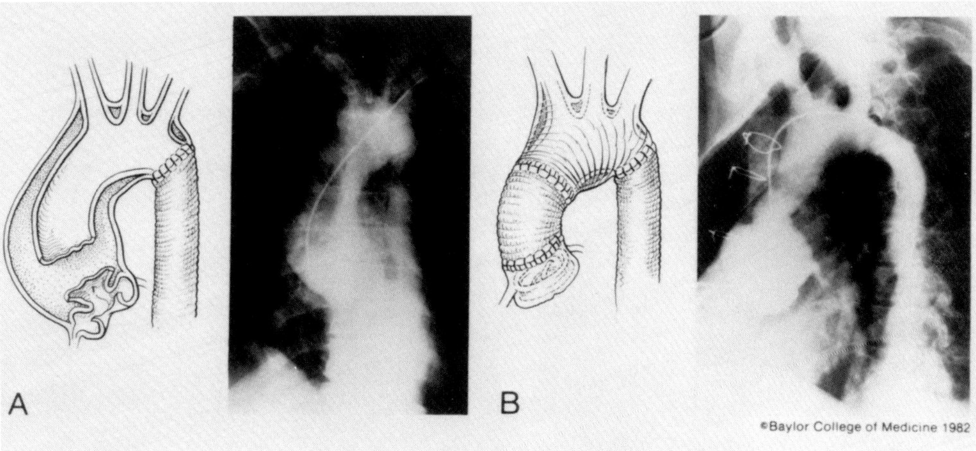

Figure 4.2. Illustrations of a patient with type I dissection in whom the technique illustrated in Figure 4.1 was employed. Aortograms and drawings made before (*A*) and after (*B*) operation showing the location and extent of dissection and a separate valve and graft in place after operation. Note the enlarged coronary sinuses.

dissection has extended into the annulus, the heart, or has ruptured into the pericardium at the aortic root. It is believed that this technique decreases blood loss, shortens operative time, lowers mortality, and decreases late complications. Our results with this technique have been very gratifying, improving patient survival from 74% in earlier years to 92% with the composite graft-valve technique (3).

Insertion of the composite graft-valve requires several modifications in technique (Figs. 4.3 and 4.4). Following opening of the aneurysm, if sinus dilatation or valvular insufficiency are noted, the valve is excised. Properly sized valve and graft are then sewn together with continuous polypropylene suture, and the valve end of the graft is sutured to the aortic annulus with horizontal mattress sutures. The orifices of the coronary arteries are then visualized and openings are made in the graft opposite to these structures. The origins of the coronary arteries are then sewn circumferentially to the openings in the graft with 4-0 polypropylene suture. The distal end of the graft is then sewn to uninvolved aorta or, in the case of dissection, to aorta that has been appropriately coapted between strips of Dacron felt (Fig. 4.3). The operation is then carried on to completion (as previously described). Pseudoaneurysms have been observed at the coronary graft anastomoses and attributed to tissue friability by some authors who recommend performance of these anastomoses with horizontal mattress sutures through Dacron pledgets. Fortunately, we have not encountered development of pseudoaneurysms at this level (9, 12, 13).

Further modifications are required in patients with concurrent coronary artery disease, or in those in whom the dissecting process has extended into the coronary arteries. In such cases, the orifices of the

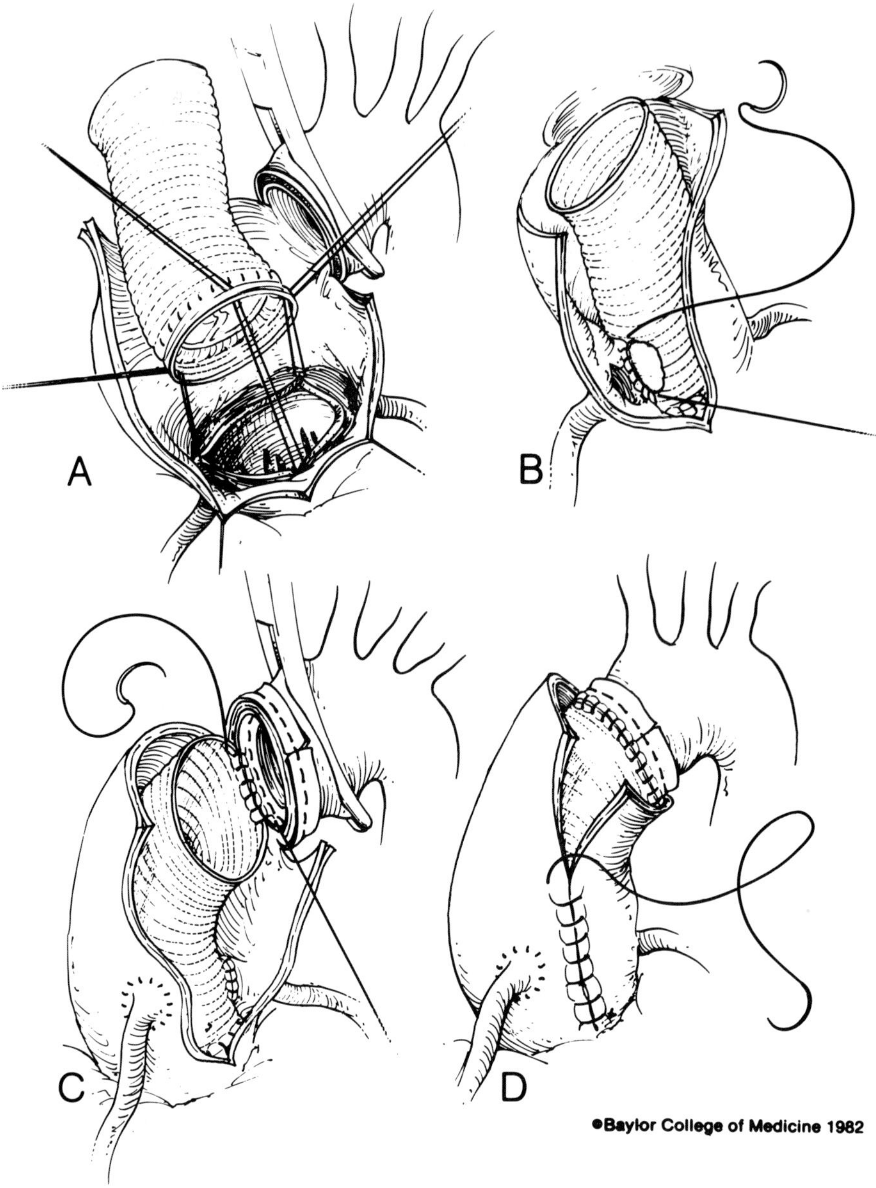

Figure 4.3. *A* to *D*, drawings showing a technique of composite valve-graft insertion for treatment of a dissecting aortic aneurysm producing either aortic insufficiency or rupture at the base of the aorta.

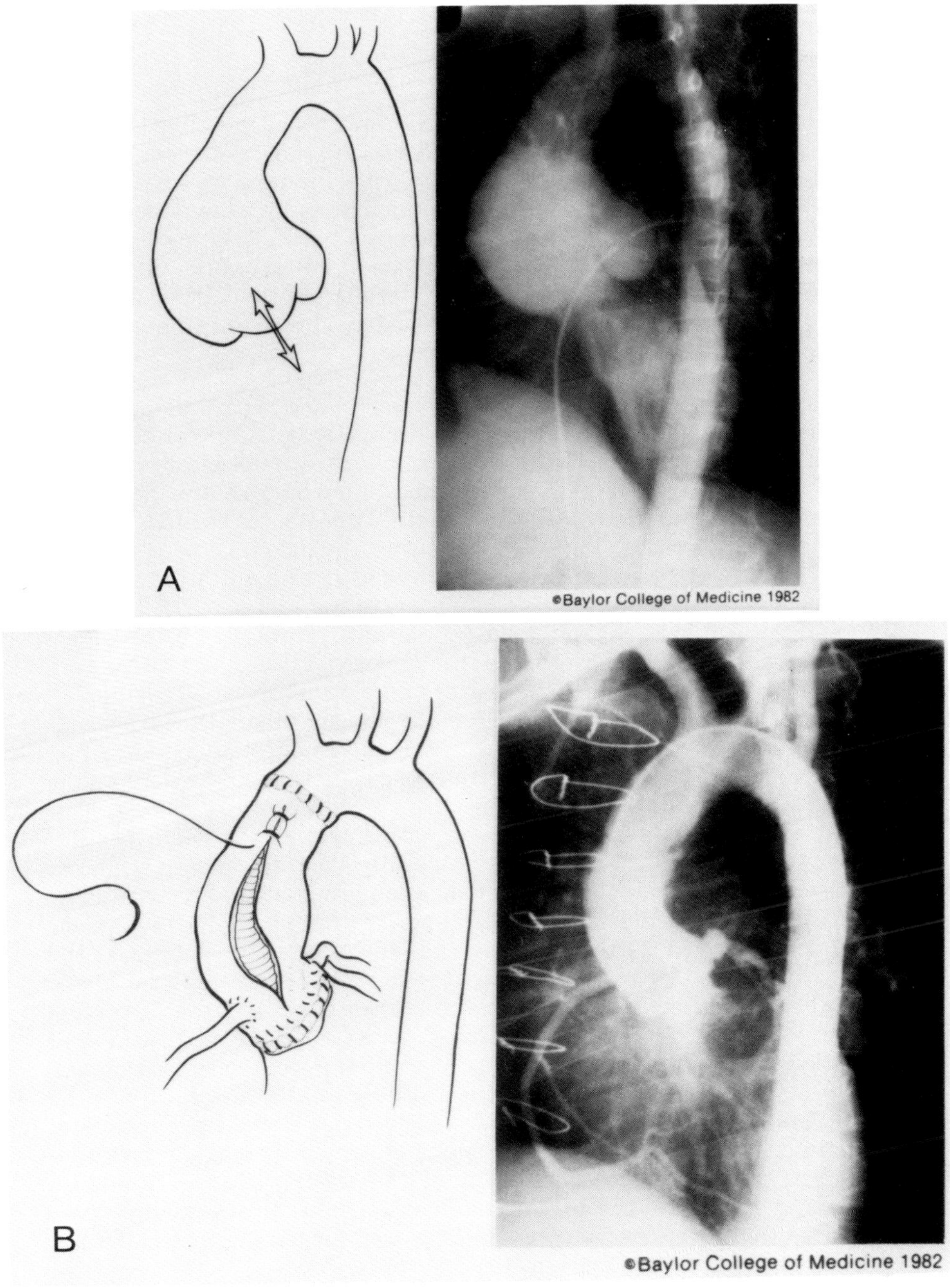

Figure 4.4. Illustrations of a valve-graft replacement in the treatment of annuloaortic ectasia from cystic medial necrosis (Erdenheim's disease) producing aortic valvular insufficiency. *A,* drawing and aortogram made before operation showing the extent of the disease. *B*, drawing and aortogram made after operation showing the valve-graft in place and functioning.

coronary arteries are obliterated by suture and occlusions bypassed by insertion of saphenous vein grafts (attached distally in a routine manner). Proximally, however, graft attachment to the innominate, carotid, or subclavian artery is preferred so that the aneurysmal wall may be tightly closed over the aortic graft, assuring hemostasis. If it is necessary to attach the vein grafts to the aortic graft, openings are made into both the aneurysmal wall and aortic graft; vein grafts are then attached after the aneurysmal wall has been circumferentially sutured to the openings in the aortic graft (1–3, 10, 11).

Aortic Arch Aneurysms

Aneurysmal involvement of the aortic arch may be quite variable and, for this reason, provides the ultimate challenge to the cardiovascular surgeon. Sacciform aneurysms, in particular, may involve only a portion of the aortic circumference usually directly opposite the orifices of the brachiocephalic vessels (Fig. 4.5). Fusiform aneurysms, on the other hand, usually involve the entire circumference of the aorta for variable distances. In association with aneurysms of the ascending aorta, only the proximal arch into the region of the innominate artery may be involved; whereas in the case of descending aortic aneurysms, only the distal arch in the region of the left subclavian artery may be involved. Occasionally, only the arch is involved in the disease process, sparing both the ascending and descending aorta, while in others involvement may extend from, or include, the aortic annulus proximally to, or including, the descending thoracic aorta distally (3, 4, 14).

Until recently, operative correction in this area of the aorta has not been as successful as in other areas. Operative therapy in this segment imposes unique technical and physiologic requirements most specifically concerning cerebral and myocardial preservation. Various techniques have been employed for this purpose and have been dependent upon the nature, location, and extent of aneurysmal involvement of the aortic arch. Early operative techniques for aneurysms in this area, involving the innominate and left common carotid artery, utilized the insertion of temporary or permanent bypass grafts from the uninvolved ascending aorta proximally to the distal cut ends of these vessels distally. Once the grafts were functioning, the aorta was cross-clamped proximal and distal to the aneurysm and graft replacement performed. While the insertion of bypass grafts prior to correction of the actual aneurysm reduced myocardial strain and cerebral ischemia, their presence in the operative field often increased the technical difficulty of the operation and did not eliminate cerebral complications (4).

With the advent of extracorporeal cardiopulmonary bypass as a support means for open heart surgery, further operative techniques evolved. Cardiopulmonary bypass with separate brachiocephalic perfusion became the method of choice for treatment of patients with transverse aortic arch aneurysms. Early in the experience, however, problems with excessive cerebral perfusion due to high flow rates and pressure were encountered, resulting in capillary damage, cerebral swelling, and hemorrhagic

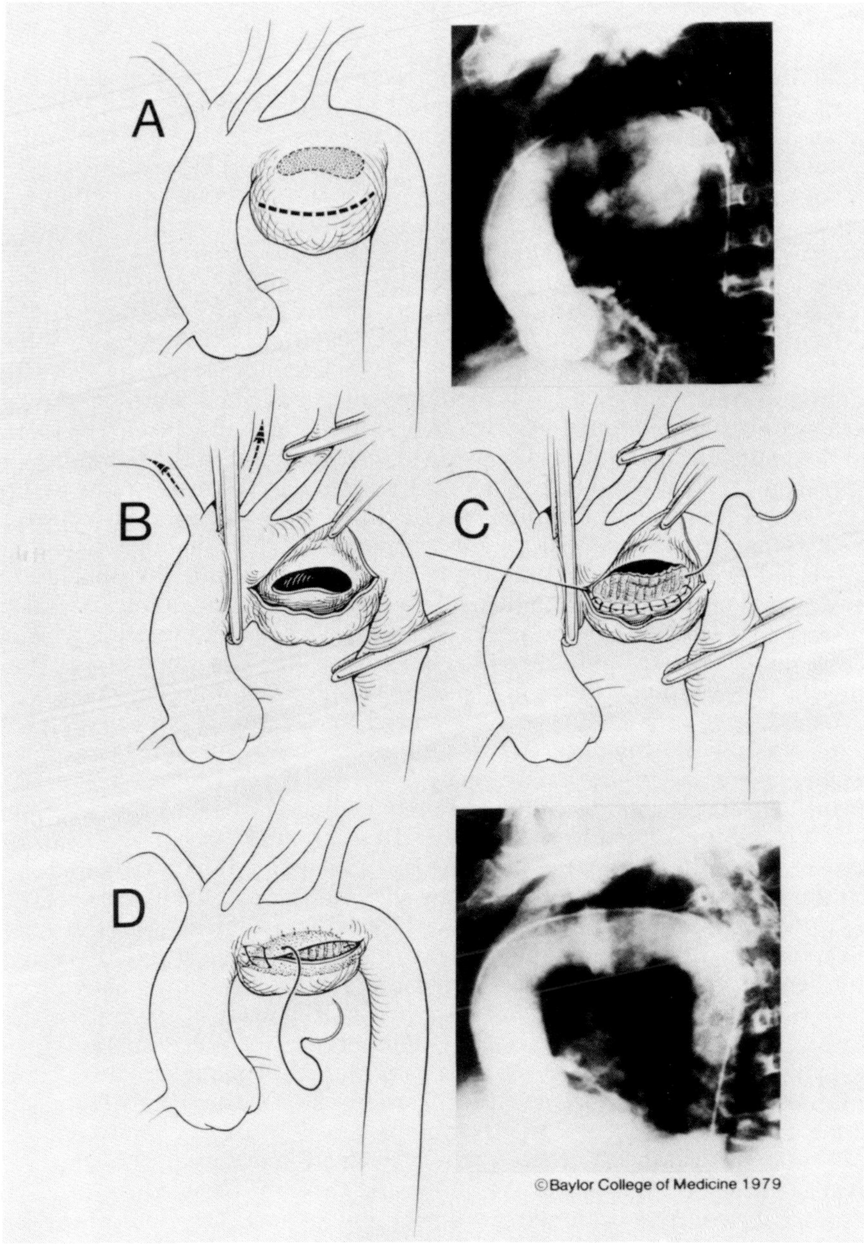

Figure 4.5. Illustrations of treatment of an aneurysmal distal aortic arch by a simple cross-clamp technique, using nitroprusside to maintain normal blood pressure and cardiac function. *A*, drawing and aortogram made before operation showing the location and extent of the disease. *B* to *D*, drawings showing the technique of aortic reconstruction using a patch-graft and aortogram made after operation, showing final appearance of the repaired aorta.

infarcts. Adjustments were made by reducing flow rates and perfusion pressure, but, although reduced, cerebral complications were still encountered. Utilizing these various shunting and bypass techniques, the senior author treated 20 patients with a 75% survival in earlier years (3).

On the other hand, aneurysms of the distal aortic arch involving the segment of aorta from which the subclavian artery arises do not present such difficult technical and physiologic demands for operative treatment. Most have been treated by simple proximal and distal aortic cross-clamping using sodium nitroprusside to control blood pressure and cardiac hemodynamics (Fig. 4.5). The operative approach is through a left posterolateral thoracotomy overlying the bed of the 5th or 6th rib. Proximal control is usually obtainable between the left common carotid artery and subclavian artery, but, occasionally in more extensive distal arch aneurysms, clamping is performed just proximal to the left common carotid artery. Cerebral flow is maintained through the innominate artery in all cases and the left common carotid artery in most cases, with cardiac hemodynamics controlled as previously described. The distal cross-clamp is placed at the level of uninvolved thoracic aorta and the subclavian artery is likewise cross-clamped. If the proximal aortic clamp is placed proximal to the left common carotid artery, this vessel must likewise be cross-clamped to avoid bothersome back bleeding. The aneurysm is then incised longitudinally on its anterior surface and the walls retracted with sutures. Sacciform aneurysms are closed by Dacron patch aortoplasty, with the aneurysmal sac imbricated over the repair for hemostasis. Fusiform aneurysms are corrected by inserting woven Dacron tube grafts, utilizing the inclusion technique as previously described. In the event the aorta is cross-clamped between the innominate and left common carotid arteries once the proximal anastomosis is completed, flow is reconstituted to the left common carotid artery by moving the proximal aortic clamp to a more distal location, which is usually directly across the graft itself just beyond the proximal anastomosis. Proximal anastomosis is performed in such a fashion as to keep the subclavian orifice above it, if possible—this technique is aided by cutting the graft at an appropriate angle to allow an increase in the circumference for anastomosis. If the subclavian artery orifice cannot be maintained proximal to this suture line, it is reattached to the graft using a separate Dacron graft. The distal anastomosis is then done in a routine manner. Prior to completing this anastomosis, the head of the table is lowered and appropriate flushing techniques employed to remove all air and thrombus from the graft. The anastomosis is then completed and the aneurysmal sac closed over the graft in a hemostatic fashion after flow is reconstituted. The senior author has treated 37 patients with this type of lesion utilizing this technique with only one death, although the left common carotid artery was cross-clamped in five patients.

A major advance in the treatment of extensive arch lesions involving the innominate and left common carotid arteries occurred in 1974 with the introduction of profound hypothermia and circulatory arrest by

Griepp and associates (11), who showed a 75% survival in their first report. This new approach alleviated the need for continued cerebral perfusion, clearing the operative field of cumbersome bypass grafts and perfusion catheters. Although not completely eliminated, the number of cerebral complications was reduced. The most troublesome complication of this new technique was bleeding during the rewarming period, occasionally extending into the postoperative period. Subsequently, modifications have been adopted which essentially eliminate the bleeding problem and have now been successfully applied in 29 of 30 patients by the senior author without complications.

Exposure is obtained through a standard median sternotomy incision, with arterial perfusion achieved through the common femoral artery and venous cannulation through the right atrium. Left-sided heart sumping is obtained by insertion of a separate cannula into the left ventricle *via* the right superior pulmonary vein. Perfusion is controlled at a rate of 55 ml/kg and temperature modified by a disposable hypothermic heat exchanger attached to the venous return system. Temperature is monitored by three separate probes inserted into the rectum, esophagus, and nasopharynx which measure surface, core, and cerebral temperature, respectively. With the onset of cardiopulmonary bypass, cooling is begun at a rate of 1°C/min and, following graft insertion, rewarming is commenced at a rate that should not exceed 1°C every 3 minutes to avoid possible gas vaporization. During the cooling and rewarming periods, sodium nitroprusside is administered to promote better perfusion and reduce skin-core temperature differential. Hemoconcentration and cellular sludging have been shown to occur during cooling and, consequently, hemoglobin and hematocrit values are diluted by 25 to 30% of normal during this period. Myocardial protection is afforded by the combination of systemic cooling and intermittent cardiac surface cooling with cold saline solution (7, 10, 12).

The ascending aorta, transverse aortic arch, and brachiocephalic vessels are exposed anteriorly with minimal dissection. Once the desired level of hypothermia is obtained (usually 12°–15°C core temperature), the head of the table is lowered and brachiocephalic vessels clamped. Prior to opening the aneurysm, the rate of perfusion is reduced to 50 to 150 ml/min, but never completely stopped. The aneurysm is incised longitudinally and the walls retracted with suture (Figs. 4.6 and 4.7). Gauze sponges are then inserted into the proximal and distal openings of the aorta to collect debris as the thrombus in the aneurysmal wall is removed, avoiding potential embolization when flow is reconstituted. Debris is, likewise, removed from the orifices of the brachiocephalic vessels proximal to the cross-clamps by saline irrigation. Blood flow at the opening of the descending aorta is controlled with the pump aspirator at all times. An appropriately sized, woven Dacron tube graft is chosen and the distal anastomosis performed to the descending thoracic aorta via the inclusion technique, with two rows of running 4-0 polypropylene suture. The graft is then occluded manually and the suture line checked

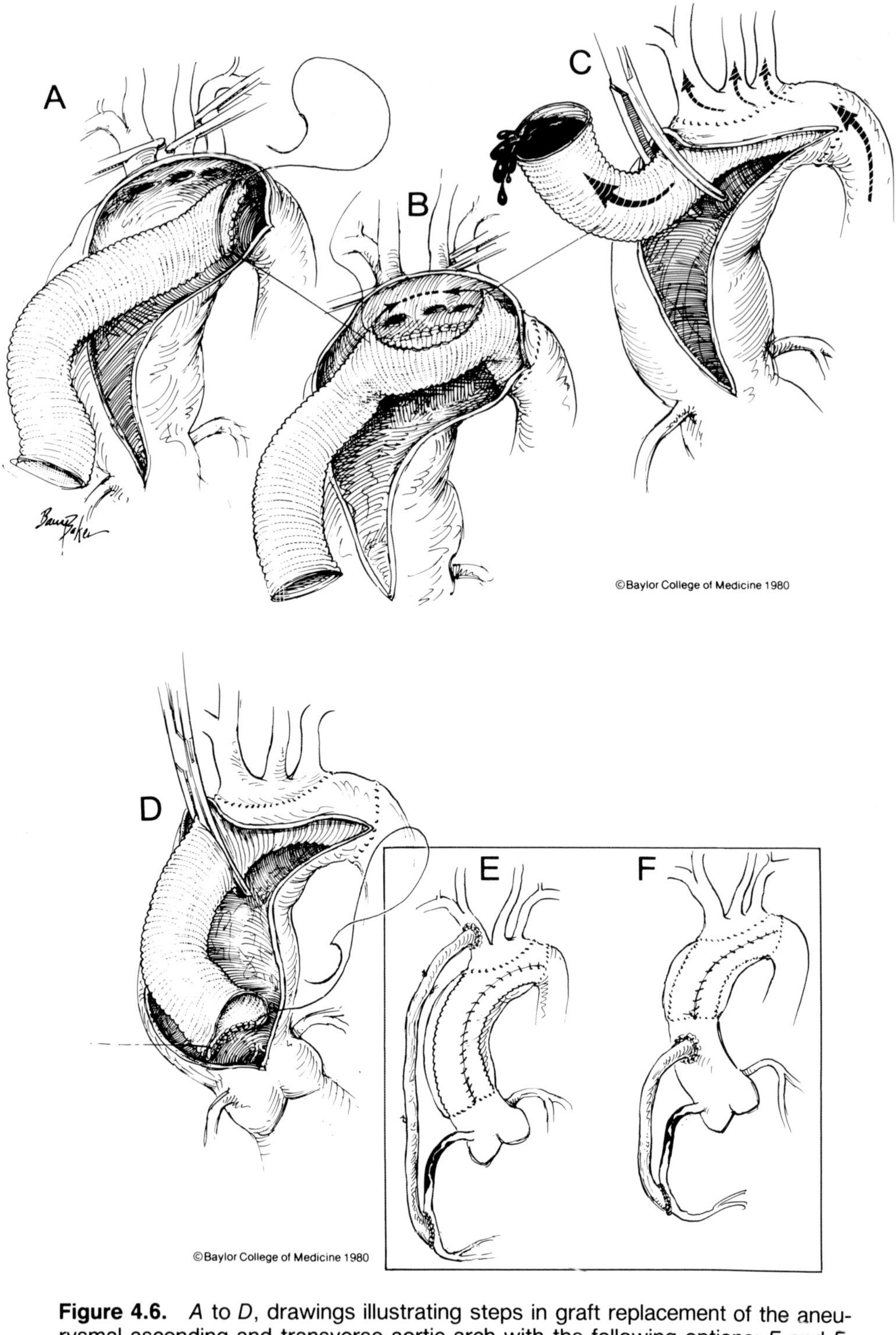

Figure 4.6. *A* to *D*, drawings illustrating steps in graft replacement of the aneurysmal ascending and transverse aortic arch with the following options: *E* and *F*, proximal coronary artery bypass graft attachment, depending upon extent of the ascending aortic involvement.

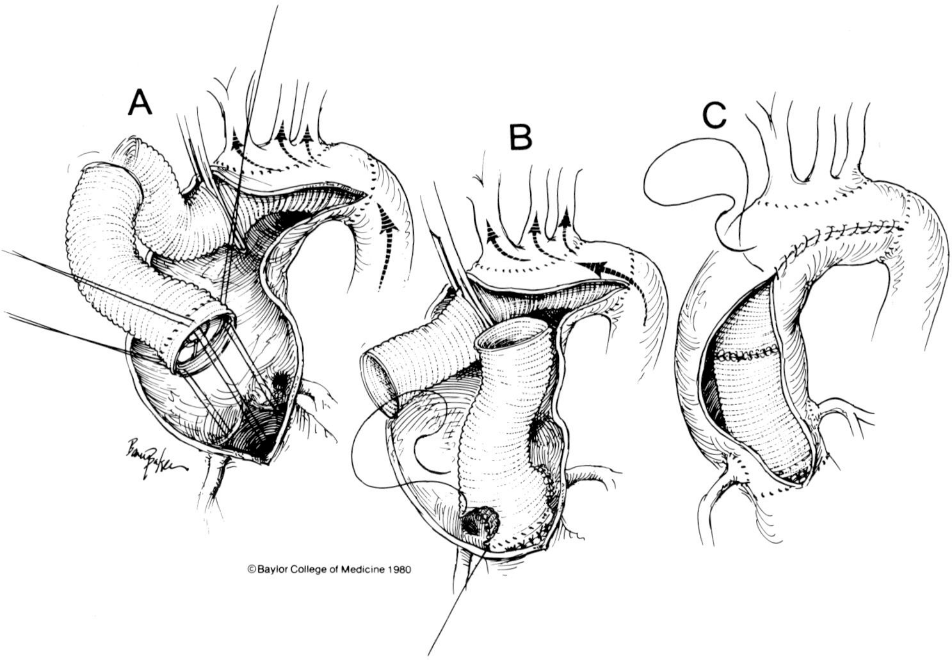

Figure 4.7. *A* to *C*, drawings showing steps of a composite valve-graft replacement in patients in whom an arch aneurysm extends proximally to involve the aortic root.

for leakage by temporarily increasing the perfusion rate. Interrupted sutures are used to control any bleeding sites. Appropriate tension is applied to the graft and an oval opening made in the graft opposite the origins of the brachiocephalic vessels. The opening is then sewn circumferentially around these origins from within the opened aorta, as described for the distal anastomosis. The graft is manually compressed proximal to the suture line and the perfusion rate again temporarily increased to check for leaks, which are appropriately suture-ligated. The patient's head is lowered and the proximal end of the graft elevated and allowed to fill with blood for evacuation of any air; brachiocephalic vessels are unclamped and milked proximally to remove any air. The graft is cross-clamped proximal to this anastomosis and normal perfusion is restored and rewarming begun. The position of the proximal anastomosis depends upon the extent of aneurysmal involvement. If the aortic annulus is not involved, the proximal anastomosis is done to the closest normal-appearing part of the ascending aorta and is performed in a similar fashion (as described for the distal anastomosis). However, if the annulus is dilated and aortic insufficiency presents, the valve is excised and replaced by a composite valve-graft (as described previously for isolated aneurysms of the ascending aorta) (Fig. 4.7). The coronary arteries are then sutured to the openings in the graft from within the

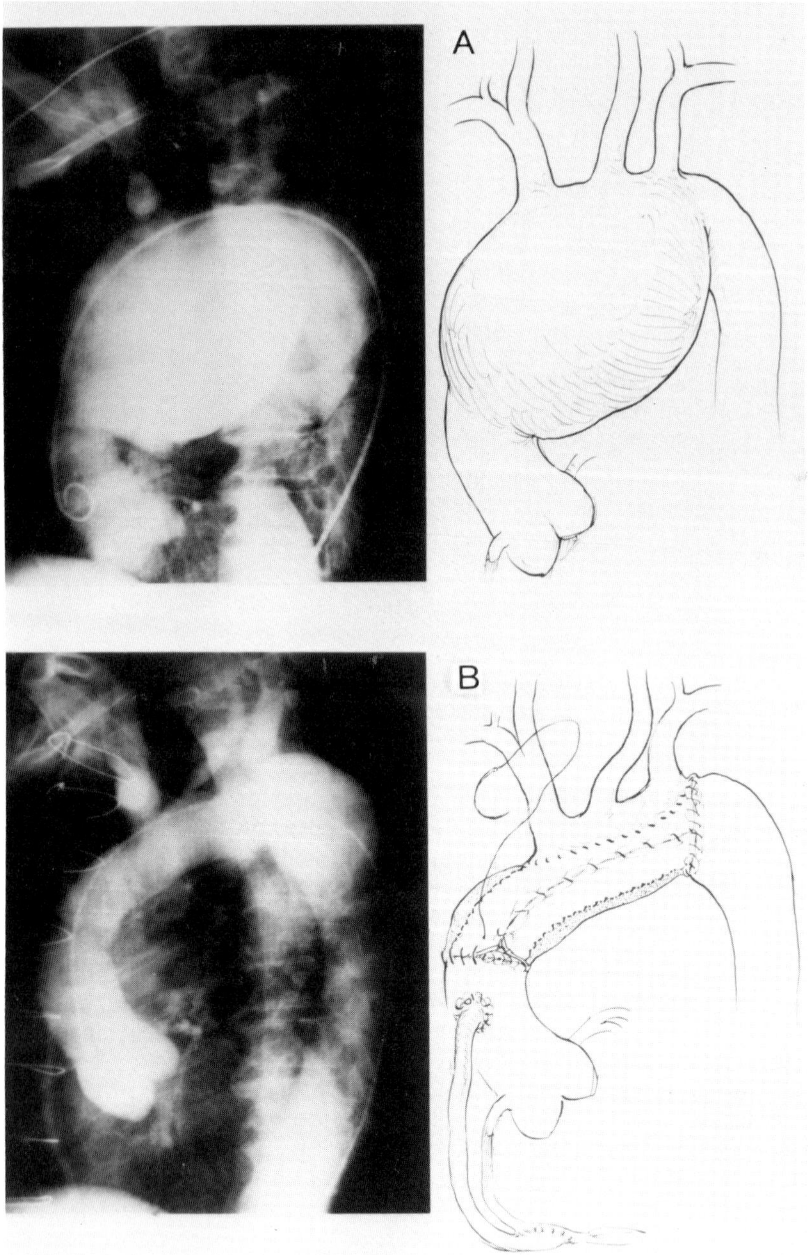

Figure 4.8. Illustrations of the treatment of a patient with coronary artery disease and a large arch aneurysm that compressed and ruptured into the pulmonary artery. *A*, aortogram and drawing made before operation showing the location and extent of the disease. *B*, aortogram and drawing made after operation showing the aortic and coronary artery bypass grafts in place and functioning. *C*, pulmonary

opened aorta and the proximal and distal grafts cut to appropriate length and sutured together with running 3-0 polypropylene suture. Prior to completing this final anastomosis, the heart and graft are allowed to fill completely with blood to fully evacuate any air and the anastomosis is completed. At this point in the operation, bleeding (troublesome to others in the past) is avoided by securely reapproximating the aneurysmal walls over the reconstruction with running 3-0 polypropylene suture. A watertight closure is performed and complete hemostasis obtained. In our experience, graft compression has not been a problem (Fig. 4.8).

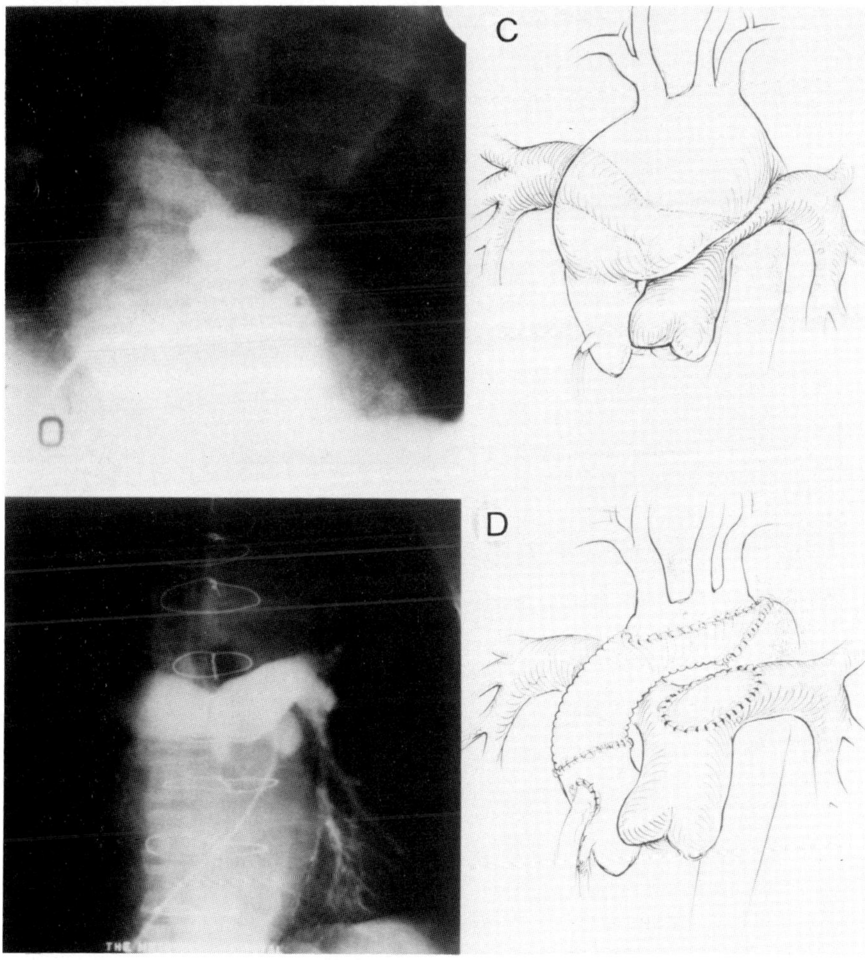

Figure 4.8 (*C* and *D*)

---

angiogram and drawing made two weeks before operation showing compression of the pulmonary artery. *D*, pulmonary angiogram and drawing made after operation showing the normal pulmonary artery after repair. [Reproduced with permission from Crawford and Saleh (5).]

In the event it has been determined preoperatively that the patient will also require coronary artery grafting, the grafts may be attached during the cooling period. Distal anastomoses are performed in the standard fashion, while the proximal anastomosis is performed to the

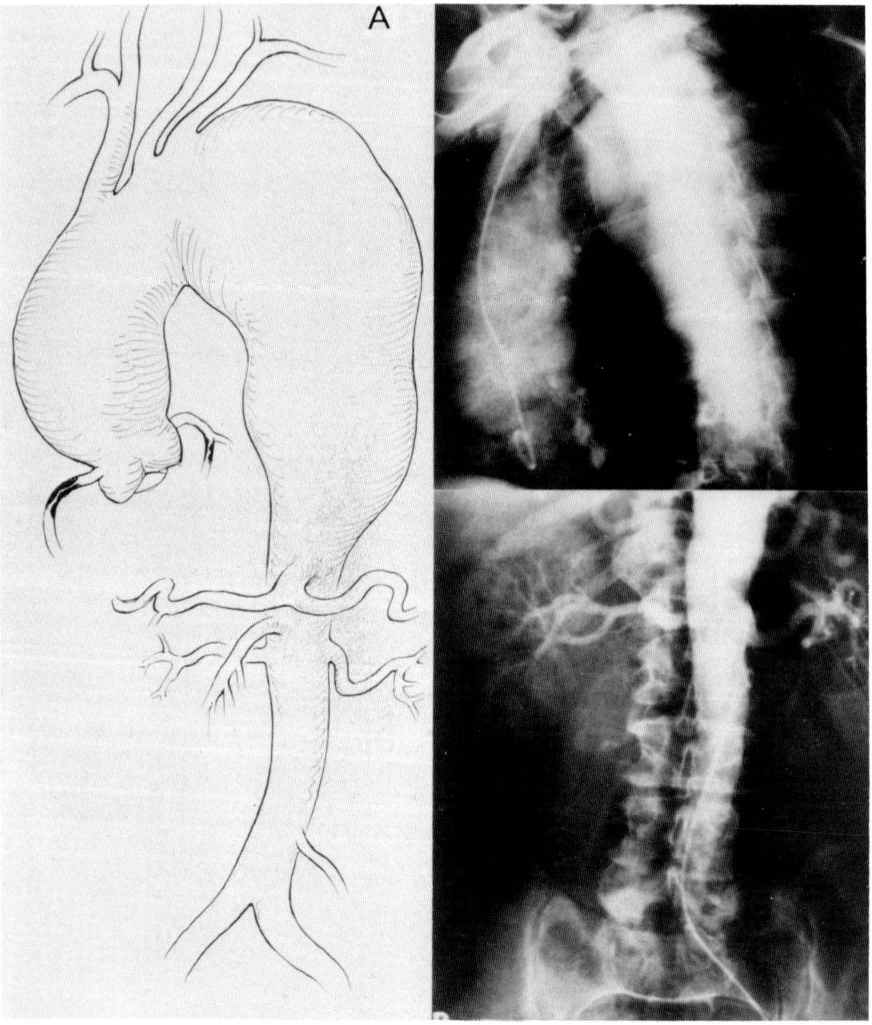

Figure 4.9. Illustrations of treatment of a patient with coronary artery disease and extensive aneurysmal disease of the ascending arch and descending thoracic aorta. Coronary artery bypass graft and replacement of the ascending and transverse arch replaced first at one operation and then, six weeks later, the aneurysm descending thoracic aorta replacement at a second operation. *A*, drawing and aortogram made before operation showing the location and extent of the disease. *B*, drawing and aortogram made after second operation showing the location and extent of the grafting. [Reproduced with permission from Crawford and Saleh (5).]

ascending aorta if uninvolved, or to brachiocephalic vessels in instances in which the ascending aorta is also aneurysmal (Figs. 4.6*E* and *F* and 4.9). Only if these techniques are not feasible should the coronary artery bypass grafts ever be attached directly to the aortic reconstruction (this technique has been described previously in the "Ascending Aortic Aneurysms" section).

The cooling period generally lasts from 30 to 60 minutes, while the rewarming interval is substantially longer, lasting from 78 to 138 minutes. Thrombocytopenia has been observed during profound hypothermia and, during the rewarming period, the platelet count does not completely

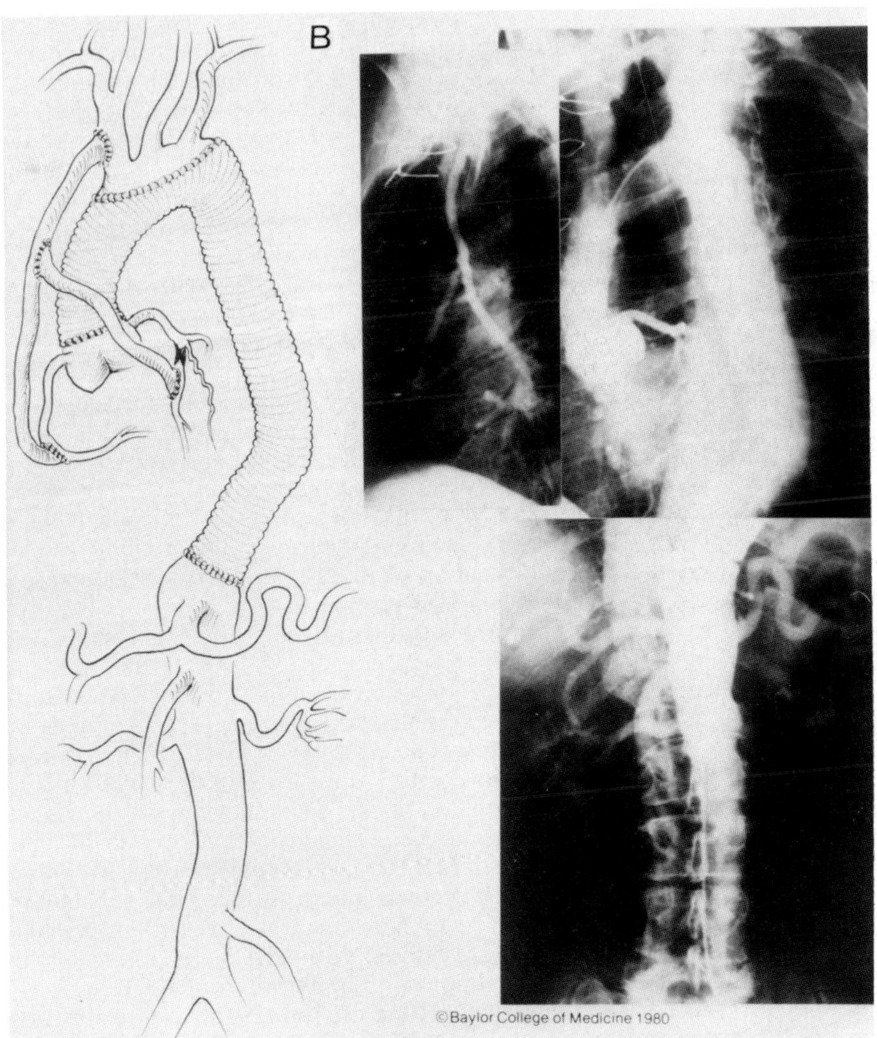

Figure 4.9 (*B*)

return to its preoperative level. For this reason, 10 to 12 units of platelets are administered, along with protamine and blood components, to normalize the clotting mechanism and stabilize cardiovascular hemodynamics. Once hemostasis is complete, the chest is closed in a routine fashion. As a result of our experience, we now prefer profound hypothermia and circulatory arrest in treatment of all patients with extensive arch aneurysms. Those patients whose lesions are confined to the distal transverse arch are still managed by simple aortic cross-clamping (as previously described) (3, 4, 7, 10, 12).

Descending Thoracic Aortic Aneurysms

Paraplegia, renal failure, and acute left ventricular strain have been major complications in the operative repair of descending thoracic aortic aneurysms and, for this reason, various techniques have been employed to avoid these problems. Earliest attempts utilized surface hypothermia, extracorporeal circulation, and temporary extravascular shunting to decompress the proximal aortic segment and perfuse the distal aorta during operation. Utilizing such a technique, mortality ranged from 11 to 22% and paraplegia varied from 1 to 11%. From 1956 to 1967, the senior author treated 36 patients with aneurysms of the descending thoracic aorta using various bypass and shunting techniques, with a mortality rate of 22% and incidence of paraplegia of 6%. However, during the interval from 1962 to 1967, patients underwent graft replacement by simple proximal and distal aortic cross-clamping because bypass or shunts had to be abandoned at the onset of replacement for technical reasons or the aneurysm ruptured, necessitating rapid control of bleeding. A reduction in both mortality and morbidity, including paraplegia, was noted in this group and the operation was greatly simplified. For these reasons, since 1967 simple aortic cross-clamping and pharmacologic control of cardiac and circulatory hemodynamics (as previously described) have been exclusively employed in 140 patients, with mortality of 9% and incidence of paraplegia of 3% (1, 6, 8).

Exposure is obtained through a left posterolateral incision made through the bed of the 6th and 7th ribs and the lung is deflated (as previously described). Minimal dissection is employed to circumferentially expose the aorta proximal and distal to the area of involvement for application of aortic cross-clamps. The posterior aspect of the aorta is mobilized by digital dissection and great care is exercised to avoid injury to the esophagus, intercostal arteries, or left pulmonary artery. In most cases, proximal aortic clamping can be performed just distal to the left subclavian artery. However, in approximately 30% of cases, the proximal clamp was applied between the left common carotid and left subclavian arteries because of the proximity of the aneurysm to the subclavian artery. The application of the distal clamp varied with the extent of the lesion, but was very near to the diaphragm in over half of the cases.

No attempt is made to dissect the lung off the aneurysmal wall, thus avoiding the occurrence of pleural stripping from the lung parenchyma and development of troublesome bleeding. The proximal aortic clamp is first slowly applied in concert with hemodynamic manipulations performed by the anesthesiologist. Following application of the distal clamp, the aneurysm is longitudinally incised through the pleura and aneurysmal wall, using electrocautery, and the edges of the aneurysmal wall are retracted with stay sutures (Figure 4.10). Laminated clot and thrombus in the aneurysmal sac are then manually removed. While extensive sacciform aneurysms may require replacement by tube grafts, most can be closed by simple Dacron patch-graft aortoplasty without the need for ligation of intercostal arteries (Fig. 4.11). The aneurysmal wall is then imbricated over this repair forming a watertight seal (as previously described).

All fusiform arteriosclerotic aneurysms are replaced with woven Dacron tube grafts (Fig. 4.12). Bleeding intercostal arteries are suture-ligated from within the aorta, minimizing the potential for interruption of collateral vessels. Transverse incision is then made at the proximal and distal ends of the longitudinal incision in the anterior half of the aortic circumference to facilitate graft insertion by inclusion technique. Appropriately sized, woven Dacron tube graft is then chosen and a proximal anastomosis is performed with continuous 3-0 polypropylene suture. Suture-line bleeding is checked by manually compressing the graft just beyond the anastomosis and temporarily releasing the proximal clamp, and is controlled with interrupted suture. The graft is placed under appropriate tension and cut to the desired length to reach the distal aorta; the distal anastomosis is performed in a similar fashion using continuous suture. Prior to completing this anastomosis, the patient's head is lowered and the proximal and distal aortic segments are flushed by temporarily removing the aortic clamps for the evacuation of air and thrombus which may have occurred, since heparin is not used. The distal anastomosis is completed while back bleeding from the distal aortic segment is allowed to continue. The proximal aortic clamp is removed in concert with the activities of the anesthesiologist (as described in a previous section), and the reconstruction completed by suturing the aneurysmal wall in a watertight fashion around the graft, securing hemostatis and preventing erosion of the graft into adjacent structures. The chest is closed in a routine fashion. This same operative technique is utilized to replace chronic traumatic and false aneurysms in this segment of the aorta.

Aortic cross-clamp time averaged 30 minutes in most cases but varied from 9 to 91 minutes, depending upon type and extent of the aneurysm, with sacciform aneurysms requiring the shortest clamp times. Urine flow ceases during the period of aortic occlusion and usually appears within an interval equal to the period of clamping, unless the patient has had inadequate volume replacement (1, 6, 8).

Thoracoabdominal and Abdominal Aortic Aneurysms Involving Celiac, Superior Mesenteric, and Renal Arteries

Aneurysms involving both the thoracic and abdominal aorta, or the abdominal aorta from which the visceral arteries arise, pose special

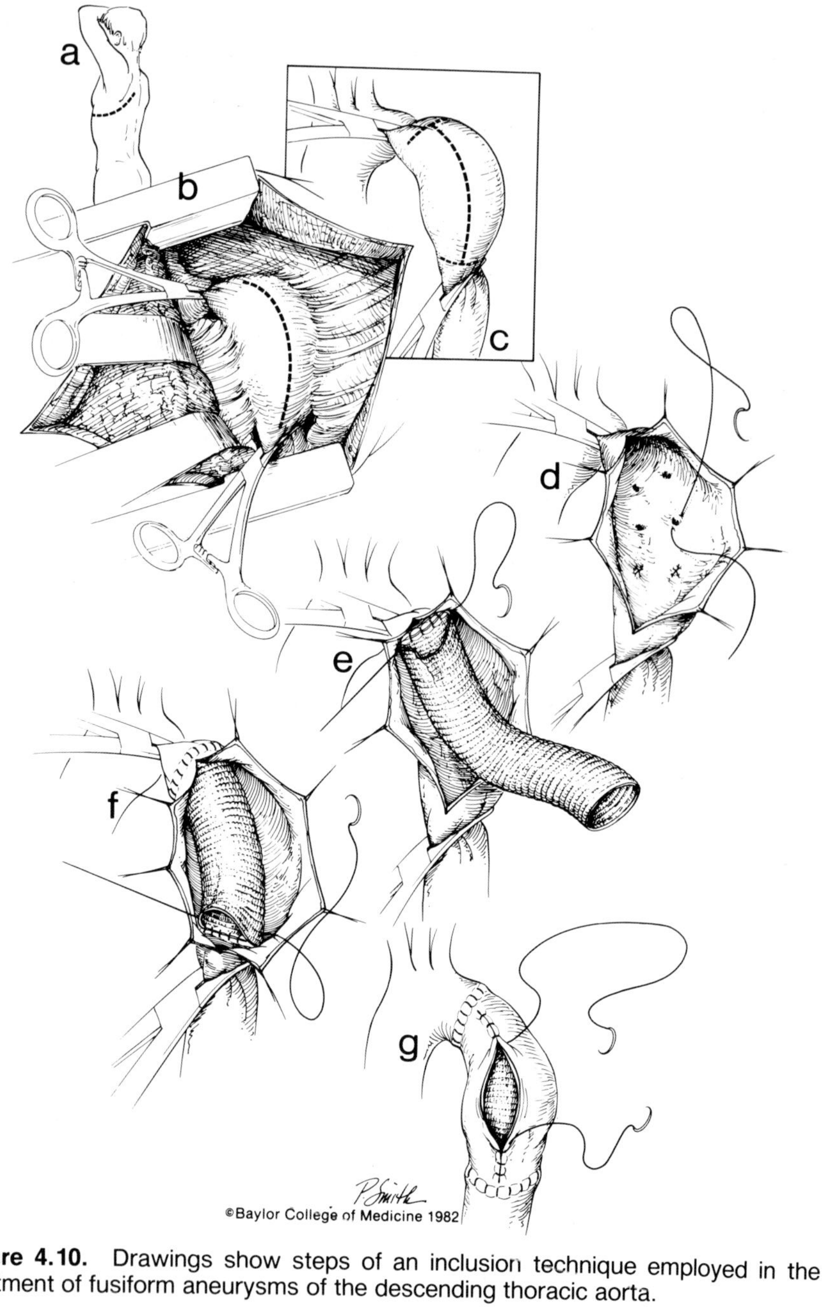

Figure 4.10. Drawings show steps of an inclusion technique employed in the treatment of fusiform aneurysms of the descending thoracic aorta.

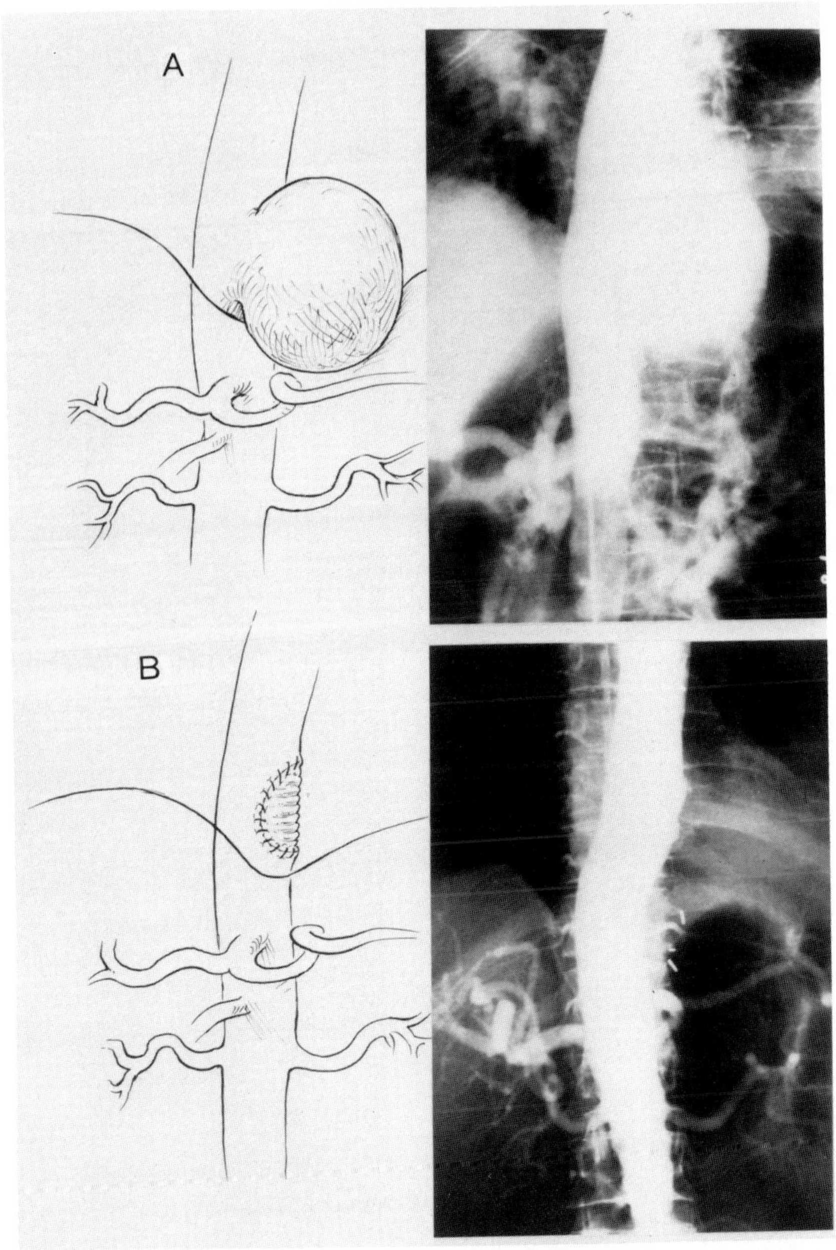

Figure 4.11. Illustrations of the treatment of a sacciform aneurysm in the lower end of the descending thoracic aorta using a patch-graft. *A*, drawing and aortogram made before operation showing the location and extent of the lesion. *B*, drawing and aortogram made after operation showing the location of the patch and aortic appearance after reconstruction.

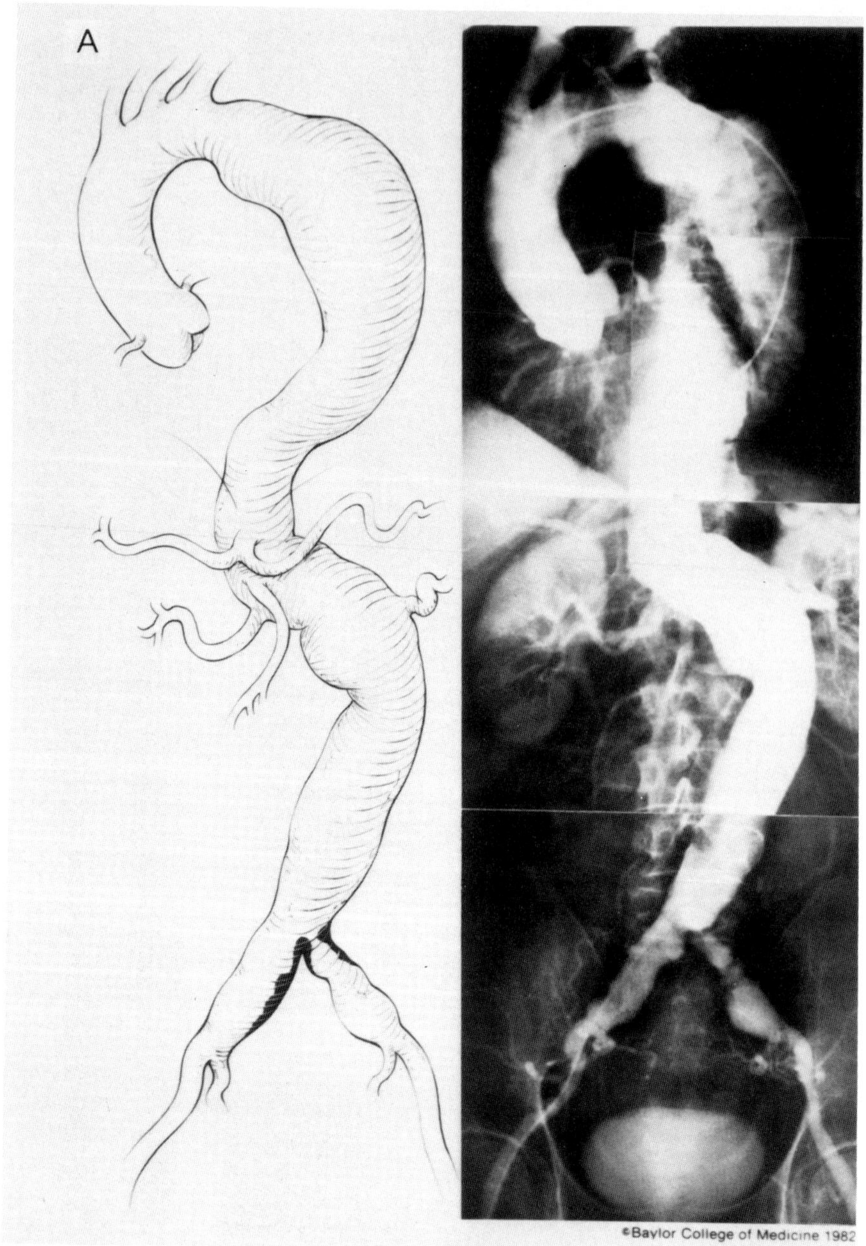

Figure 4.12. Illustrations of a graft replacement of a separate aneurysm of descending thoracic and abdominal aorta performed at the same operation to prevent rupture during the interval required for a staged operation. The aneurysms were asymptomatic and the thoracic aneurysm was removed first through a posterolateral chest incision. Then after closure of this wound, the abdominal aortic aneurysm was replaced through the standard midline abdominal incision. *A*, drawing

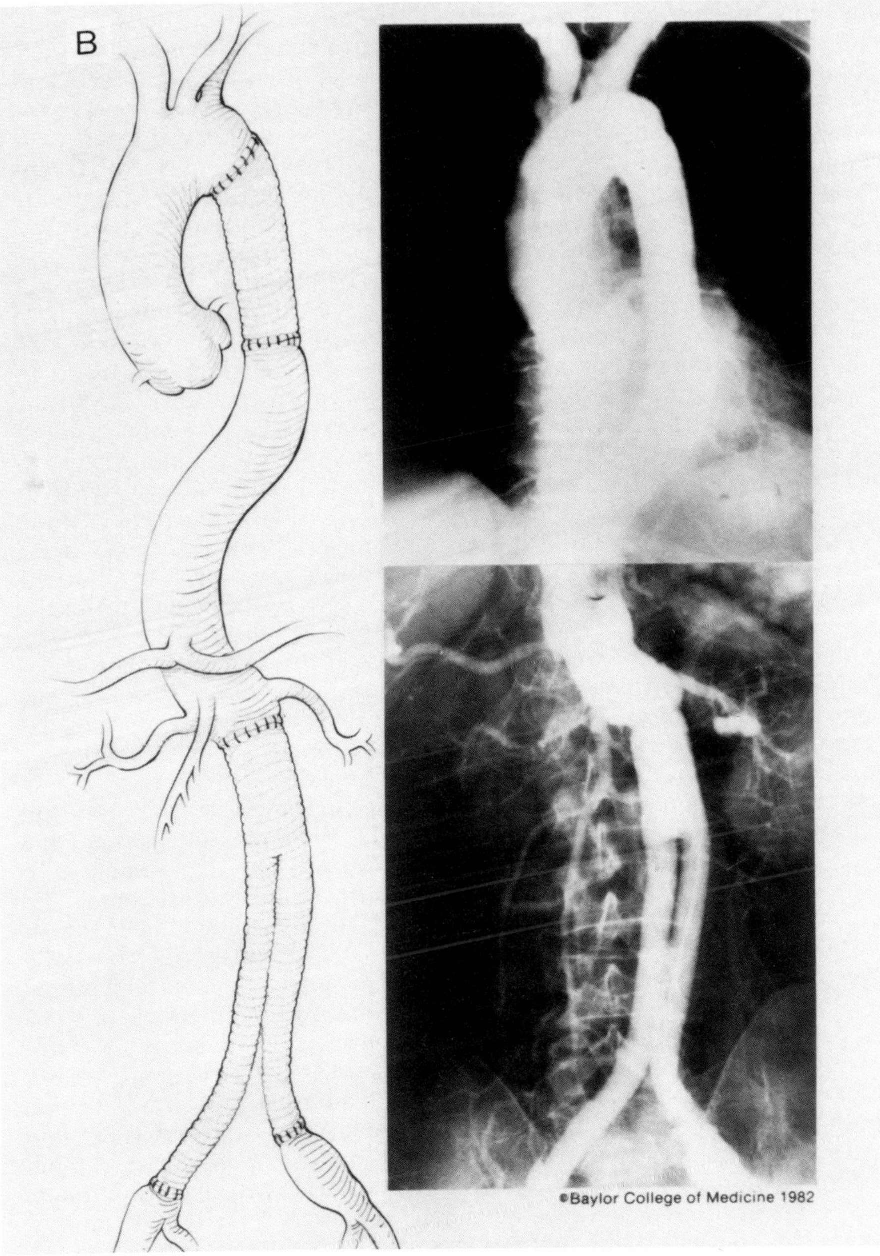

Figure 4.12 (*B*)

and aortogram made before operation showing the location and extent of the disease. *B*, drawing and aortogram made after operation showing the location and extent of the grafting.

problems in surgical management. These aneurysms usually require thoracoabdominal exposure of the aorta, reattachment of visceral vessels, and occasionally replacement of long segments of both the thoracic and abdominal aorta. Because of the refinements in surgical technique, anesthesia, medical management, and blood replacement therapy, significant progress has been achieved in the treatment of these lesions during recent years. These aneurysms can now be surgically managed in most patients with an operative survival rate of over 90% and an actuarial survival approaching that of abdominal aneurysm resection.

Thoracoabdominal aortic aneurysms can be classified into six groups according to location and extent of aneurysmal involvement. These groups are of clinical significance, as they determine the method and results of treatment, and occurrence of paraplegia after operation. In group I, the aneurysm extends from the left subclavian artery to below the diaphragm opposite the celiac axis. In group II, the aneurysm involves the entire aorta including the ascending aorta and the arch. In group III, most of the descending thoracic and abdominal aorta is involved with involvement of the celiac, superior mesenteric, and renal arteries. Group IV involves the distal thoracic aorta and most of the abdominal aorta with visceral arteries. Group V is limited to the upper part or all of the abdominal aorta with visceral arteries, while group VI involves primarily the infrarenal aorta but also involves the renal arteries (3, 5).

Aneurysms of groups I to V are best exposed through a left thoracoabdominal incision with the patient lying at an angle of about 45° on the right side. In patients with extensive aneurysms involving most of the descending thoracic aorta and all of the abdominal aorta, in whom the upper thoracic aorta and iliac arteries must be exposed for cross-clamping and reconstruction (groups II and III), the incision is started as a full midline abdominal incision which enters the abdomen and is completed by extension across the costal arch into the 6th or 7th interspace. In patients with more limited involvement to the distal thoracic aorta and upper abdominal aorta (group IV), the incision is made obliquely across the upper abdomen just above the umbilicus and extends across the costal arch into the 8th or 9th interspace. With more extensive abdominal involvement (group V), the oblique abdominal incision is made about 3 cm below the umbilicus. Patients with aneurysms involving the abdominal aorta from which the visceral vessels arise (group VI and some of group V) are best approached through a long midline abdominal incision in the supine position. For group VI aneurysms, the exposure and operation are performed anteriorly as is commonly done for infrarenal abdominal aortic aneurysms, except that the aorta is clamped proximally at the aortic hiatus of the diaphragm. For groups II, III, IV, and V aneurysms, however, the abdominal aortic segment exposure is *via* the retroperitoneal space. The peritoneum in the left gutter is incised lateral to the left colon with cautery and extended above to the esophageal hiatus and below to the pelvic brim. A relatively avascular plane in the retroperitoneal space adjacent to the body wall is entered which can be easily dissected up to the diaphragm, down to the abdominal aortic bifurcation, and medially to the posterior edge of the aneurysm adjacent to the vertebral column. This procedure is done by mobilizing and retracting to the right the abdominal viscera including the left colon, left kidney, spleen, body and tail of pancreas, and fundus of the stomach. The diaphragm is then transected radially to the aortic hiatus. The thoracic component of the aneurysm is then exposed by retracting the lung which has been collapsed by obstructing the left mainstem bronchus with the help of a previously placed double-lumen endotracheal tube. The proximal uninvolved aorta is exposed by minimal dissection for proximal circulatory control.

With the aneurysm exposed and without use of heparin, hypothermia, or organ perfusion, the clamp is slowly placed proximally to allow the anesthesiologist sufficient time to decrease peripheral vascular resistance to avoid significant elevation in proximal blood pressure and disturbances

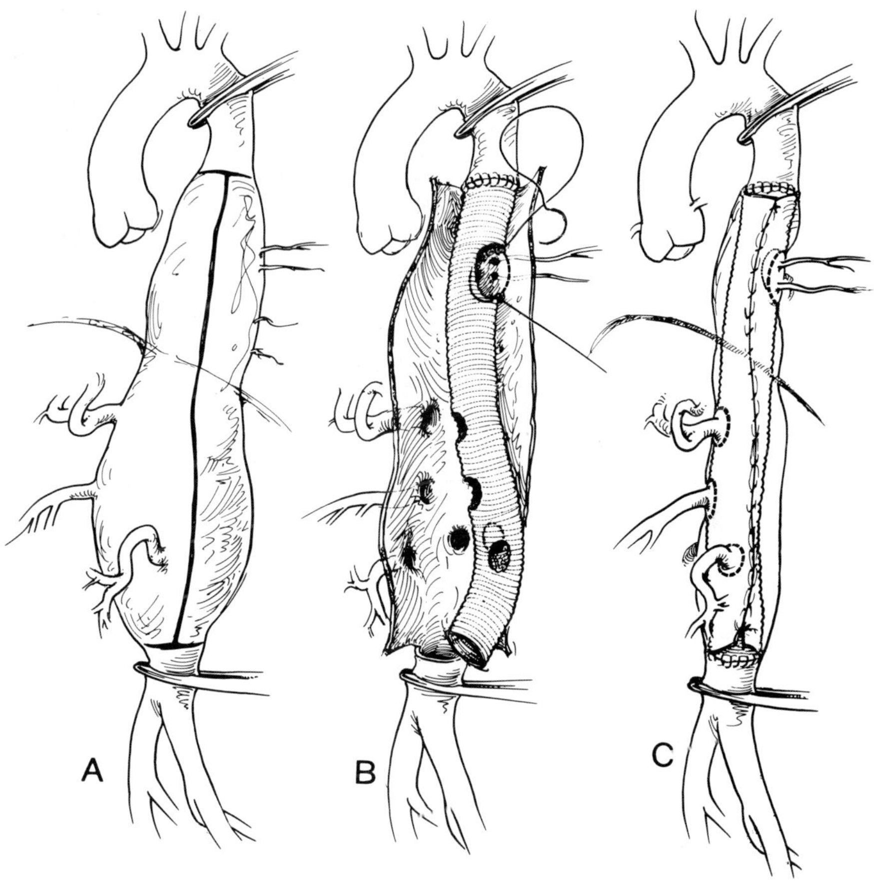

Figure 4.13. *A* to *C*, drawings showing methods of graft, a replacement of a thoracoabdominal aortic aneurysm, and vessel reattachment employing the graft-inclusion technique.

in cardiac hemodynamics (as previously discussed). The uninvolved segments are then clamped distally. The aneurysm is opened posterior to the left renal artery in the longitudinal direction, using electrocautery to prevent bleeding from the cut edges of the aneurysm (Fig. 4.13). Bleeding from major vessels (including renals, superior mesenteric, celiac,

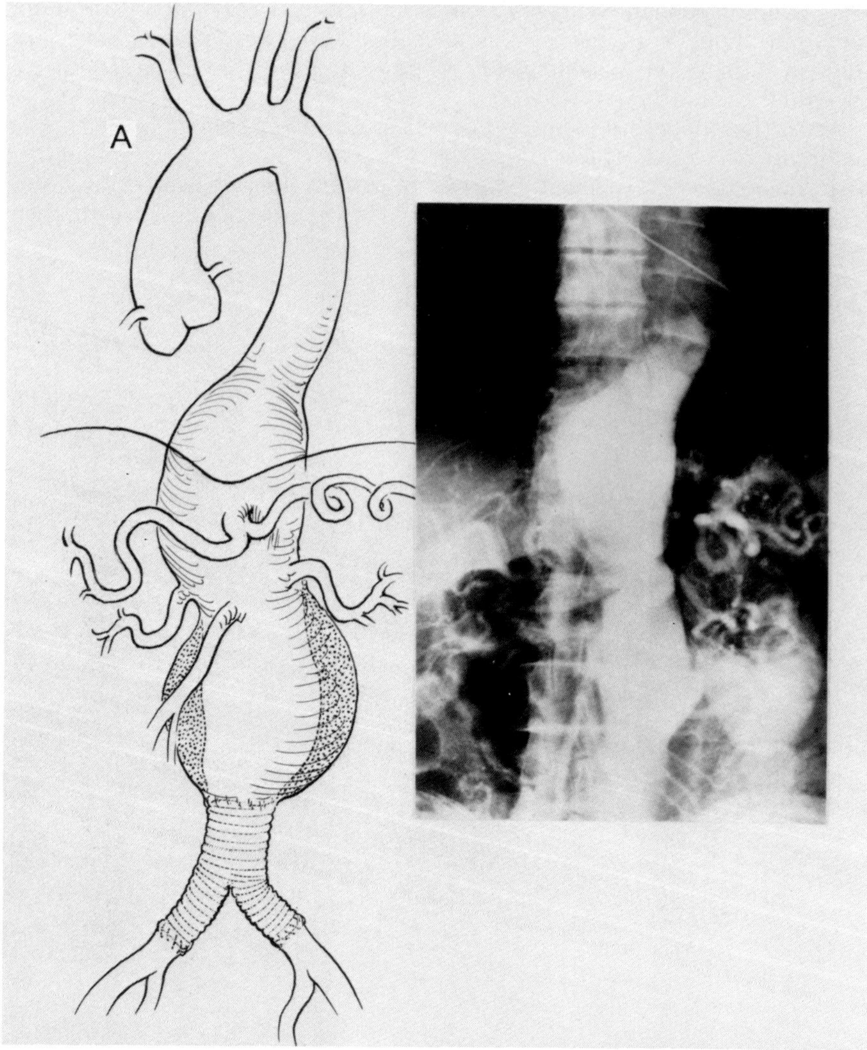

Figure 4.14. Illustrations of the method shown in Figure 4.13 in the treatment of a patient and thoracoabdominal aortic aneurysm involving the distal thoracic and abdominal aorta. *A*, drawing and aortogram made before operation showing the location and extent of the disease and location of the previously inserted graft. *B* and *C*, technique of operation and aortogram made afterwards showing the graft in place and functioning.

lumbar, and intercostal arteries to be reattached) is controlled with No. 4-gauge Fogarty catheters; remaining bleeding intercostal and lumbar arteries are sutured from within. The longitudinal incision is converted into a "T" at the junction of the aneurysm and uninvolved aorta proximally. A woven Dacron tube of appropriate size is inserted end-to-end with a continuous 3-0 polypropylene suture. In patients with extensive aneurysms (groups II and III), one pair of intercostal arteries in the middle or lower thoracic portion is reattached by suturing an opening made in the graft circumferentially around the origins of these vessels. The graft is placed under tension and openings are made for reattachment of visceral arteries and a pair of lumbar arteries. Reattachment of visceral arteries is variable and dependent upon the distance between the vessels. In some cases, these arterial orifices may be close together and reattached to one opening made in the graft; in others, reattachment may vary from two to four openings (Fig. 4.14). The left renal artery may be difficult to

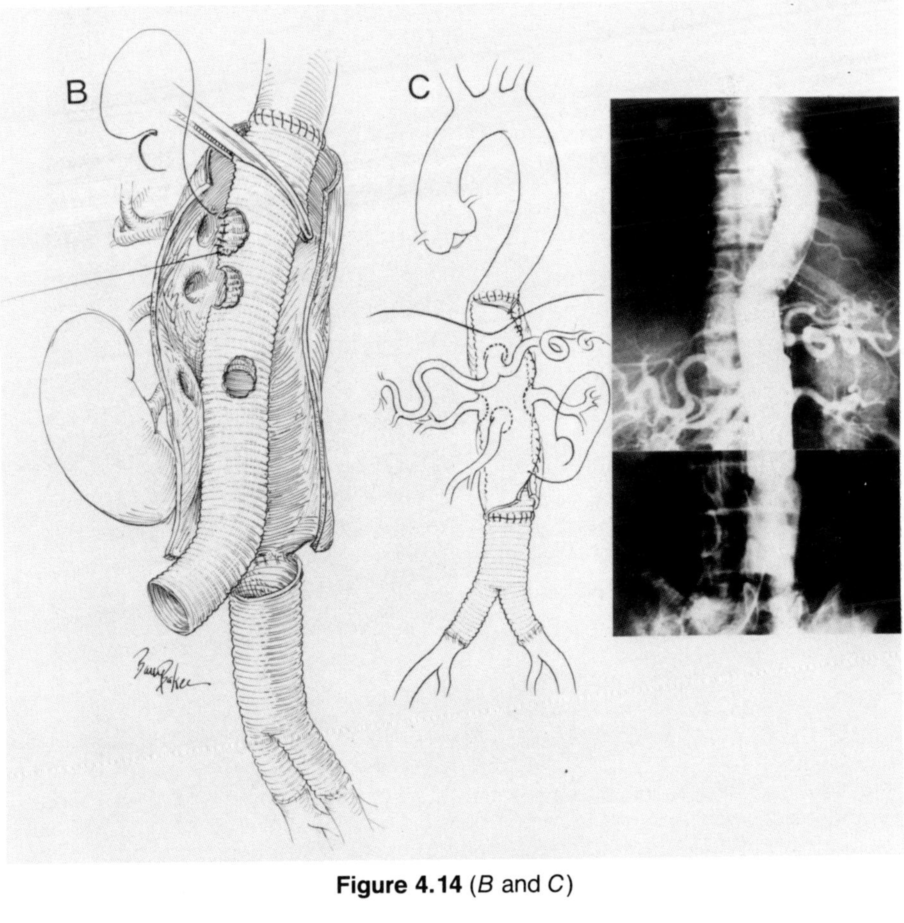

Figure 4.14 (*B* and *C*)

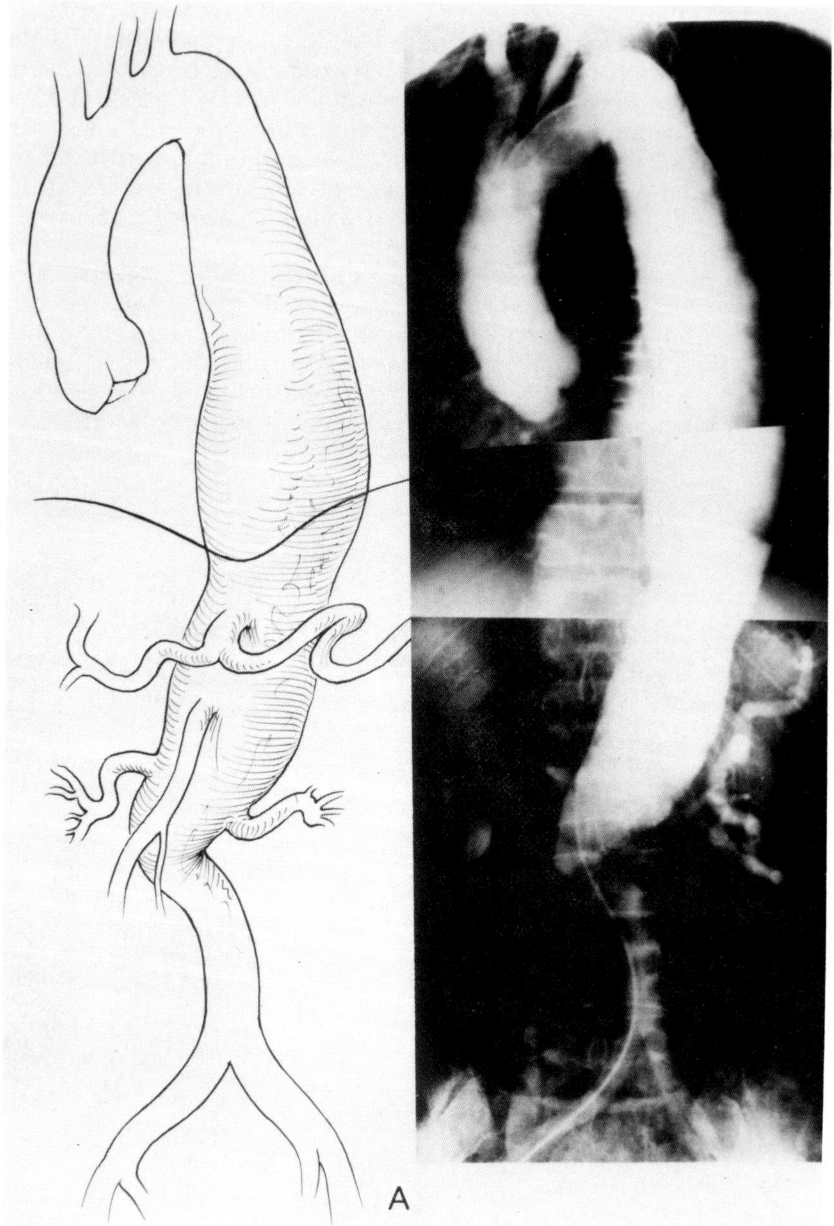

Figure 4.15. Illustration of a patient with an extremely large and diffuse thoracoabdominal aortic aneurysm treated both by direct vessel reattachment and use of branch grafts. *A*, drawing and aortogram made before operation showing the location and extent of the disease. *B*, drawing and aortogram made after operation showing the method of reconstruction and functioning grafts and vessel reattachments.

reattach, due either to involvement by associated disease or wide separation resulting from the large size of the aneurysm. Reattachment in those cases is best achieved by graft method, employing either the splenic artery or Dacron graft (Fig. 4.15). After completion of vessel reattach-

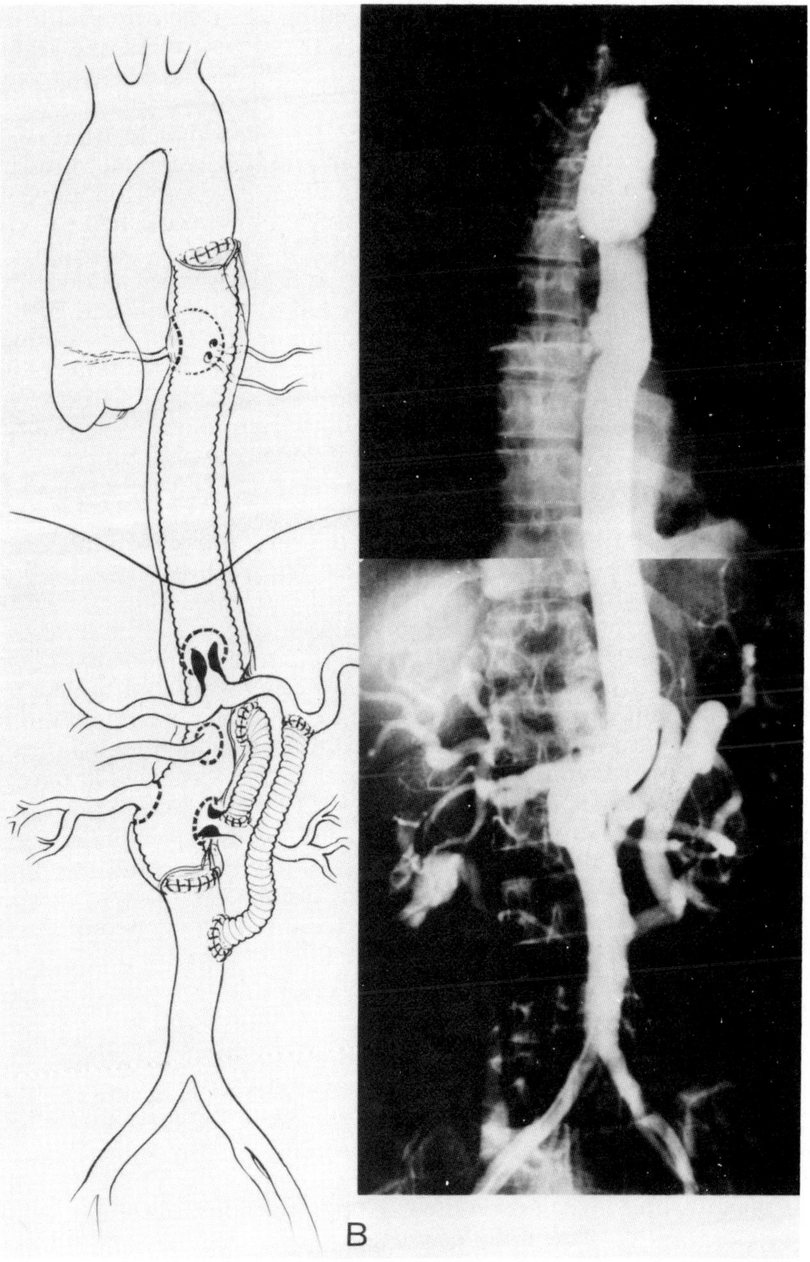

Figure 4.15 (*B*)

ment, the graft is flushed by temporary removal of the proximal clamp. The Fogarty catheters are removed and the graft is clamped distal to the renal arteries. Circulation is restored to the abdominal viscera by gradual removal of the proximal clamp. Distal reconstruction is accomplished by tube or bifurcation graft insertion, depending upon the extent of involvement. The aneurysmal wall is then tightly sutured about the graft. By the use of this technique, a survival rate of 93% has been achieved in 239 patients.

The principle areas of complication are disturbances of renal and spinal cord function. Approximately 9% of patients not already on chronic hemodialysis can be expected to develop signs of renal dysfunction in the form of either creatinine elevation or acute tubular necrosis, which tend to be transient and reversible although hemodialysis is occasionally required to tide them through the critical period. These complications occur regardless of the period of renal ischemia, although the greatest incidence of severe dysfunction occurs with long periods of occlusion. Cord ischemia manifested by neurologic deficits of the lower body occurs in about 8% of patients and usually in those with extensive involvement of both the descending and abdominal aorta; however, it is unpredictable and may occur with less extensive replacements. Deficits may be permanent or transient, may occur immediately, or may be delayed up to four years following surgery.

In recent studies, two factors appear very important in both the prediction and prevention of this complication. Well-developed collateral circulation appears to prevent spinal cord ischemia. This circumstance is manifested angiographically by the relative absence of intercostal and lumbar arteries arising from the aorta, large internal mammary-epigastric arterial systems perfusing intercostal arteries obstructed by the aneurysm, prominent collateral circulation to the lumbar artery system from the internal iliac arteries by way of the midsacral and iliolumbar arteries, and, finally, by encountering large arteries in the chest wall at operation (as in coarctation of the aorta). Collateral circulation studies are still preliminary; but, as progress is made, the incidence of paraplegia decreases because efforts are made to reattach intercostal and lumbar arteries in the patients with extensive lesions and poorly developed collateral circulation. Successful reattachment seems to reduce the incidence and severity of paraplegia by 50% (3, 5, 6).

Aortic Dissections

There are two accepted classifications of aortic dissection: DeBakey types I, II, and III and Shumway's A and B; both may be described as acute or chronic. Practically, however, irrespective of the site of entry or extent of dissection, the management approach is dictated by whether the ascending aorta is involved. There are two principle therapeutic modalities involved in the management of aortic dissection: 1) *medical* treatment by pharmacologic control of hypertension and cardiac impulse; and 2) *surgical* treatment by correction of the dissection. Controversy over which is the optimal initial treatment modality has persisted for the past 20 years. There is now a consensus among surgeons, however, that all *acute dissections* involving the ascending aorta are best treated by operation to relieve or prevent dreaded, and possible lethal, complications of aortic insufficiency and rupture into the heart or pericardium (Figs. 4.1 to 4.3). It is also generally agreed that acute dissections arising in and involving the descending thoracic aorta should be initially treated medically. If they respond with relief of pain and no deterioration of organ function, acute dissections may be treated medically on a long-term basis and converted to chronic dissections. If they do not respond and are associated with evidence of continued dissection, occlusion of distal vessels, and aortic dilatation and rupture, acute dissections are treated by operation (Fig. 4.16). Chronic dissections of both the ascending and descending aorta should be surgically corrected if they are symptomatic and/or expanding (Fig. 4.17). All patients should be continued on medical therapy following surgery (9, 11, 13).

Medical therapy refers to the use of pharmacologic agents to decrease the cardiac impulse (dP/dT maximum) and lower the systolic blood pressure. Two classes of drugs are used: Arfonad and nitroprusside dramatically lower the blood pressure with very little effect on the heart itself, while propranolol has a selective, negative, inotropic effect with minimal peripheral effect. Use of these agents in combination can achieve the desired effect of decreasing the steepness of the pulse wave (dP/dT maximum) and dramatically lowering blood pressure.

All patients suspected of having aortic dissection should be managed in a cardiovascular intensive care unit with continuous monitoring of the electrocardiogram, arterial blood pressure, pulmonary artery wedge and pulmonary artery pressures, and hourly urine output. The blood pressure should be reduced within an hour and then maintained at a mean arterial pressure of 80 to 90 mm Hg by continuous Arfonad or nitroprusside infusion and intermittent 1- to 2-mg boluses of propranolol. Careful monitoring of renal function by repeated serum BUN, creatinine, and potassium levels ensure one is alerted early to renal dysfunction. Pulsus paradoxus may be noted on the arterial tracing and indicates pericardial tamponade. These complications are indications for urgent operation.

The pain which the patient experiences is due to stretching of the adventitia that occurs with propagation of the dissecting hematoma. Hence, relief of the pain, which indicates arrest and stabilization of the dissecting process, is a very important clinical point in the management of these patients. Once the patient is stabilized in the cardiovascular unit, he should be transferred to the angiography suite for angiographic confirmation of the diagnosis. Subsequent management is determined by the location and extent of dissection (as previously described).

When the dissection involves the ascending aorta, operation is directed to the ascending aorta regardless of origin of dissection (Figs. 4.1 to 4.3). This procedure prevents the possible lethal complications that occur with dissection of the ascending aorta and either allows the distal dissection

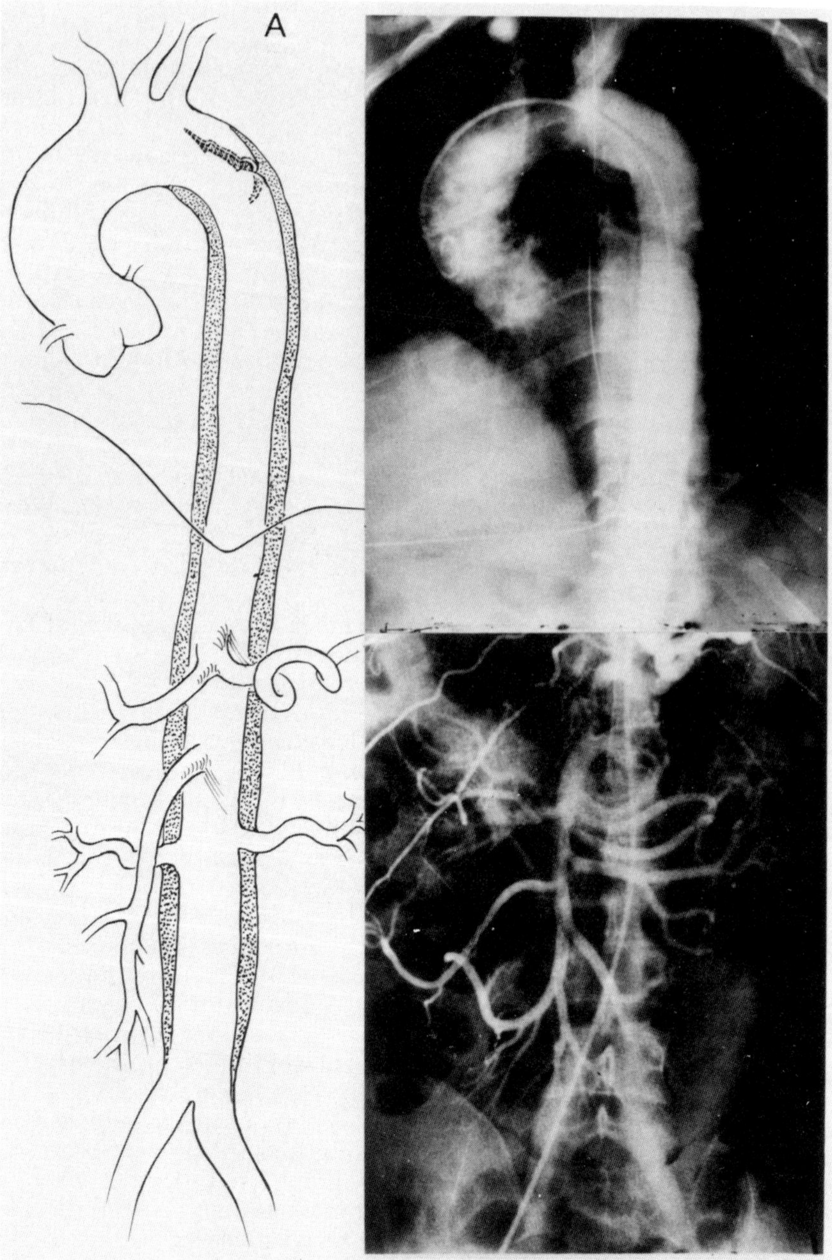

Figure 4.16. Illustrations of the treatment of an acute type III aortic dissection for distal artery occlusion. *A*, drawing and aortogram made before operation showing the location and extent of the dissection. *B* and *C*, drawings and aortogram showing the technique of replacing the origin of dissection and rediversion of blood flow into true lumen to take pressure off distal vessel origins and appearance of the reconstructed aorta after operation.

to clot off or become chronic and be treated at a later date with better survival rates. The surgical approach is similar to that of ascending aortic aneurysms (described under that section). Choice of method depends upon the presence or absence of aortic insufficiency and disruption of the aorta near the annulus, as indicated by the presence of hematoma, bleeding at the site, bleeding in the pericardium, or thinning of the aorta. A graft of woven Dacron is used in all cases to interrupt the dissection, replace the ruptured segment of aorta, and take tension off the suture lines of the repair.

In patients with advanced aortic root injury with leakage, disruption, or excessive weakening of the aortic wall, the entire aortic root is replaced with a composite graft-valve prosthesis which is sutured proximally directly to the aortic annulus (Fig. 4.3). The coronary arteries are reattached by techniques described previously (14).

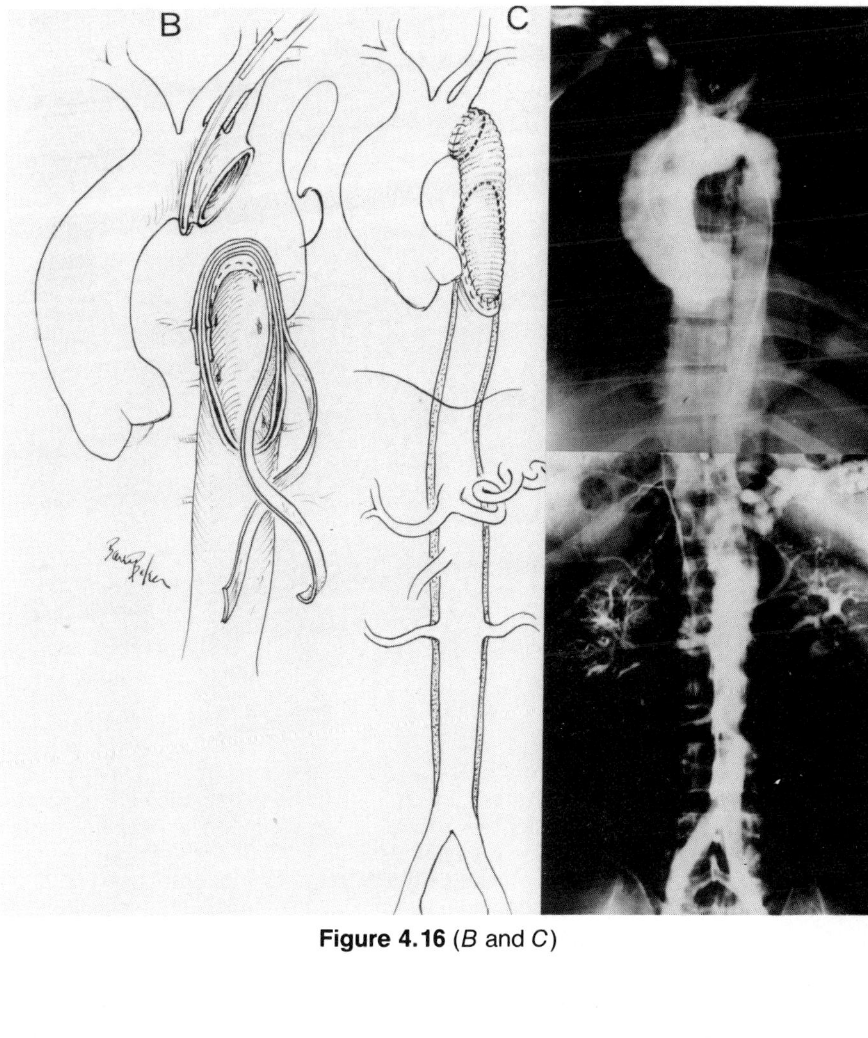

Figure 4.16 (*B* and *C*)

The method of treating acute undilated dissections involving the descending thoracic aorta unresponsive to medical therapy is by operation, resecting origin of dissection proximally and diverting flow distally into the true lumen (Fig. 4.16). With the patient in the right lateral

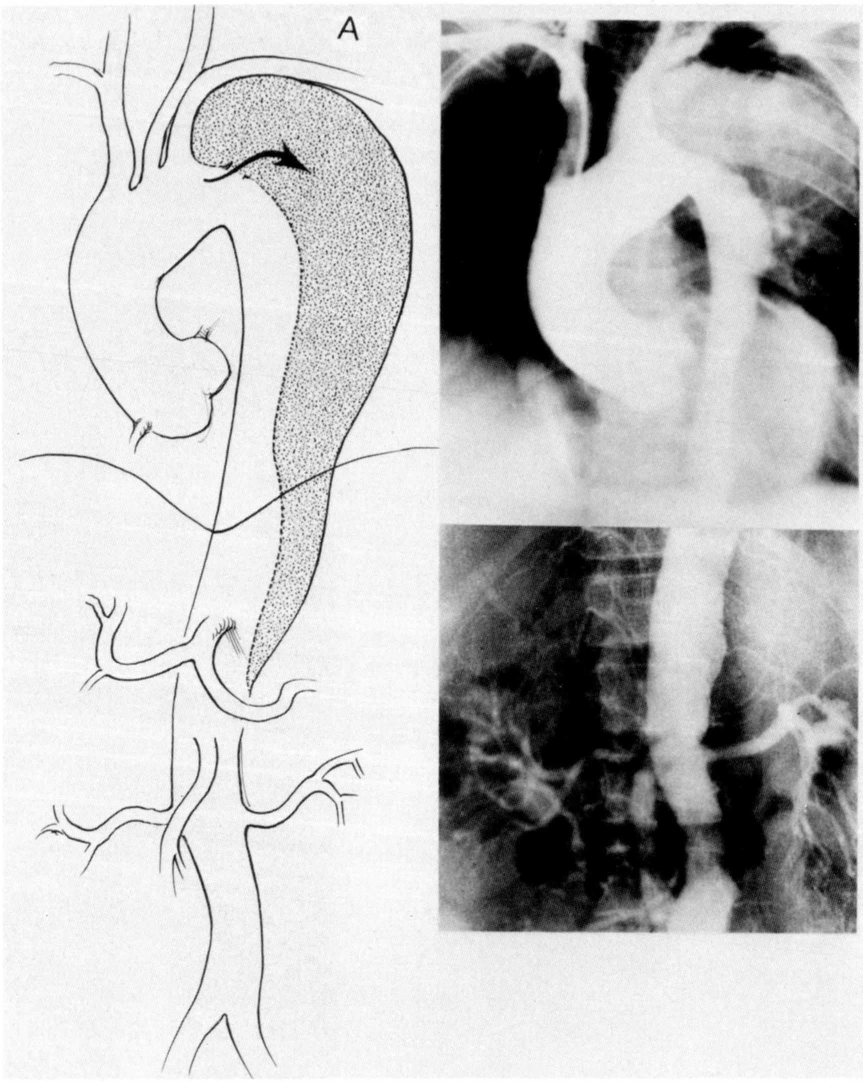

Figure 4.17. Illustrations of a graft replacement of a large, chronic type III aortic dissection using the graft-inclusion technique. *A*, drawing and aortogram made before operation showing the extent of the disease. *B* to *D*, drawings and aortograms made of and after operation showing the techniques of graft insertion and functioning graft after the operation.

position, posterior thoracotomy incision through the 5th or 6th interspace is made; removal of the 6th rib facilitates the procedure. Dissection around the aorta is kept to a minimum to just allow for placement of proximal and distal clamps. The proximal clamp must be placed proximal to the entry site of the dissection to prevent acute retrograde dissection on cross-clamping, which would invariably lead to a catastrophic result. Occasionally, it is necessary to place the proximal clamp between the innominate and left common carotid artery to obtain proximal control. The clamp is placed slowly as the anesthesiologist controls peripheral vascular resistance and blood pressure, followed by application of the distal clamp. No heparin or shunts are used and the operation is limited to eliminating the point of entry. The aortic false and true lumen are opened longitudinally and the distal false lumen is closed by opposing both aortic walls between two strips of Dacron felt, applied so as to bevel the distal aorta to preserve the origins of all possible intercostal arteries.

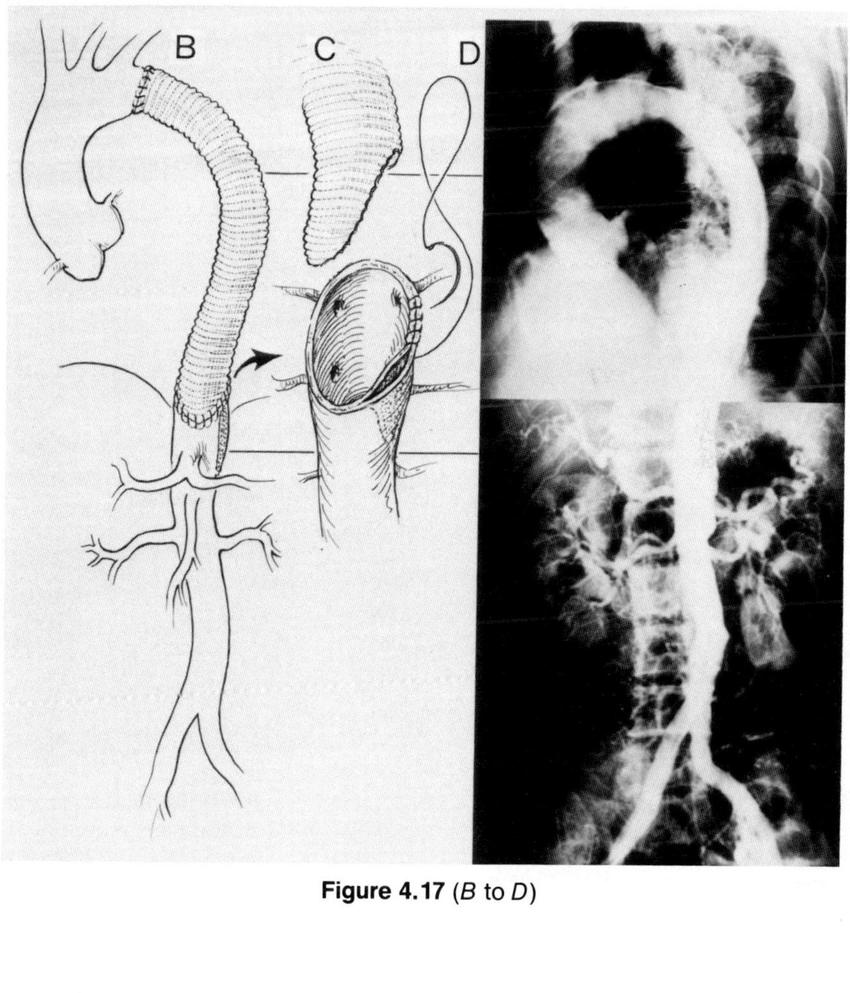

Figure 4.17 (*B* to *D*)

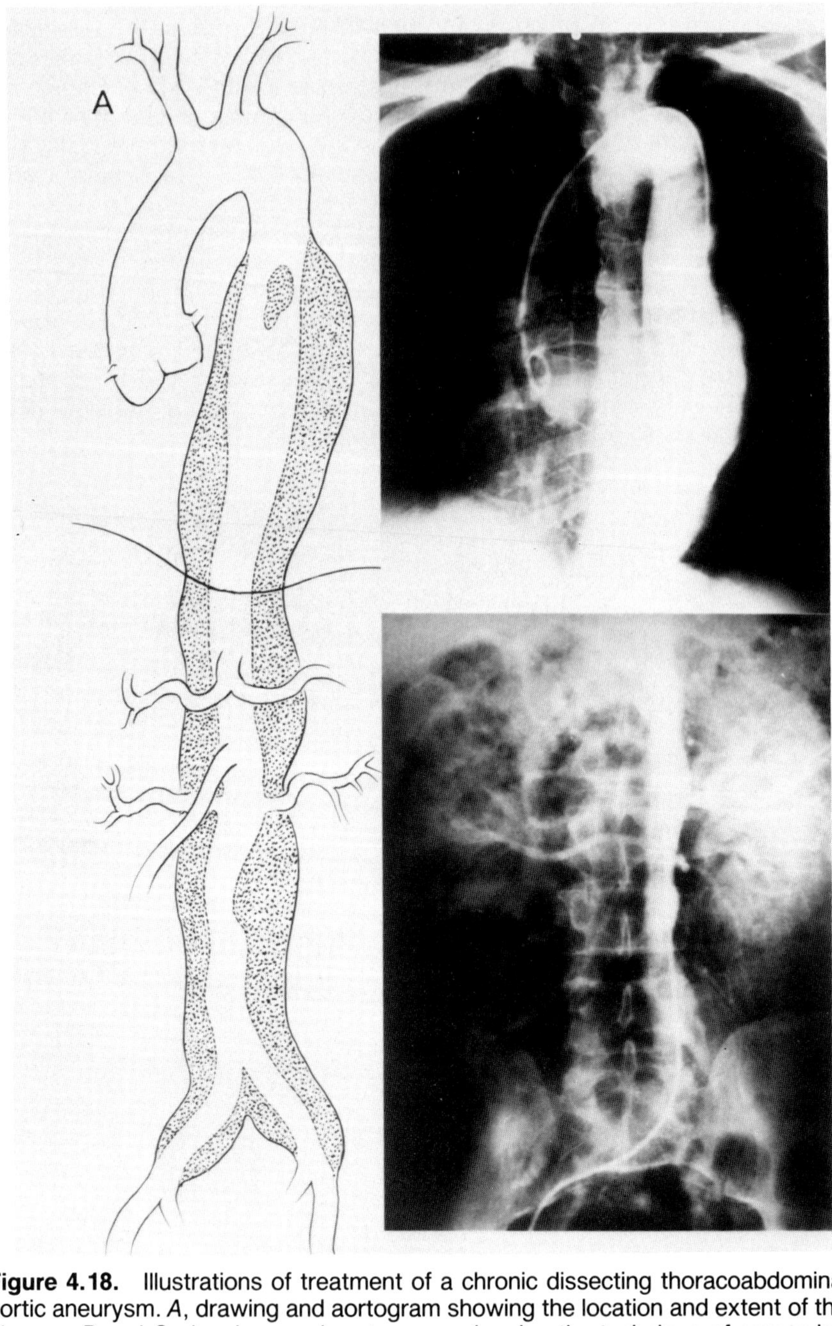

Figure 4.18. Illustrations of treatment of a chronic dissecting thoracoabdominal aortic aneurysm. *A*, drawing and aortogram showing the location and extent of the disease. *B* and *C*, drawings and aortograms showing the technique of preserving intercostal and upper lumbar circulation by replacing only the dissected aortic

The end of a woven, tubular, Dacron graft is attached proximally and the distal end beveled to fit the distal reconstructed aorta. The distal anastomosis is then performed, rediverting all blood flow through the normal lumen, arresting the dissection and taking pressure off origins of the distal branches, and permitting resumption of normal blood flow. This type of operation is very effective in restoring circulation in patients

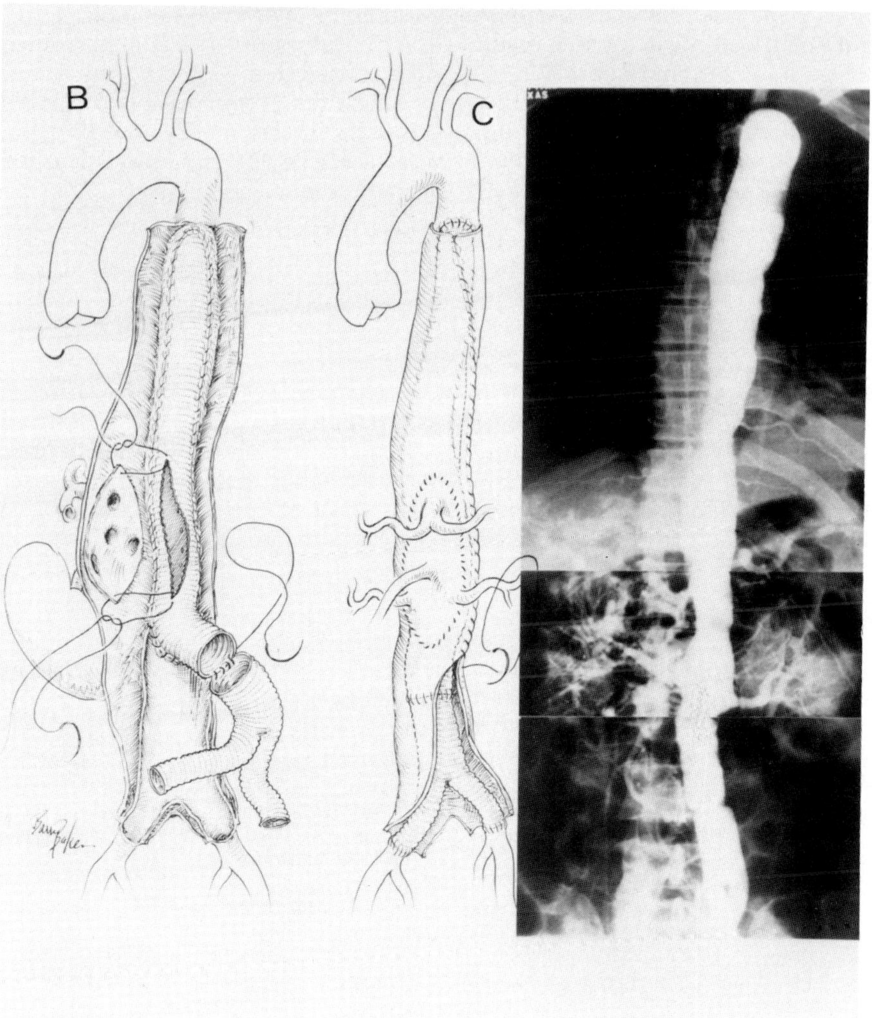

Figure 4.18 (*B* and *C*)

circumference in the chest and upper abdomen, with reattachment of visceral arteries to one opening made in the graft. The aortogram made after operation shows the preservation of intercostal circulation and satisfactory perfusion of the visceral vessels.

with renal, mesenteric, and iliac artery obstruction. Rarely, abdominal operation is necessary when the proximal operation fails to relieve distal obstruction. The method of treating acute or chronic dilated dissections is by appropriate tube graft replacement using the inclusion technique (as previously described) (Fig. 4.17).

If dissections, either acute or chronic, involving the thoracic and abdominal aorta become aneurysmal while being medically treated, or during the late follow-up period, they should be operated upon (Fig. 4.18). An aneurysm in such cases results from dilatation of the weakened outer or false lumen, and operation should be centered at replacing the *aneurysmal* portion and not eliminating the entire dissection process. Rupture is the dreaded complication and occurs only in the aneurysmal portion. The approach to the thoracoabdominal aorta is the same as described previously, limiting resection only to the dilated segment (9–11, 13).

SUMMARY

Improved surgical and anesthetic techniques, monitoring, and volume replacement with a cell saver have provided the milieu upon which thoracic aortic operations have become increasingly successful. All aneurysms of the aorta are surgically accessible.

Presenting most often with pain, aneurysms are confirmed through roentgenologic means. Arteriography is required for anatomic definition and associated pathology. Detailed treatment is outlined in the chapter, including the approach to composite graft-valve modifications, dissections, multiple aneurysms, associated disease of the arch, and visceral arteries arising from the aneurysm.

References

1. Applebaum, A., Karp, R. B., and Kirklin, J. W. Ascending vs. descending aortic dissections. *Ann. Surg. 183:* 296–300, 1976.
2. Bentall, H., and DeBono, A. A technique for complete replacement of the ascending aorta. *Thorax 23:* 338–339, 1968.
3. Crawford, E. S., Palamara, A. E., Saleh, S. A., and Roehm, J. O. F., Jr. Aortic aneurysm: current status of surgical treatment. *Surg. Clin. North Am. 59:* 597–636, 1979.
4. Crawford, E. S., Saleh, S. A., and Scheussler, J. S. Treatment of aneurysm of transverse aortic arch. *J. Thorac. Cardiovasc. Surg. 78:* 383–393, 1979.
5. Crawford, E. S., and Saleh, S. A. Transverse aortic arch aneurysm: improved results of treatment employing new modifications of aortic reconstruction and hypothermic cerebral circulatory arrest. *Ann. Surg. 194:* 180–188, 1981.
6. Crawford, E. S., Snyder, D. M., Cho, G. C., and Roehm, J. O. F., Jr. Progress in treatment of thoraco-abdominal and abdominal aortic aneurysms involving celiac, superior mesenteric, and renal arteries. *Ann. Surg. 188:* 404–422, 1978.
7. Crawford, E. S., Walker, H. S. J., III, Saleh, S. A., and Normann, N. A. Graft replacement of aneurysm in descending thoracic aorta: results without bypass or shunting. *Surgery 89:* 73–85, 1981.
8. DeBakey, M. E., Crawford, E. S., Cooley, D. A., and Morris, G. C., Jr. Successful resection of fusiform aneurysm of aortic arch with replacement by homograft. *Surg. Gynecol. Obstet. 105:* 657–664, 1957.
9. DeBakey, M. E., McCollum, C. H., and Graham, J. M. Surgical treatment of aneurysms of the descending thoracic aorta. *J. Cardiovasc. Surg. 19:* 571–576, 1978.
10. Edwards, S. W., and Kerr, A. R. A safer technique for replacement of the entire ascending aorta and aortic valve. *J. Thorac. Cardiovasc. Surg. 59:* 837–839, 1970.

11. Griepp, R. B., Stinson, E. B., and Hollingsworth, J. F. Prosthetic replacement of the aortic arch. *J. Thorac. Cardiovasc. Surg. 70:* 1051–1063, 1975.
12. Hufnagel, C. A., and Conrad, P. W. Dissecting aneurysms of the ascending aorta: direct approach to repair. *Surgery 51:* 84–89, 1962.
13. Kouchoukos, N. E., Karp, R. B., and Lell, W. A. Replacement of the ascending aorta and aortic valve with a composite graft: results in 25 patients. *Ann. Thorac. Surg. 24:* 140–148, 1977.
14. Najafi, H., Dye, W. S., Javid, H., Hunter, J. A., Goldin, M. D., and Serry, C. Aortic insufficiency secondary to aortic root aneurysm or dissection. *Arch. Surg. 110:* 1401–1407, 1975.

CHAPTER 5

Renal and Visceral Artery Aneurysms

WILEY F. BARKER, M.D.

Most of the aneurysms arising in other parts of the body are relatively easy to identify, and many have a simple etiology. Aneurysms of the visceral arteries, however, are small, frequently asymptomatic until some complication occurs, and are caused by a variety of etiologic processes. The basic patterns of the natural history they share indicate that the lesions may rupture, thrombose, cause peripheral emboli, and only on rare occasions will they cause symptoms because of their size alone. In general, the small, asymptomatic aneurysms may be followed carefully, whereas the larger or symptomatic lesions are best treated by excision with vascular reconstruction if necessary and if possible. Preservation of the tissue nourished by the artery in question is of great importance, especially in the kidney. Very highly specialized techniques are available to preserve tissue.

As a matter of convenience, renal and other visceral lesions will be discussed separately.

ANEURYSMS OF THE RENAL ARTERIES

The true incidence of renal artery aneurysms is unknown, but an approximation can be made. Tcherdakoff *et al.* (24) report an incidence of 1.32% in patients undergoing arteriography during the evaluation of possible renovascular hypertension. The experience of Hageman and coworkers (8) indicates 0.3% of patients undergoing arteriography for all reasons are found to have renal artery aneurysms. The incidence of renal aneurysms identified in patients undergoing arteriography for non-renal lesions was only 0.09% (22); this is a slightly different group than that of the Henry Ford Hospital. It is likely many small aneurysms remain asymptomatic during life and are overlooked at autopsy.

RENAL ARTERY ANEURYSMS AND RENOVASCULAR HYPERTENSION

Although 70 to 80% of renal artery aneurysms are associated with arterial hypertension (10, 20, 22), the nature of the relationship is not clear. It is unlikely there is sufficient reduction of arterial flow because of the turbulence in the aneurysm to produce hypertension through the mechanism of renal ischemia. To some degree, the relationship may be the reverse; arterial hypertension, for whatever cause, may provoke the expansion of the small, established aneurysm because of simple hydrodynamic principles. The occurrence of symptomatic stenosis is a more likely cause of true associated renovascular hypertension. Cortical infarct from embolized clot is another possible cause of renovascular hypertension (22).

Several of the lesions associated with renal artery stenosis are also associated with aneurysms, especially arteriosclerosis and fibromuscular dysplasias. The classification of renal artery disease of a nonatherosclerotic nature published by Harrison and McCormack (9) indicates aneurysmal dilatations may be found in three of their combined diagnostic categories that involve medial disease: fibromuscular dysplasia, perimedial fibroplasia, and medial dissection. Arteriosclerotic aneurysms are often associated with the larger main trunk rather than with the smaller branches, but stenosis at the inlet or outlet of the aneurysm may cause a serious reduction in flow. All of these lesions carry the possibility of an associated medial or subintimal dissection and acute occlusion. Furthermore, polyarteritis nodosa, a cause of multiple, small aneurysms, is also commonly associated with hypertension.

ETIOLOGY

The large series from the Mayo Clinic (10) and from Michigan (22) indicate that roughly one-half of renal artery aneurysms are due to one of the forms of fibromuscular dysplasia, best summarized by Harrison and McCormack (9).

Medial fibroplasia with mural aneurysms is probably the most common form. It is usually found in the distal portion of the main renal artery and often extends into the primary branches. The aneurysmal or bead-like dilatations exist between thickened fibromuscular ridges; in these, the muscle is largely replaced by fibroplasia with loose collagen. In between these circular ridges there is almost complete loss of smooth muscle, and the internal elastic lamella is missing.

Perimedial fibroplasia is the second most common form. In this form, the media varies in thickness; thus, the "chain of beads" may be quite small and, indeed, smaller than the proximal normal artery. It would appear that this variety, although truly an aneurysm in anatomic terms, should have little importance clinically except for its relationship to a reduction of flow. A third aneurysmal type is the form in which dissection occurs within the media, but under the external elastic lamella. It would appear that the above lesions are, for the most part, aneurysms by definition, but, in fact, have more importance clinically because of the concomitant stenoses and are unlikely to rupture.

Atherosclerotic aneurysms tend to involve only the major trunk of the renal artery. There are three possible anatomic variants. In the first form are the aneurysms at the very origin of the artery; these are more truly aneurysmal bulges on the aortic wall from which the vessel takes origin. Often these are densely calcified and, at the very least, thoroughly fibrotic, and progression in size is slow. Figure 5.1 shows such an aneurysm, which has not changed in 15 years. The second site is the

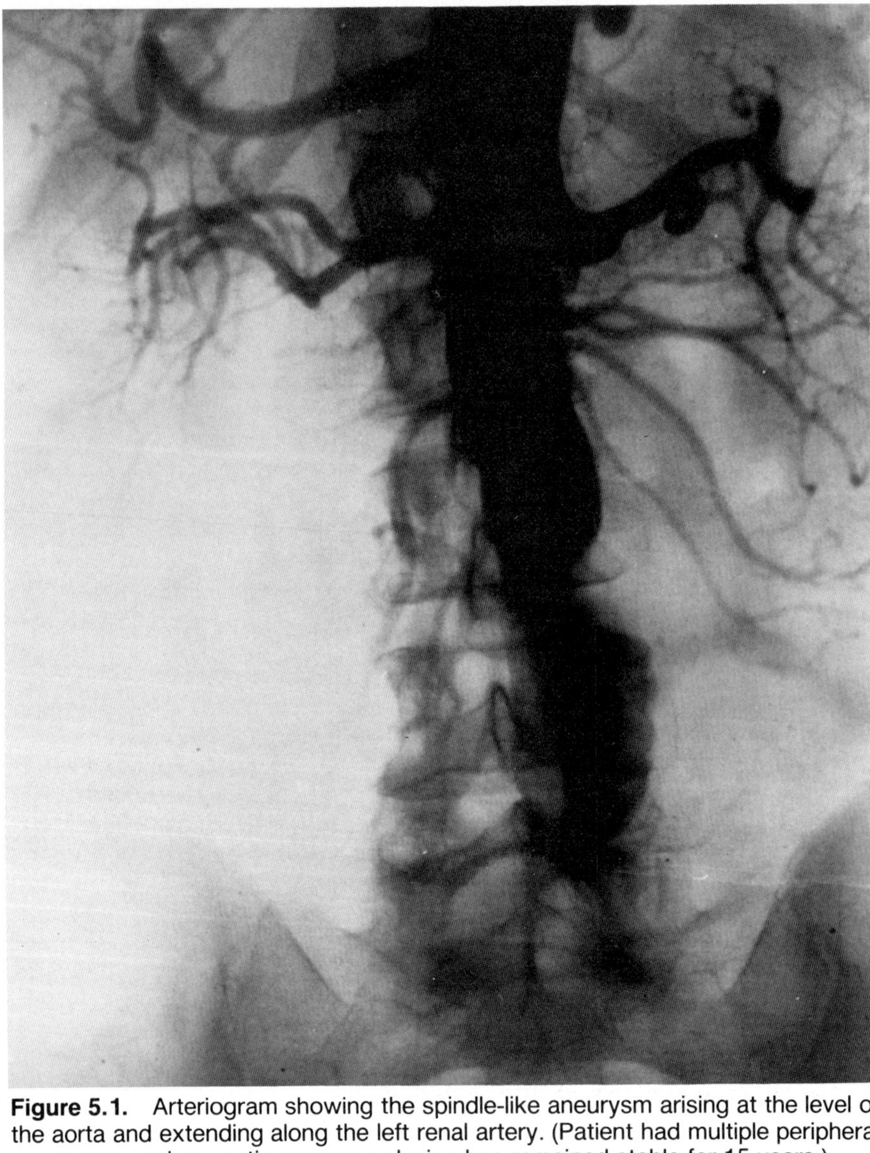

Figure 5.1. Arteriogram showing the spindle-like aneurysm arising at the level of the aorta and extending along the left renal artery. (Patient had multiple peripheral aneurysms and an aortic aneurysm; lesion has remained stable for 15 years.)

main portion of the artery. The third form includes the distal portion of the artery and the origin of the primary branches.

It has been suggested (16) that if these are calcified with a complete shell of calcium they may be followed safely, but the proof that calcification is complete in all areas is almost impossible. Fracture of the shell and either rupture or subintimal dissection can occur in all of these lesions.

Another category of aneurysms are those which are similar to the congenital *berry aneurysms* of the intracranial vessels (7). These berry aneurysms may derive from a weakness where elements of structural importance fail to enclose the actual "carina" of the bifurcation, allowing for the formation of what amounts to a false aneurysm, since those circular musculofibrous elements are lacking. These may occur at the primary division of the renal artery or at secondary or even tertiary branches. Secondary atherosclerosis and calcification may make the distinction between these aneurysms and true atherosclerotic aneurysms difficult.

Trauma from various penetrating missiles, including renal biopsy needles, may also provoke either false aneurysms or arteriovenous fistulas, with or without concomitant aneurysmal formation. In addition, the larger aneurysms due to atherosclerosis or of the congenital defects may rupture into the renal vein and create arteriovenous fistulas.

The lesions of Kawasaki's syndrome (the mucocutaneous lymph node syndrome), Ehlers-Danlos syndrome, or Behçet's syndrome may produce aneurysms. The matter of importance to be remembered is that some solitary lesions of Kawasaki's syndrome may be amenable to surgical reconstruction; the adjacent artery is often of good enough quality to hold sutures. Where multiple aneurysms exist, the lesion often appears much like the multiple aneurysms of polyarteritis nodosa. The other inflammatory lesions or degenerative processes are usually unsatisfactory for surgical management. Figure 5.2 shows an anatomic specimen from a child who had Kawasaki's syndrome; a small aortic aneurysm is present as well (5).

The multiple aneurysms of polyarteritis similarly are unsuitable for reconstruction and should not be treated unless rupture occurs. Such small, multiple aneurysms are a finding pathognomonic of polyarteritis nodosa. Kaufman (11) described the problems of cirsoid aneurysms, which are substantially arteriovenous malformations. Saccular elements may appear and undergo thrombosis or rupture and, thus, require treatment.

CLINICAL COURSE

Three papers have contributed much to the understanding of the course of renal aneurysms. Hubert *et al.* (10) focused on the solitary renal aneurysm. In their series of 67 patients, sex distribution was substantially equal. The right renal artery was involved more frequently than the left; two-thirds were calcified and, in a large number of patients, this served as the means of making the diagnosis. Major associated aneurysmal or arteriosclerotic occlusive disease was present in only 2.5%. The average size was slightly over 15 mm. Over three-fourths of the patients had normal renal function; two-thirds did have hypertension but the exact origin of the hypertension was not apparent. Hematuria was present in only 10%.

Physical findings similarly were not helpful in the diagnosis. Three patients had an abdominal mass, but none of these was the aneurysm;

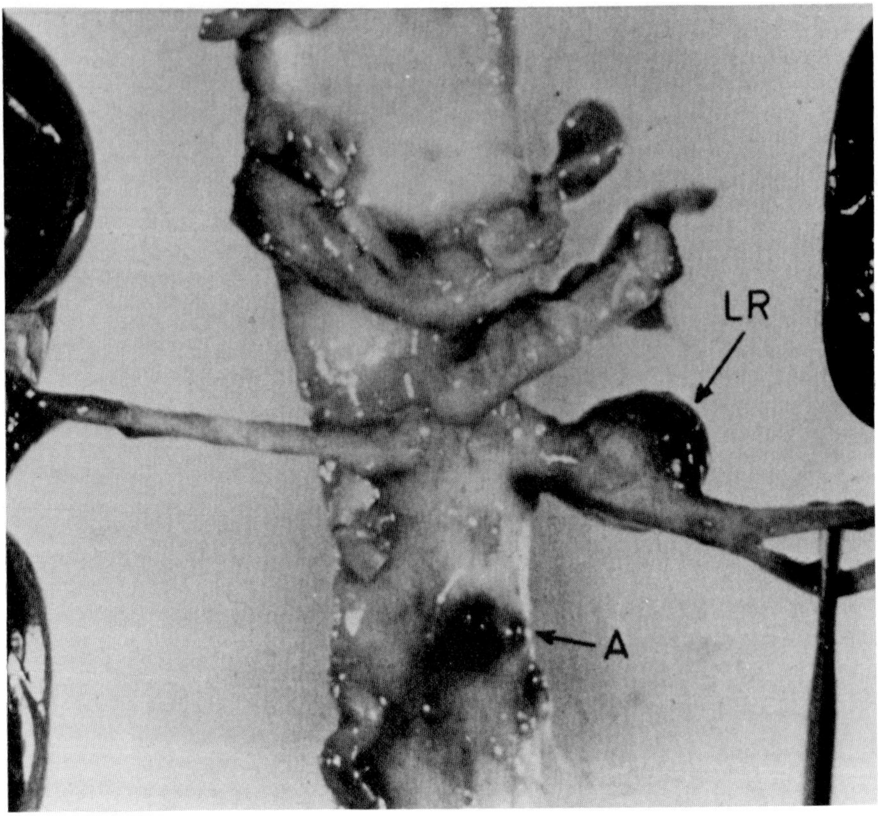

Figure 5.2. Photograph of an anatomic specimen of the aorta and its branches from an 8-year-old child who died of Kawasaki's syndrome. [Reproduced with permission from Fukushige *et al.* (5).]

the largest aneurysm in this series was only 4 cm in diameter. Fewer than 10% had abdominal pain, but the pain could not be related to the aneurysm; a similar number exhibited an abdominal bruit. Operation was performed in only one patient in this series for a complication of the aneurysm.

Hageman *et al.* (8) reported a series of 29 patients. Nineteen patients whose aneurysms were considered asymptomatic and stable in size were observed without operation. Ten patients were operated upon, but only three because of symptoms directly due to the aneurysm. One of these had formed an arteriovenous fistula, one was very large, and one was causing pain thought to be due to expansion of the aneurysm.

Stanley and his associates (21) described a series of 72 patients which they believed to exhibit a slightly more ominous course. Two patients experienced frank rupture of the aneurysm and, in two, the covert rupture into the renal vein had caused an arteriovenous fistula. In three patients, emboli produced cortical infarcts thought to be the cause of renovascular hypertension.

Eleven patients suffered flank or abdominal pain consistent with expansion of the aneurysm; 2 of these had, indeed, ruptured, but the remaining 9 were intact. Fifty-nine patients were totally asymptomatic. Operation was deferred in 28 of the 72 patients. The ages of the patients in these reported series were highly variable, extending from 8 to 90 years. The most common involvement occurred in the third and fourth decades, reflecting the large component of nonatherosclerotic lesions.

OPERATIVE INDICATIONS

Given the above information, appropriate indications for operation begin to emerge.

1. Any symptomatic aneurysm producing pain, hematuria, or renovascular hypertension should be excised.
2. Any aneurysm judged capable of producing renal parenchymal loss through embolization, pressure, or thrombosis should be operated upon.
3. On the basis of the axiom that patients do not get younger and aneurysms do not become smaller, solitary aneurysms larger than 15 mm (8) or 20 mm (10) should be excised.
4. Patients who have aneurysms and are either pregnant or may become pregnant should be operated upon because of changes in the fibromuscular elements of the arterial wall which may lead to rupture.
5. Multiple aneurysms due to systemic processes, such as polyarteritis, should be approached with utmost conservatism.

As a practical matter, it appears that the number of patients operated upon for their renal aneurysms is relatively small. Stanley (20), in the discussion of the paper by Hubert *et al.* (10), noted his agreement with the conservative approach of the latter authors and mentioned that he had deferred operation in 38 of 72 patients with renal aneurysms and these non-operated patients have been followed for a mean of 58 months without event. Hageman *et al.* (8) operated upon only 10 of 29 patients.

TECHNICAL CONSIDERATIONS

Correction of lesions of the main renal artery or its primary bifurcation should pose no major technical problem for the vascular surgeon. Exposure is best obtained through a long, midline incision so as to allow full control of the aorta. The direct approach through the base of the small bowel mesentery as one would approach the infrarenal aorta is satisfactory; but, at times, concomitant exposure of the hilum of the kidney by reflection of either the splenic flexure of the colon with the tail of the pancreas or mobilization of the duodenum and hepatic flexure can be helpful.

Management of lesions of the main renal artery is usually best done by a bypass to a normal vessel beyond the lesion. The origin of the bypass graft is usually taken off the distal aorta, the iliac artery, or comparable segments of the aortofemoral or aortoiliac prosthesis. End-to-end anastomoses are preferable when the size of the prosthesis or graft and the distal renal artery are comparable (20, 21).

As a rule, aneurysms involving the primary bifurcation can be handled similarly. The standard procedure involves creation of a common orifice of the distal branches by sewing their apposing sides together. An alternative method makes an end-to-end anastomosis with the larger branch and a side-to-end anastomosis between the graft and the smaller branch. When either the hypogastric artery or a branched segment of the saphenous vein is used, direct Y-shaped grafts can also be fashioned (Figs. 5.3 to 5.5).

Under most circumstances, arterial flow can be re-established within the hour of warm ischemia time which is ordinarily tolerated by the kidney. Where any doubt exists, cooling the kidney with saline ice slush is desirable. This can be done directly or by means of slush-filled plastic bags or by utilizing a special kidney-shaped container, such as that designed by Cockett *et al.* (3). Under any circumstances, the use of some optical magnification is desirable, but when one must work with the smaller branches (such as the secondary bifurcations), the use of the operating microscope is mandatory. The operation may be carried out *in situ* (15) or totally *ex vivo*, as described by Gelin (6), using workbench

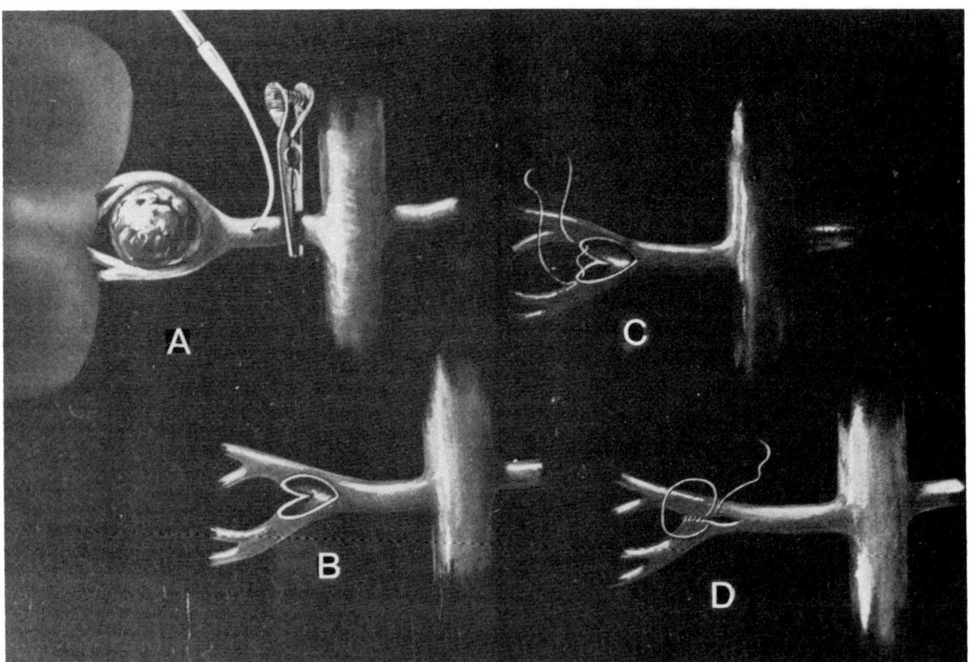

Figure 5.3. Technique of reconstruction of the renal artery: resection and arteriography. [Reproduced with permission from Hageman *et al.* (8).]

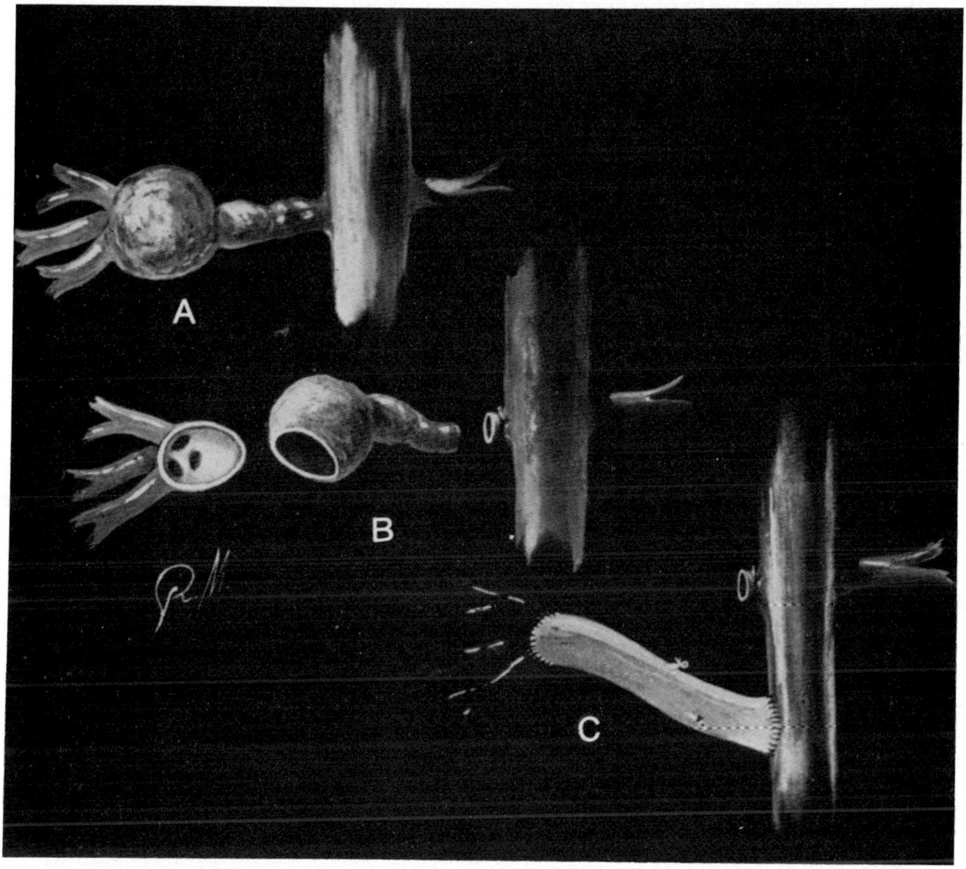

Figure 5.4. Technique of reconstruction of the renal artery: resection and graft replacement. [Reproduced with permission from Hageman *et al.* (8).]

methods. The ureter may be left intact to obviate the problems of ureteric anastomosis, but some surgeons divide the ureter as well. When either form of *ex vivo* surgery is carried out, perfusion of the kidney by some mechanism is important to assure minimal parenchymal dysfunction. The Belzer perfusion technique (18), or simple perfusion with a modification of Simmonds solution (15), is effective; the latter is much simpler and more readily available in most operating rooms.

Repairs under the microscope can be performed using standard arterioplastic techniques. Saccular aneurysms can be obliterated with lateral suture. Grafts and anastomoses can be placed in these small, secondary vessels. The technique is demanding, however, and should never be undertaken without considerable experience working with small vessels under the operating room microscope.

The choice of graft materials for the renal artery substitution deserves

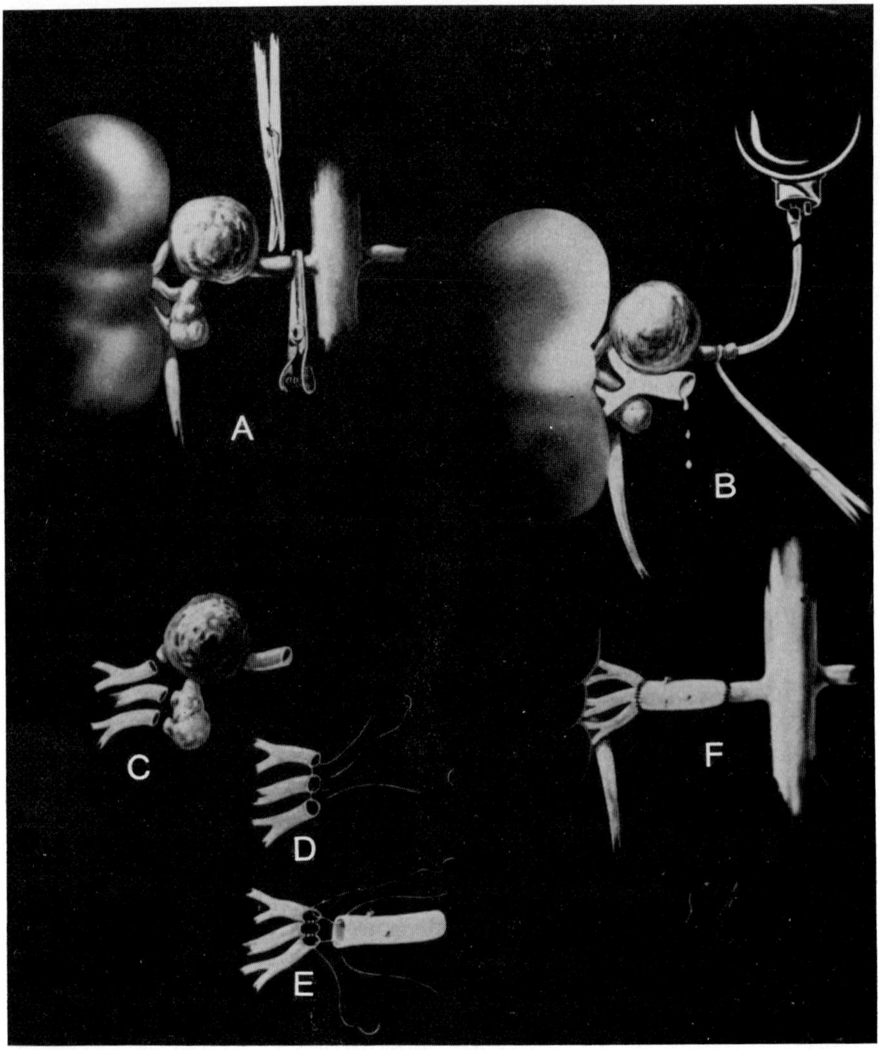

Figure 5.5. Technique of reconstruction of the renal artery: resection and creation of one common orifice of distal vessels; replacement with segmental graft. [Reproduced with permission from Hageman *et al*. (8).]

special attention. The saphenous vein would seem to be the most obvious choice, especially since one can fashion a bifurcation for use in secondary branches and carry out a variety of procedures. Stanley *et al.* (22), however, indicated that at least 6% of renal grafts underwent significant aneurysmal dilatation in the long-term follow up. At least partly for this reason, Lye and his associates (13) have commonly used autologous arteries harvested from the patient's own hypogastric system. In the older patients, a thrombosed and endarterectomized, superficial, femoral artery may be used, a choice rarely available in younger patients.

RESULTS

The fate of surgically treated patients is not made clear in most series. Figures are often combined with the results of surgical treatment of renovascular hypertension. The following estimates are derived from the papers of Hageman *et al.* (8), Soussou *et al.* (19), and Stanley *et al.* (22). Soussou and co-workers described 30 renal aneurysms in 25 patients, all of whom were hypertensive (19). Two calcified aneurysms were not resected. There were two patients who required early nephrectomies: one had severe distal renal artery disease which produced reconstruction, and the other suffered severe and unremitting hypertension following reconstruction. Hypertension was relieved initially in 13 patients, and the kidneys preserved in 19 patients. Four late nephrectomies were performed in the subsequent 36 months. Seventy percent of the patients in whom the kidney was preserved were relieved of their hypertension.

The series of Hageman *et al.* (8) and Stanley *et al.* (22) present a clearer picture of the overall pattern of renal aneurysm disease. As previously noted, only 10 of 29 patients were operated upon in the Hageman *et al.* series: 2 had specific symptoms due to the aneurysm (1 had formed an arteriovenous fistula causing congestive failure, and the other was suffering pain from the expansion of the aneurysm); 1 was free of symptoms, but was a female in the childbearing years; 2 had no reason for operation except the size of the aneurysm; and the remainder were operated upon because of renovascular hypertension.

Eight patients underwent successful reconstruction. The patient who had formed the arteriovenous fistula and a patient with an 8-cm aneurysm were treated by nephrectomy. In one of the patients undergoing reconstruction, the late aneurysmal failure of a vein graft from the inferior mesenteric artery caused a late nephrectomy. Of those patients not operated upon, all remained totally free of complications due to the renal aneurysm, but nine died of miscellaneous, unrelated causes. Data from the Stanley *et al.* (22) series indicated similar results. Twenty-eight of the 72 patients were treated without operation and during a follow-up period of a mean of 36 months had presented no problems from their aneurysms. Some form of reconstruction following aneurysmectomy was carried out in 31 patients. Thirteen primary and 4 late nephrectomies were performed. There was no operative mortality. The effect on the renal hypertension is not stated. No patients required extracorporeal surgery.

DISCUSSION

The renal artery aneurysm is a very uncommon lesion; it occurs in all age groups and is due to a variety of lesions. The larger aneurysms from any cause are prone to rupture. Those related to fibromuscular dystrophy are more likely to be associated with renovascular hypertension, but the majority of all renal aneurysms occur in patients who also have some form of hypertension. The multiple microaneurysms of systemic disease should not ordinarily be treated unless hemorrhage forces a nephrectomy or partial nephrectomy.

Indications for operation should be based on symptoms or potential symptoms related to the aneurysm: pain, frank rupture, arteriovenous fistulation, embolism, or renovascular hypertension. Although nephrectomy is at times necessary, it should be carried out only when all other technical methods have been tried and failed.

A large proportion of aneurysms do not justify operation. Stable, asymptomatic aneurysms smaller than 15 mm in diameter should ordinarily be followed conservatively. The effect of pregnancy on the musculofibrous elements of the aneurysm is such that all aneurysms identified in pregnant women, or women who may conceivably become pregnant, could be operated upon. The modern techniques of vascular surgery are exacting, whether carried out *in situ* or extracorporeally, but in the hand of the experienced surgeon excellent results will be obtained.

ANEURYSMS OF THE VISCERAL ARTERIES

Aneurysms of the many branches of the abdominal visceral arteries present an even wider spectrum of anatomic and etiologic patterns of natural history than do those of the renal vessels. In the long run, the therapeutic principles in those patients who can be treated entail excision or obliteration of the aneurysm and restoration of the flow to the involved tissue, if possible. The categorization of aneurysms by site, etiology, and propensity for complications may provide a clarification of the general understanding of these processes.

Etiology

It is apparent the pathologic patterns are not only varied but are also changing. Luetic aneurysms, common in the past, have become exceedingly infrequent. Mycotic aneurysms due to bacterial endocarditis caused by streptococcus are rare, but mycotic aneurysms due to various septic agents acquired by drug addicts are becoming relatively commonplace. Deterling's collected series (4) of over a thousand visceral aneurysms gives the best perspective of the anatomic sites and etiology. In his summary are included the case reports of Stanley and his associates (23), who provide an excellent picture of the course of these aneurysms. Deterling's tabulation is presented in modified form in Table 5.1.

It would seem from Deterling's compilation that the pathologic processes involving splanchnic aneurysms are more clear-cut than those of the renal arteries. Medial degeneration, however, plays a large role in splenic aneurysms, which constitute almost one-half of the total number of aneurysms. Mycotic aneurysms appear to be most common in the superior mesenteric artery (SMA), but large, mycotic aneurysms have been found commonly in the other intestinal vessels and in all of the arteries mentioned. Fibromuscular dysplasia has also rarely been encoun-

Table 5.1
Aneurysms of the Renal and Visceral Arteries: Type, Number, anc

Arterial Site	Number	Major Etiologic Process
Gastric	25	Arteriosclerosis
Celiac	50	Arteriosclerosis
Splenic	665	Arteriosclerosis or medial degeneration
Hepatic or cystic	230	Arteriosclerosis
Gastroduodenal	7	Arteriosclerosis
Pancreaticoduodenal	18	Arteriosclerosis
Superior mesenteric	90	Mycotic
Jejunal, ileal, or colic	29	Arteriosclerosis or medial degeneration
Total	1114	

tered in these vessels; Stanley *et al.* (23) present a case of splenic artery involvement, and a case of celiac and SMA involvement will be presented below.

Congenital lesions and lesions due to medial degeneration often occur in younger patients. There is also a scattering of Kawasaki's syndrome, Ehlers-Danlos syndrome, and polyarteritis. Erosion and aneurysmal formation occur acutely in serious local sepsis or pancreatitis, but whether these acute lesions deserve to be categorized as true aneurysms is questionable. Because so many of these lesions seem to behave according to established patterns predicated upon their location, the several anatomic sites will be discussed separately.

Splenic Aneurysms

This lesion makes up almost one-half of the reported splanchnic aneurysms. The incidence among routine autopsies is reported by Moore and Lewis (14) as 0.05% and as 0.07% by Stanley *et al.* (23); it is at least twice as common in women as in men. There is a biphasic age distribution with peaks in the third decade associated with pregnancy and in the sixth or seventh decades in both sexes related to arteriosclerosis. The occurrence of either secondary or concomitant atherosclerosis and calcification confuse the pathologic picture.

The expansion and rupture of aneurysms due to medial degeneration in females during pregnancy are accompanied by thinning of the media, fragmentation of elastic tissue, and loss of the internal elastic lamella. These changes are consistent with, but an exaggeration of, similar vascular changes seen in other vessels during pregnancy. Stanley *et al.* (23) described an 8% incidence of rupture with a mortality of one-fourth of those undergoing rupture. In 65 patients whose rupture was associated with pregnancy, the mortality rate was 68%. A large number of these aneurysms are asymptomatic, but Deterling (4) notes that almost one-half show splenomegaly and a large number are associated with portal hypertension. Nonspecific complaints, such as upper abdominal discomfort, nausea, and vomiting, do occur; many are identified by the charac-

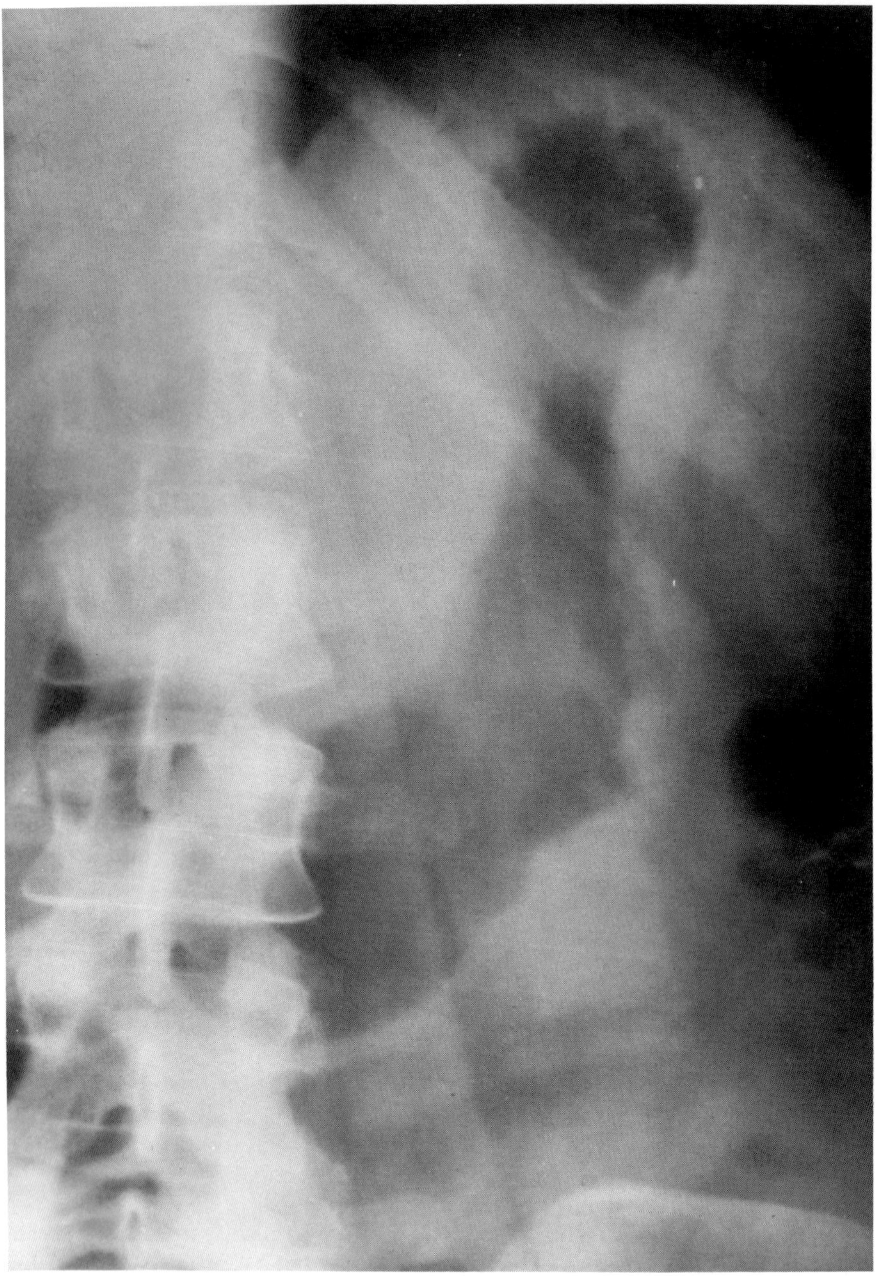

Figure 5.6. Calcified splenic artery aneurysm seen on plain abdominal X-ray; patient was a 30-year-old multipara.

teristic ring shadow on plain abdominal X-rays (Fig. 5.6). A loop in a tortuous, calcified, splenic artery can be mistaken for an aneurysm.

Free intra-abdominal rupture of any major vessel, such as the splenic artery, presents with a picture of severe pain and hemodynamic collapse described as "abdominal apoplexy." Local infiltration of the hemorrhage may control the blood loss by tamponade before final eruption of blood occurs into the free peritoneal cavity. A special form of splenic rupture of this nature occurs as the aneurysm leaks into the lesser sac, thus obtunding the symptoms of bleeding somewhat. Evacuation of the tamponaded clot then allows the surgeon to see the smaller bleeding points from the bed of the artery itself (2).

The high risk of fatality from the rupture of a splenic aneurysm makes resection of the lesion mandatory, especially in young females, and even more so during pregnancy. Stanley *et al.* (23) state that an overwhelming proportion of aneurysms encountered during gestation have ruptured. Resection of the aneurysm may require resection of the spleen if rupture has occurred. It would be desirable to trap the aneurysm and resect it between ligatures and preserve the spleen, if at all possible. The aneurysm should be opened and obliterated by endoaneurysmorrhaphy if resection is not feasible. This operation is associated with minimal risk if performed electively. There is no reason for arterial reconstruction.

Hepatic Aneurysms

Aneurysms of the hepatic or cystic artery occur about one-half as frequently as those of the splenic artery, constituting roughly 20% of splanchnic aneurysms. They are commonly arteriosclerotic, but the average age at which they occur is only 38, which is unusual among the visceral aneurysms and for patients with atherosclerosis. A likely explanation of this age distribution is that medial degeneration, congenital aneurysmal formation, or mycotic aneurysms make up a larger proportion than is usually recognized. In addition, some lesions may be formed on the basis of being bathed in pancreatic secretions during the course of acute pancreatitis. The term mycotic is sometimes misused; "mycotic" is the Oslerian term for the aneurysms which form in the shape of a mushroom at the site of septic emboli (1) in bacterial endocarditis and should not necessarily be used for those infection-related lesions that develop, for instance, in the liver in connection with major hepatic trauma.

Lipson *et al.* (12) described a case of multiple, large aneurysms of the common hepatic and branches of the right and left hepatic arteries in a 14-year-old boy. These were probably congenital in origin. The symptoms of an hepatic artery aneurysm may mimic biliary tract disease with pain, a mass, jaundice, and even hepatic dysfunction. Rupture into the hepatic parenchyma may occur, producing dramatic hemobilia. Diagnosis may be suspected on clinical grounds, but arteriography is the most accurate diagnostic tool. Computerized axial tomography (CAT) scan and ultrasonography may demonstrate blood-filled masses, but the arteriogram still is the most important tool in identifying the vascular relationships. Aneurysms of the hepatic artery which occur proximal to the gastroduodenal branch may often be treated by ligation; distal to that the collateralization of the liver is less secure and, if the vessels are accessible, reconstruction should be undertaken (2).

Reconstruction of the proper hepatic artery can be done, but the exposure is difficult and the branches may be quite small. Bypass procedures using a distal end-to-side anastomosis with origin of the prosthesis or arterial graft from any large vessel may be effective. Intrahepatic aneurysms may be successfully treated by transarterial embolization. Placement of the embolus should be as carefully done as possible to assure minimal hepatic parenchymal ischemia.

Celiac Aneurysms

Celiac aneurysms are considerably less common than the hepatic or splenic aneurysms previously discussed; they account for approximately 4% of Deterling's series (4) and are usually arteriosclerotic in nature. In the past, they have been identified most commonly because of rupture, for they otherwise produce few symptoms. Males are most commonly afflicted. Symptoms, if any, are vague, with the rare presentation of a mass or symptoms of intestinal ischemia. Anatomic definition is best done by arteriography, although identification may be made on the basis of CAT scan or ultrasonography.

Treatment by ligation or resection without reconstruction is possible. If restoration of flow to the hepatic system is necessary, a bypass from a portion of the aorta can be done. The proximal splenic artery and the left gastric artery may usually be sacrificed with impunity. The most convenient site from which to take the bypass is often the thoracic aorta just as it enters the diaphragm. This exposure can be obtained through the diaphragm without entering the chest; at times, splitting the lower portion of the sternum will yield better exposure. This part of the aorta is often free of disease and the course of the graft is direct, rather than the errant course necessary if the graft is taken from the main infrarenal aorta.

The importance of specific delineation of the arterial anatomy is a point made by Stanley *et al.* (23), who encountered an aneurysm of the celiac axis in which the SMA arose from the axis. During the preparation of this manuscript, Dr. William Mikkelsen of Los Angeles (personal communication) provided me with an arteriogram of a patient he had recently treated. This elderly male had experienced upper abdominal pain and was found to have the lesion shown in Figure 5.7. A 3-cm aneurysm arose from the celiac axis just beyond the point at which an anomalous SMA left the main axis. The lesion was treated by ligation of the vessel proximal and distal to the aneurysm with no ischemic complications. Failure to recognize this anomaly and observe the possible ischemia of the small bowel could be catastrophic.

Another uncommon lesion was encountered by the author in 1959. A

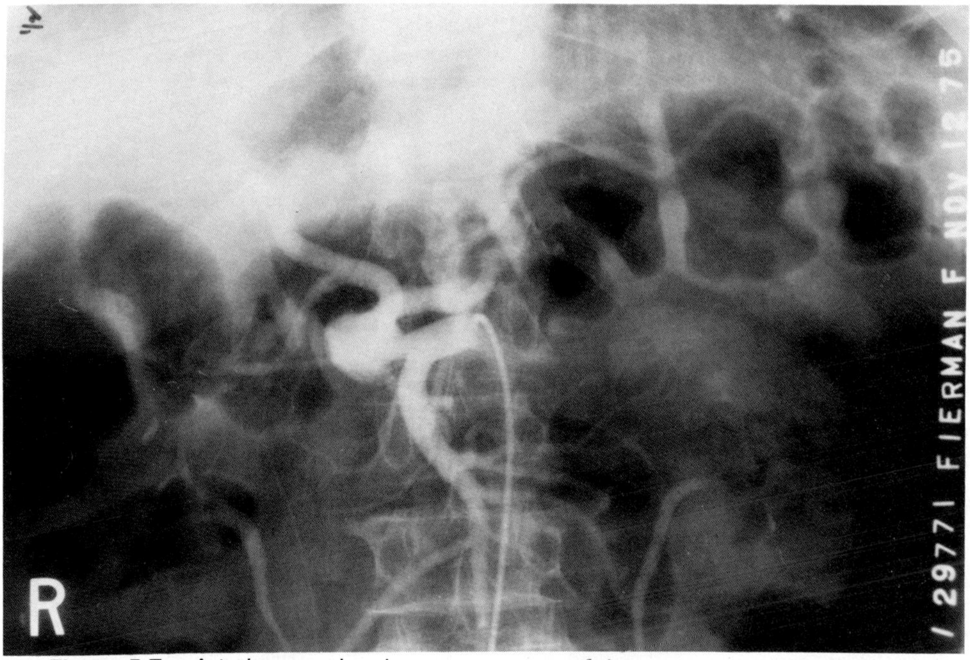

Figure 5.7. Arteriogram showing an aneurysm of the anomalous celiac axis; the superior mesenteric artery arises from the common trunk just before it gives rise to the aneurysm; the left gastric artery, splenic artery, and hepatic artery arise just beyond the aneurysm. (Used with permission of W. P. Mikkelsen; personal communication.)

40-year-old woman, known to have fibromuscular lesions of the right kidney and carotid arteries, developed signs of intestinal ischemia. Arteriogram revealed only an absence of the celiac axis and superior mesenteric trunks; the distal vessels were patent and a large, meandering, mesenteric artery was present (Fig. 5.8). At operation, the celiac axis and superior mesenteric vessels at their origin were represented by a thrombosed "chain of beads" consistent with a series of thrombosed fibromuscular aneurysms. The SMA was revascularized by a short Dacron graft directly from the adjacent aorta.

Superior Mesenteric Artery Aneurysms

The SMA aneurysms are twice as common as the celiac axis aneurysms. The majority of these lesions are described as mycotic in nature. In the past they were usually found as classical Oslerian mycotic lesions in the presence of subacute bacterial endocarditis. It is not clear why the SMA should be such a favorite target for septic emboli, except that the flow into the artery is large in volume and there is a direct access anatomically. The modern drug culture and the many associated infections continue to be associated with many mycotic aneurysms.

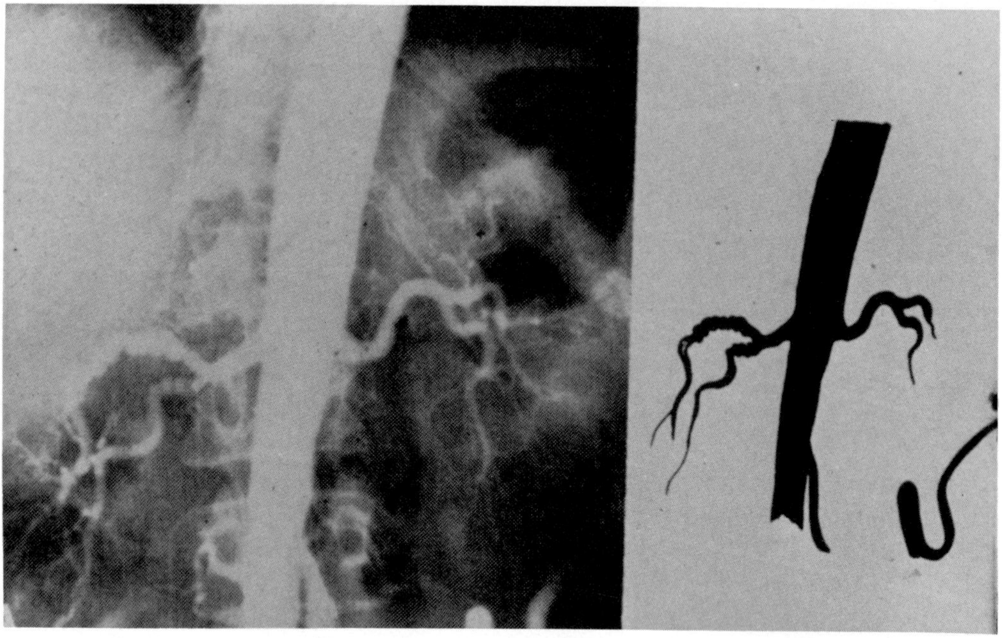

Figure 5.8. Arteriogram showing renal artery fibromuscular dysplasia and absence of the superior mesenteric artery and celiac axis; the large inferior mesenteric artery has a proximal stenosis and gives rise to a large central anastomotic arcade.

The complex of symptoms is not particularly specific: upper abdominal or periumbilical pain, nausea, and vomiting; if there is an associated arterial stenosis, intestinal angina may be present. These symptoms take on much more importance in the face of endocarditis or other vascular infections. In some instances a bruit can be heard and, rarely, the aneurysm is large enough to be felt as an abdominal mass. This pattern of signs and symptoms alone may well justify an arteriogram. A preliminary ultrasonic study or CAT scan will occasionally find a mass that cannot be felt. Arteriographic evaluation usually follows.

The non-mycotic aneurysms will usually be seen in older patients with extensive arteriosclerosis; in these patients, calcification may be seen on plain abdominal films. Rupture of these arteriosclerotic aneurysms is a hazard that justifies elective resection or ligation of the aneurysm.

Collateralization may be sufficient to allow simple ligation, but if the lesion lies in the proximal portion of the artery, ischemia and a serious threat to a large portion of the small bowel may exist. Under these circumstances, a bypass graft into the artery beyond the aneurysm from the infrarenal aorta will be satisfactory. If the lesion is mycotic in origin, it is probably wise to use an autologous artery.

Aneurysms of the Gastric, Jejunal, Ilial, and Colic Vessels

Aneurysms of these smaller abdominal arteries are often discussed separately, but they share many traits in common. Frequently, they are multiple and, although they show calcification and secondary atherosclerosis, it is believed that most are congenital in origin. Some are mycotic in origin, as well.

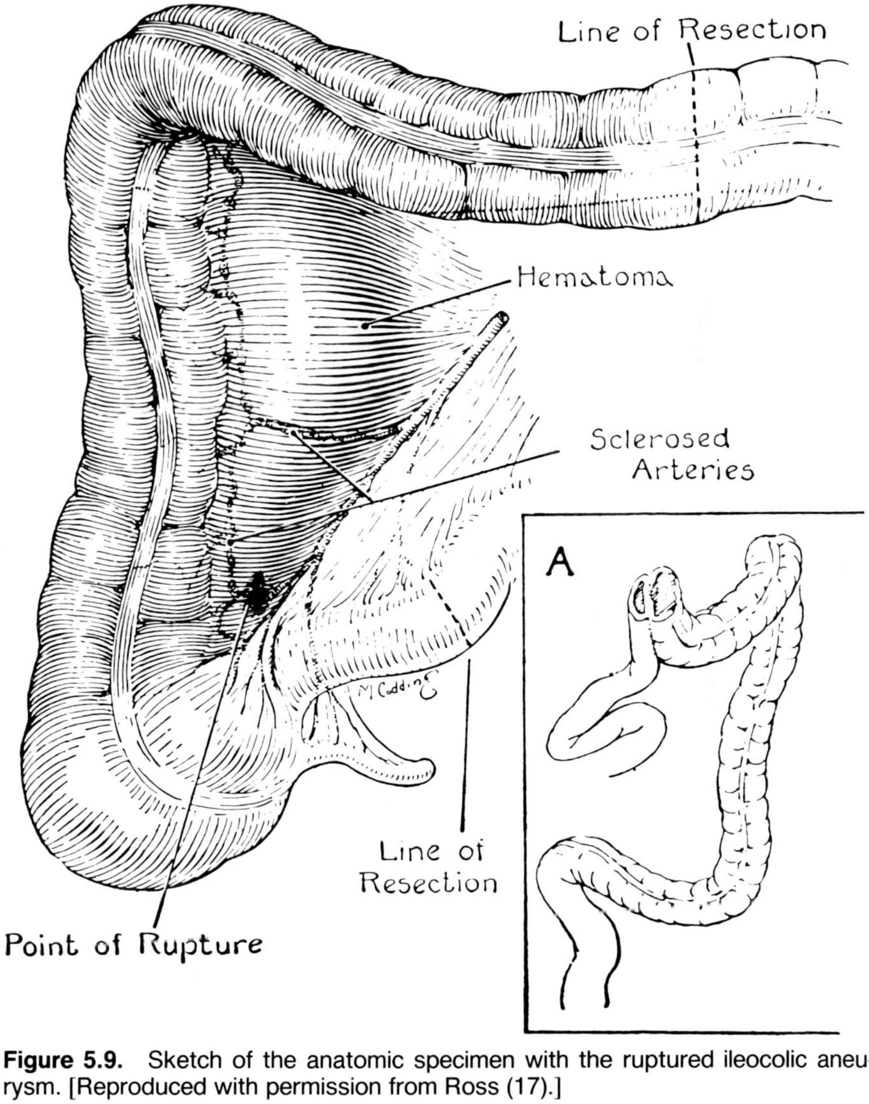

Figure 5.9. Sketch of the anatomic specimen with the ruptured ileocolic aneurysm. [Reproduced with permission from Ross (17).]

Symptoms are apt to be minimal unless there is growth to a considerable size. Under these circumstances, vague pain and a mass may be identified. Approximately one-half of splanchnic aneurysms announce themselves by rupturing either freely or into an adjacent viscus. Resection of the aneurysm and of any tissue rendered ischemic thereby is the treatment of choice. The author's first experience with visceral aneurysms occurred in 1948, when as a fellow in pathology he was presented with an unusual specimen by Dr. Frederick Ross (17). The patient was a 61-year-old man who had developed some vague right abdominal pain which led to more severe pains, with signs of serious blood loss consistent with abdominal apoplexy. At operation, the surgeon encountered a discolored and hemorrhagic right colon with extensive hematoma in the mesentery. Multiple calcifications were felt in the mesentery, and the bleeding was found to be coming from a 7-mm aneurysm which had ruptured (Figs. 5.9 and 5.10). The right colon was resected as the primary treatment.

SUMMARY

Splanchnic aneurysms are an unusual presentation of arterial disease. The splenic artery is most commonly involved, but no artery is spared. Arteriosclerosis, medial degeneration, possible congenital defects, and mycotic lesions comprise the pathologic background.

Pain, nausea and vomiting, and distal ischemia may be the only signs

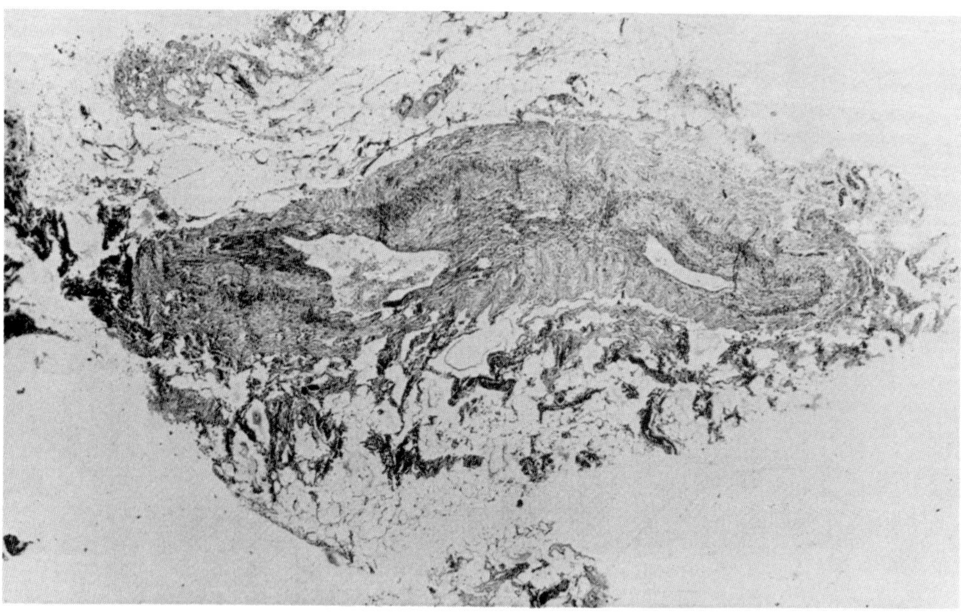

Figure 5.10. Microscopic picture of the ruptured 7-mm aneurysm. [Reproduced with permission from Ross (17).]

preceding the frequent tendency to rupture. Hemorrhage may occur into an adjacent viscus or the free peritoneal cavity.

Reconstructive repair of the larger vessels can often be accomplished successfully. In smaller vessels, resection of the aneurysm or even simple ligation may be all that is required. Where hemorrhage has occurred, obliteration of the anatomy often prevents repair and may, therefore, require resection of the ischemic tissue.

It is likely that newer diagnostic methods, such as ultrasonography, CAT scan, and even arteriography, will identify more of these lesions at earlier stages and allow treatment before the stage of rupture.

References

1. Barker, W. F. Mycotic aneurysms. *Ann. Surg. 133:* 84–88, 1954.
2. Busuttil, R., and Brin, B. J. The diagnosis and management of visceral artery aneurysms. *Surgery 88:* 619–624, 1980.
3. Cockett, A. T. K., Lai, M-K., Davis, R. S., Mandour, W. A., and Youssef, A. M. R. Intrarenal and *in situ* kidney work bench surgery under hypothermia. *Urology 15:* 112–114, 1980.
4. Deterling, R. A. Aneurysm of the visceral arteries. *J. Cardiovasc. Surg. 12:* 309–322, 1971.
5. Fukushige, J., Nihill, M. R., and McNarmara, D. G. Spectrum of cardiovascular lesions in mucocutaneous lymph node syndrome: analysis of eight cases. *Am. J. Cardiol. 45:* 98–107, 1980.
6. Gelin, L. E. Extracorporeal surgery for renal problems. *Surg. Annu. 9:* 351–379, 1977.
7. Glynn, L. E. Medial defects in the circle of Willis and their relationship to aneurysm formation. *J. Pathol. Bacteriol. 51:* 213–222, 1940.
8. Hageman, J. H., Smith, R. F., Szilagyi, D. E., and Elliott, J. P. Aneurysms of the renal artery: problems of prognosis and surgical management. *Surgery 84:* 563–572, 1978.
9. Harrison, E. G., Jr., and McCormack, L. J. Pathologic classification of renal arterial disease in renovascular hypertension. *Mayo Clin. Proc. 46:* 161–167, 1971.
10. Hubert, J. P., Jr., Pairolairo, P. C., and Kazmeir, F. J. Solitary renal aneurysm. *Surgery 88:* 557–564, 1980.
11. Kaufman, J. J. Renal artery aneurysms. *Contemp. Surg. 3:* 19–25, 1973.
12. Lipson, M. H., Fonkalsrud, E. W., and Ament, M. E. Hepatic aneurysms in a 14-year-old boy. *J. Pediatr. 98:* 933–936, 1981.
13. Lye, C. R., String, S. T., Wylie, E. J., and Stoney, R. J. Aortorenal arterial autografts. *Arch. Surg. 110:* 1321–1326, 1975.
14. Moore, S. W., and Lewis, R. J. Splenic artery aneurysm. *Ann. Surg. 153:* 1033–1043, 1961.
15. Novich, A. C., Straffon, R. A., and Stewart, B. H. Surgical management of branch renal artery disease: *In situ* versus extracorporeal methods of repair. *J. Urol. 123:* 311–316, 1980.
16. Poutasse, E. F. Renal artery aneurysms. *J. Urol. 113:* 443–449, 1975.
17. Ross, F. P. Abdominal apoplexy complicated by mesenteric venous thrombosis. *Ann. Surg. 131:* 592–598, 1950.
18. Salvatierra, O., Jr., Okott, C. V., and Stoney, R. J. Ex vivo renal artery reconstruction using perfusion preservation. *J. Urol. 119:* 16–19, 1978.
19. Soussou, I. M., Starr, D. S., Lawrie, G. M., and Morris, G. C., Jr. Renal artery aneurysm. Long-term relief of renovascular hypertension by *in situ* operative correction. *Arch. Surg. 114:* 1410–1415, 1979.
20. Stanley, J. C. In discussion of Hubert, J. P., Jr., Pairolairo, P. C., and Kazmeir, F. J. Solitary renal aneurysm. *Surgery 88:* 557–564, 1980.
21. Stanley, J. C., Ernst, C. B., and Fry, W. J. Fate of 100 aortorenal vein grafts: characteristics of late graft expansion, aneurysm dilatation and stenosis. *Surgery 74:* 931–944, 1973.

22. Stanley, J. C., Rhodes, E. L., Gerwertz, B. L., Chang, C. Y., Walter, J. F., and Fry, W. J. Significance of macroaneurysms exclusive of dissections and fibrodysplastic mural dilatations. *Arch. Surg. 110:* 1327–1333, 1975.
23. Stanley, J. C., Thompson, N. W., and Fry, W. J. Splanchnic artery aneurysms. *Arch. Surg. 101:* 689–697, 1970.
24. Tcherdakoff, P., Maillet, R., Ecoiffier, J., Vaysse, J., and Milliez, P. Aneurysm of renal artery in hypertensive patients. *Presse Med. 79:* 123–128, 1971.

CHAPTER 6

Abdominal Aortic Aneurysms

STEVEN A. BLAU, M.D.
MORRIS D. KERSTEIN, M.D.
RALPH A. DETERLING, Jr., M.D.

HISTORY

The history of the treatment of abdominal aortic aneurysms is, in many respects, the history of vascular surgery. From accurate clinical observations came an accumulation of cases and descriptions leading to an understanding of the etiology and pathophysiology. Subsequently, there were a series of operative interventions—each owing its increased success to advancing technology—until the modern surgical approach was developed.

Diagnosis

The term "aneurysm" is probably derived from the Greek "aneurysma" (to dilate), although some scholars claim it owes its origin to another Greek root meaning "to leap forth" or "to pour forth" (185). Despite this Hellenic etymology, Hippocrates did not mention arterial aneurysms (185). Credit for their description goes to Galen, who wrote that "... when the arteries are enlarged, the disease is called an aneurysm ... If the aneurysm is injured, the blood gushes forth and it is difficult to staunch it" (122). But Galen seemed ignorant of abdominal aneurysms, as did a number of ancient authors including Paul of Aegina, Oribasius, Aetius, Acturius, and Avicenna. Commenting upon what was probably the first museum specimen of an aortic aneurysm, Elsner, in 1670, stated that aneurysms were never, or rarely, found in the larger arteries "... so it seems strange that it could have occurred in the aorta" (186). The first clinical diagnosis of an abdominal aortic aneurysm, though, was made over a century before by Vesalius (184), who asserted in 1555 that a pulsating tumor in a patient's back near the vertebrae was a "... dilation of the aorta." He was proven correct at the patient's autopsy two years later.

The reported frequency of aortic aneurysms changed within a century and by 1760 the case histories of aortic aneurysms were "... almost equal to if not greater than those observed in all other parts of the body together" (184). Lancisi's brilliant treatise *De Motu Corids et Aneurysmatibus* (185) was published in 1728 and provides a strikingly modern discussion on the etiology (echoing Pare's earlier observations on syphilis) and pathology of abdominal aortic aneurysms, recognizing rupture as the cause of death in several cases.

The 19th century saw further work on the clinical aspects of the disease, with Hodgson and Guthrie emphasizing the course towards rupture and death. In 1847, Crisp (75) provided an almost definitive analysis of the biometry of the disease in his monograph on vascular surgery. By this time, considerable effort had also gone into the therapy of aneurysms.

Therapy

The principles of therapy advanced during this time may be divided into three broad groupings: 1) those designed to promote thrombosis and fibrotic organization, 2) endoaneurysmorrhaphy, and 3) extirpation of the lesion, with or without restoration of blood flow through the parent vessel. To effect the first goal, Matas (208) classified the techniques as those: "... (a) diminishing the blood pressure, (b) retarding the velocity of circulation, (c) increasing the coagulability of blood, and (d) provoking thrombus formation within the sac by agents which act directly on the aneurysmal tissues from within and from without."

COMPRESSION

The simplest technique of producing thrombosis was the application of digital pressure on the vessel (sometimes with relief teams of medical students over several days) and the use of tourniquets. This technique was applied to abdominal aortic aneurysms in 1864 (175). In 1875, a similar case was reported (175) using a combination of general anesthesia and Esmarch bandaging of the abdomen.

LIGATION

Ligation of the parent artery is the oldest surgical technique employed. Its application to non-aortic aneurysms illustrates medicine's curious habit of rediscovering forgotten inventions. John Hunter is most closely associated with arterial ligation, but his work dates from the late 18th century. The first description of the procedure was that of Antyllus, who, in the 2nd century, combined proximal and distal ligation with the packing of the aneurysmal sac (78). This was next described by Paul of Aegina in the 7th century. The concept was rediscovered by Guillemeau (187) in the early 1500's and again by Anel (201), who in 1710 described ligation of the artery proximal to the aneurysm. Brasdor (175) modified the operation by placing the ligature distal to the aneurysm. Pasquin (175), however, placed ligatures both proximally and distally.

The abdominal aorta was not approached in this manner until 1817. Earlier, Sir Astley Cooper had demonstrated the efficacy of proximal ligation of both extremity arteries and the common carotid artery. He had also demonstrated that the dog survived total occlusion of the distal aorta. The first patient to be operated on in this manner was suffering from a bleeding iliac artery aneurysm. Cooper ligated the distal aorta with a single silk suture and, although the patient did well initially, he developed thrombosis of the ipsilateral iliac artery and died 40 hours postoperatively (51). Bigger (35) provides a good review of the further status of aortic ligation finding that none of the 18 patients operated upon prior to 1920 lived to hospital discharge. With medical improvements, however, the period from 1920 to 1940 is characterized by survival and "improvement" in 7 of 12 patients. A patient of Matas, in fact, survived nearly a year and a half, dying of tuberculosis with autopsy proof of almost complete obliteration of the aneurysmal sac (206).

THROMBOSIS

A variety of substances has been introduced into the aneurysmal sac to induce thrombosis (194). These techniques have included galvanopuncture (Philetus), needling (Valpeau), and insertion of horsehair (Levis, 1876) (14). The most persistent method has been the use of wire. In 1865, Moore introduced lengths of silver wire into an aneurysm and left them *in situ*. His patient died of sepsis, presumably from the unsterilized material (16). This technique was modified by Corradi, who added an electric current to the methodology. Power and Colt (247), in 1903, constructed a gold-plated wire wisp, or umbrella, which could be introduced into the artery and advanced into the aneurysm. They had a few brilliant successes with this technique and, as recently as 1950, a series of nine syphilitic thoracic aortic aneurysms included five successes (43). Blakemore and King (38) added a more sophisticated technique with the application of an electric current to insulated copper wire within the sac, providing a temperature of 80°C for 10 seconds. The last publication describing a significant series of patients treated with wire was that of Linton (199) who, on the eve of the modern era in 1951, described in detail his procedure for inserting hundreds of feet of stainless steel wire into the aneurysm (204). Of 25 patients, he reported 10 living from one month to two and one-half years after the procedure. Another 7 had been successfully discharged from the hospital only to have their aneurysms rupture from one month to more than two years later. There is convincing evidence (16) that this technique resulted in at least a marked reduction in pain, if not an actual increase in patient survival. An occasional long-term survivor is reported (13).

Attempts to induce intra-aneurysmal thrombosis also utilized extra-aneurysmal techniques. After Page (236) discovered that cellophane could induce fibrosis secondary to chemical irritation, Pearse (239) utilized this material to gradually occlude flow in large arteries in experimental dogs. This technique was applied to aneurysms of the subclavian artery by Harrison and Chandy (154) and then to syphilitic aneurysms of the thoracic aorta (1, 244, 245). Other workers used skin grafts placed around the aneurysm to cause this same gradual occlusion. Although there were many reported successes with these wrapping techniques, many of these same patients are represented in the early series of homografts and heterografts of both the thoracic and abdominal aorta.

ENDOANEURYSMORRHAPHY

Matas' technique (207) of endoaneurysmorrhaphy developed nearly a century ago was a classic innovation in vascular surgery. It was attempted for repair of aortic aneurysms by a number of surgeons without success until Bigger (35) reported a single cure in 1940.

EXCISION

A fourth avenue of approach to aneurysmal management was excision of the aneurysm itself. Prior to the modern age of surgery, this would be impossible except for a saccular aneurysm. The first attempt was made in 1902 by Tuffier, who apparently suffered a change of heart in the middle of the procedure and, after freeing the sac, decided merely to ligate the neck of the aneurysm. The patient exsanguinated when the aneurysmal sac became gangrenous (16). Alexander and Byron (12) reported the first successful use of the procedure in 1944 on a thoracic aortic aneurysm. Bahnson (15) presented the largest series of successful excisions—all six apparently performed on syphilitic abdominal aortic aneurysms.

REPLACEMENT

In addition to the work already described, Blum (41), in his review of abdominal aortic aneurysms, cites an additional four pillars upon which the modern operative therapy is based: 1) the early experimental arterial repairs of Alexis Carrel; 2) the development of angiography by Dos Santos; 3) the availability of a stable, nontoxic, measurable, anticlotting agent—heparin; and 4) the use of human homograft as conduit.

Estes' 1950 paper (111) focused attention on the clinical problem of abdominal aortic aneurysms, demonstrating a three-year survival of less than 50% with nearly two-thirds of the patients dying of aneurysmal rupture. The "history" of abdominal aortic aneurysms ended and the modern era began with the Dubost *et al.* replacement of M. LeG.'s distal aorta with a human homograft in 1951 (100). This was followed by another dozen homografts by DeBakey and Cooley in 1952 and 1953.

It was soon apparent that homograft replacement was not completely satisfactory. All hospitals could not maintain sufficient vessel banks for the possibility of surgery. The graft had to resemble in size that of the patient's own vessels, which was frequently difficult with normal donors. Although there were improvements in control of contamination, and storage time of the homograft was extended by the use of freeze-drying techniques, a search was made for an artificial substitute. Moreover, the aortic homografts were subject to progressive degenerative changes characterized by mural calcification, thinning, and patchy loss of the elastic framework (62).

Alexis Carrel (54, 55) had unsuccessfully sought a vessel substitute nearly four decades earlier. His experiences with tubes of glass, aluminum, and silver were marred by thrombosis. Polyethylene tubing achieved minor success, though it too was thrombogenic (222). Hufnagel (163) introduced methyl methacrylate as an aortic substitute. The first satisfactory material was Vinyon "N" cloth, the clinical application of which was initially reported by Blakemore and King (38) and Voorhees *et al.* (300). Schumacker's group extended the experience with this material (264, 265).

Deterling and Bhonslay (88) evaluated a number of materials including Nylon, Vinyon "N", Orlon, Dacron, Teflon (polytetrafluoroethylene, PTFE), and Saran. They concluded that only the first four were adequate and that Dacron appeared to have the best overall qualities. Simultaneously, Edwards and Tapp (103) examined chemically treated Nylon tubes, focusing less on the quality of the material than on the structure of the woven graft. Moreover, they succeeded in building a Y-shaped tube for use as a bifurcation graft without the longitudinal seams, resulting from sewing two tube grafts together.

The 1950's experience defined the necessary characteristics of both the fabric material and the graft. The fabric material should have the following characteristics (257): 1) not be physically modified by tissue fluids; 2) be chemically inert; 3) not excite inflammatory or foreign-body cell response in the tissues; 4) be noncarcinogenic; 5) not produce a state of allergy or hypersensitivity; 6) be capable of standing up to mechanical strains imposed on it; 7) be capable of being fabricated in the form required with reasonable ease and at relatively low cost; and 8) be capable of being sterilized without alteration. In addition, the graft should have these qualities (103): 1) be braided (knitted) or woven into tubes of various sizes so that the longitudinal seam could be eliminated; 2) be designed in such a way that the tube could be cut to any desired length at the operating table, yet arterial sutures would not cause fraying or unraveling at the cut ends; 3) be unwettable to prevent blood loss, yet not impermeable to fibroblastic penetration through the fibers; 4) be constructed to maintain flexibility of the tube so that it would not kink if used in flexion areas; and 5) be woven or braided into Y-tubes to replace bifurcations such as the abdominal aorta.

The most commonly employed fabric today is this same polyester Dacron, which is available in both a fairly porous knitted fabric and a tightly woven form. It is available as both a straight and a Y-tube. PTFE is also available, though the technology to achieve a Y-graft is relatively recent. But the "ultimate" arterial substitute for aortic surgery still does not exist. Today, investigators are dealing with the problems of infectivity and thrombogenesis. Graham *et al.* (139–141) have seeded Dacron prostheses with autogenous endothelial cells, demonstrating increased clot-free surfaces. Voorhees (299) described a technique for forming sulfadiazine silver-impregnated Dacron prostheses, but the drug is apparently rapidly leached from the fabric. The most successful technique was reported by Moore *et al.* (223), who bound amikacin to collagen and then coated Dacron grafts with the collagen. Not only was infection controlled, but the rate of formation of neointima was accelerated.

Summary

The logical development of therapy for abdominal aortic aneurysms is impressive, whether one views this over the last three centuries or just the last three decades. Tomorrow's history will probably be written by those who discover and understand the underlying disease process which leads to formation of aneurysms (303). Prevention will allow this and similar volumes to gather dust on library shelves.

PATHOLOGY AND PATHOPHYSIOLOGY

Aneurysms may be described and characterized by a number of different criteria, including their anatomy, morphology, and etiology. Anatomically, an aneurysm is a true aneurysm (much like a true diverticulum) if the expansion includes all of the layers of the original vessel wall, thinned out but still surrounding the arterial lumen. The false or pseudoaneurysm is "incomplete" in that the attenuation does not involve all layers. The true aneurysm is secondary to a process which results in generalized tissue weakening; whereas, the false aneurysm is consequent to a more localized event, such as trauma or infection. There is a third type of aneurysm which is uncommon in the abdominal aorta—a dissecting aneurysm. In this condition there is a defect in the media and, consequently, an intramural channel through which blood passes. The blood may regain entrance into the lumen *via* another medial defect, but this is not necessary.

Aneurysms may also be described by their external morphology. The more common abdominal aortic aneurysm is fusiform in shape, extending along a considerable distance. Aneurysms may also be saccular in that they have relatively narrow necks and need not involve the whole of the vessel circumference. This difference plays a role in surgical management.

Finally, aneurysms may be described according to their etiology (136). The major source of abdominal aortic aneurysms today is atherosclerosis, which accounts for an estimated 96% of current cases. They may also result from trauma, syphilitic aortitis, a variety of infectious agents (including bacteria, mycobacteria, and fungi), degenerative conditions (e.g., Marfan's syndrome, Ehlers-Danlos syndrome, and cystic medial necrosis), so-called collagen vascular diseases and various vasculitides, and congenital anomalies. The pathology and pathophysiology of aneurysmal formation are described in greater detail in Chapter 1.

Etiology

The autopsy incidence of abdominal aortic aneurysms was fairly constant at 1 to 3% from the early to the mid-20th century (137). This occurred despite a changing spectrum, with syphilitic aneurysms decreasing in significance as atherosclerotic aneurysms increased. The causes for this shift seem to have been twofold: 1) increased effectiveness of public health programs and a reliable chemotherapeutic agent that reduced the incidence of syphilis in all stages; and 2) an increasingly older population more susceptible to the effects of atherosclerosis.

This shift seems almost sudden in comparison with other pathologic processes. Maniglia and Gregory (202) reviewed 6,000 autopsies performed between 1906 and 1951 and found the predominance of atherosclerotic aneurysms only in the last three years of the study. Similarly, only during the last four years of a study running from 1932 to 1953 did Blakemore and Voorhees (39) observe atherosclerotic outnumbering syphilitic aneurysms. Barratt-Boyes (20) emphasized the abruptness of this changing etiology, noting that atherosclerotic aneurysms were three times as common in the period of 1948 to 1956 as in the preceding eight years. Wright *et al.* (312) again illustrated this phenomenon—their incidence of atherosclerotic aortic aneurysms was more than twice as great from 1950 to 1953 than in the immediately preceding five years.

This changing etiology is intimately associated with a changing anatomic localization. Syphilitic aortic aneurysms are predominantly thoracic, whereas atherosclerotic aortic aneurysms are rarely encountered above the renal arteries. Abdominal aneurysms were rare in the 17th century. Osler (234) found a 10:1 ratio of thoracic to abdominal aortic aneurysms. Thirty years later, Kampmeier (173) (admittedly describing a population with a high incidence of syphilis) found a similar ratio. By 1941, though, Ruffin *et al.* (256) noted the ratio to have decreased to only 3:1. Since 1949, abdominal aortic aneurysms have been reportedly twice as numerous as those found above the diaphragm (202).

AGE, SEX, RACE

Abdominal aortic aneurysms are described in patients as young as 33 and as old as 90, in an operative series reported by DeBakey *et al.* (87). The greatest frequency occurred in the seventh decade of life, and 20% of the patients were over 70 years old. This operative series reports somewhat younger ages (as would be expected) than the autopsy series published by Halpert and Williams (151). In their review of 4,000 male war veterans, aortic aneurysms increased in frequency from 6% in the sixth decade, to 10% in the seventh, 12% in the eighth, and 14% in the ninth. Women with aneurysms fall into the same pattern, but are generally two to eight years older than men (151). Men, however, are distinctly more susceptible to the disease than females. In large series, men comprise from 70 to more than 90% of the cases, with an average of 85% (137).

Race, as a factor in aortic aneurysm disease, poses some problems. The high incidence in a study such as Kampmeier's (173) is skewed by the high incidence of syphilitic aneurysms in an indigent black population. If one focuses on atherosclerotic aneurysms solely, though, another picture emerges. In five series reporting racial factors, 16 of 366 aneurysms occurred in blacks for an incidence of only 4.3% (137). These studies, unfortunately, do not provide a racial breakdown of the hospital population. In an autopsy series in which this could be ascertained (151), aneurysms were less than half as common (2.7%) in blacks as in whites (6%). This lower incidence of abdominal aortic aneurysms may be due to a decreased susceptibility in the black population of the aorta to atherosclerosis, as was documented by McGill (213).

Pathophysiology

Development of an abdominal aortic aneurysm results from a complex interaction between the structure of the aortic wall and the physiologic stresses placed upon it. Since normal arteries do not form aneurysms, there must either be a defect in the structural integrity of the vessel wall or, possibly, excessive demands put upon the vessel by abnormal hemodynamics. Histologic review of human abdominal aortic aneurysms, coupled with experimental work in laboratory animals and mechanical models, have produced an understanding of the clinical condition. Not only can this explain the development of the aneurysm, it can mirror its progression through further expansion leading to rupture or thrombosis (69).

STRUCTURE

To understand the pathophysiology of aneurysmal formation, the structure of the arterial system must first be reviewed. Macroscopically, it is a linear system with large vessels dividing and re-dividing into smaller ones. Microscopically, it is a circumferential system composed of elastic and structural elements, organized in response to physiologic stresses.

Though the vessel wall is divided into three layers (interna, media, and externa surrounded by an adventitia), the relevant events take place predominantly in the media. At physiologic blood pressures, the microarchitecture is composed of elastic lamellae organized circumferentially and collagen fibers aligned straight and taut. At normal pressures, the aorta is nearly maximally distended, with both elastic and inelastic elements resisting further distension. This resistance is distributed throughout the media. Medial flaws and defects tend not to be propagated and are described in greater detail in Chapters 1 and 2.

The layers of the aortic media are of similar thickness in a variety of mammals, but the number of these layers increases with mean blood pressure (309). This incidence in total wall thickness correlates with the increase in wall tension deduced from Laplace's law:

$$T = f\ (\text{radius and blood pressure})$$

Curiously, this tension per layer is remarkably constant across mammalian species. Each increment of 0.017 mm in aortic radius requires another fibrocellular layer. The average tension per layer is 2,000 dynes/cm.

Although the number of layers varies with the aortic radius, the ratio of elastic and inelastic (collagen) elements does not. Probably in response to the demands placed upon them, the abdominal aorta contains more collagen than elastin, in contrast to the thoracic aorta where the reverse is true.

The last necessary structural element which should be discussed in this brief description of the vessel wall is the vasa vasorum. These vascular channels are responsible for nutrition in aortas—such as those of man—whose thickness exceeds 30 layers. Cells within a 30-layer radius derive their nutrition by diffusion only, while those beyond this point require the vasa vasorum (311).

With this microscopic structure in mind, the previously described aneurysmal types are more comprehensible. In the true aneurysm, the attenuated arterial wall is contiguous with the normal vessel. Where the overall vessel is preserved, but the medial integrity is compromised and there is blood within the media, a dissecting aneurysm exists. Finally, where there is localized absence of the arterial wall and the bloodstream is contained by extra-arterial tissues, a false or pseudoaneurysm results.

These structural elements are part of the normal, adult, human aorta. There are a number of disease processes occurring both naturally and in the laboratory, and in both man and animals, which damage this organization and contribute to aneurysmal formation. These factors include lathyrism, copper deficiency, Marfan's syndrome, cystic medial necrosis, syphilitic arteritis, and local accumulations of collagenase and elastase.

The biochemical structure of collagen is beyond the scope of this chapter. What is important to note, however, is that the transformation from chemical collagen to a fibrous structure with tensile strength is based upon cross-linking, both within the molecule and between molecules. Similar cross-linking occurs in elastin. The copper-dependent enzyme lysyl oxidase is responsible for the formation of these cross-linkages in collagen and, probably, in elastin as well.

Marfan's syndrome is a disease of man which is not biochemically well characterized. Collagen is more easily extracted from the aortas of patient's dying of the disease, but the collagen seems both abnormal and poorly cross-linked. The relevant clinical aspects of Marfan's syndrome are related to the thoracic and abdominal aorta and are characterized by a spectrum extending from dilatation associated with aortic valvular incompetence to dissecting aneurysms (309, 310).

In 1929, Erdheim described cystic medial necrosis which is commonly but not necessarily associated with Marfan's syndrome. Microscopically, this entity is characterized by cystic accumulations of mucoid material which represents fractured elastic lamina and collagen fibrils. It, too, is not truly a disease of the abdominal aorta (213, 303).

Lathyrism occurs in man as a neurologic defect characterized by progressive paralysis resulting from an upper motor neuron lesion. It is closely associated with consumption of the seeds of *Lathyrus sativus*, the common chick pea. Osteolathyrism, however, is a disease of animals, occurring both naturally and in the laboratory setting. Here, the active toxin, β-aminoproprionitrile (BAPN), has been isolated from the sweet pea. BAPN interferes with collagen cross-linking, although some researchers have demonstrated depressed elastin synthesis in the aorta of lathyritic rats. Ponseti and Baird (243) were the first to report the development of a dissecting aneurysm of the aorta in rats. There have been many subsequent reports and the microscopic lesion has been shown to be associated with medial edema and fragmentation of elastin fibers. Again, the disease is usually confined to the thoracic aorta, especially the arch, with death commonly due to aneurysmal rupture. Rats are not the only animals subject to experimental lathyrism; this has also been caused in fish, mice, turkeys, chickens, rabbits, calves, and swine.

Copper deficiency also affects collagen metabolism in a manner separate from that of BAPN. Cardiovascular lesions are the most common lesions induced. Dissecting aneurysms have been described in chicks and swine. Rupture is most common in the aortic arch. Although the abdominal aorta is widely affected, rupture is not reported.

Mammalian collagenases are characterized by their ability to digest native collagen under physiologic conditions. Increased tissue collagenase has been demonstrated in conditions of abnormal wound healing (such as abdominal wall hernias) and in conditions where normal tissue involutes (such as the postpartum uterus). It has been shown there is increased collagenase in unruptured abdominal aortic aneurysms and Swanson *et al.* (284) have suggested collagenase induced by operative trauma may play a role in subsequent aneurysmal rupture.

Syphilitic aneurysms result from medial destruction. *Treponema pallidum* infection leads to a transmural arteritis of the vasa vasorum. Rather than replacement by a fibrous avascular band, as seen in atherosclerosis, there is an irregular atrophy of the outer media with patchy disappearance of elastic fibers. That this disease is more common in the thoracic aorta is understandable, as the thicker thoracic aorta is more dependent upon the vasa vasorum for its nutrition.

Despite extensive experimental manipulation, it has been difficult to induce abdominal aortic aneurysms which rupture in animals. There are, therefore, peculiarities in the structure of the human abdominal aorta which contribute to this condition. The human abdominal aorta is not completely consistent with those of other mammals (310). The distal aorta, because of its 0.7-mm thickness, should contain 40 fibrocellular layers and vasa vasorum, but it does not. Instead, there are only 29 layers and no vasa vasorum, so all the cells are dependent upon diffusion alone for nutrition. Moreover, the wall tension is increased to 3,200 dynes/cm per layer. The atherosclerotic aneurysm is not apparently the result of intimal plaque formation, but of other events occurring in the media itself. Hypercholesteremia is known to retard the healing of spontaneous injuries, and catecholamines and carbon monoxide have been suggested as impeding cellular recovery. The loss of one layer in the media increases the tension of those remaining.

PHYSIOLOGY

Although the structural defects have been described, they do not exist in a vacuum. The physical laws of fluid mechanics interacting with these structural defects contribute to aneurysmal dilatation and its progression (see Chapters 1 and 2).

Circumferential stress on the aortic wall increases with increasing diameter and decreasing wall thickness:

$$\text{Stress} = P \times (\text{radius/thickness})$$

Atherosclerotic changes are initially associated with increased distensibility of the vessel and, secondarily, with thinning as the fibrous elements are destroyed. This would, therefore, result in a progressive increase in wall stresses further dilating the vessel. Similarly, Tilson and Dang (296) reported increased aneurysmal disease in "megalo-arteries." They consider this increased stress as a possible explanation of the increased incidence of abdominal aortic aneurysms in males whose body habitus is usually larger than that of females.

Another factor contributing to this stress of distensibility is the presence of reflected pressure waves (281). Minimal reflected waves occur backwards from a bifurcation when the ratio of the cross-section areas of the daughter vessels to the parent vessel are greater than 1:1.15 (aorta:iliacs). The closest the distal human aorta comes to this is in the child, where the ratio is 1:1.11. With increasing age, this ratio decreases to 1:0.75 in aortas unaffected by atherosclerosis and to 1:0.65 in atherosclerotic vessels, producing reflections of more than 26% of the oscillatory pressure amplitude and a partial standing wave, as well, further stressing the distal aorta. The natural history of aneurysms includes the development of intramural thrombus. Teleologically, this may be viewed as protective against progressive dilatation, as it would increase the wall thickness. Since its mechanical properties differ from those of the parent vessel, it probably offers little protection. The prediliction for rupture at the posterolateral aspect of the aortic wall may be related to its relative fixation to the vertebral column medially.

NATURAL HISTORY

The major complication of an untreated abdominal aortic aneurysm is rupture (142, 241). Aneurysms may rupture into the retroperitoneum, into the free peritoneal cavity, or they may rupture into an adjoining viscus such as the duodenum, the left renal vein, the inferior vena cava, or the urinary system. Less commonly, the intrasaccular thrombus may propagate, resulting in an aortic occlusion, or the thrombus may embolize distally. The true risks of these complications are difficult to ascertain, complicating an analysis of natural history. Autopsy studies tend to exaggerate the mortality of aneurysms (82, 231). Studies composed of patients rejected as surgical candidates will contain a large number of seriously ill patients with associated medical problems. Some older studies, based exclusively on clinical examination, will include patients who were thought to have aneurysms but who, in fact, had none.

The first major paper delineating the natural history of abdominal aortic aneurysms was that of Estes (111) published in 1950—a 102-patient series from the Mayo Clinic which was very significant. Estes recognized the increasing role of atherosclerosis in aneurysmal disease and described both the mortality of the condition and the importance of aneurysmal rupture as a cause of death. The paper is properly credited with effecting a change in the surgical attitude towards the disease at a time when graft replacement was soon to be available.

A subsequent series of autopsied patients from the same institution was presented by Sommerville *et al.* (271), who found a five-year survival of less than 10% (3 of 38 evaluable patients). Comparing their results to Estes' earlier study, they concluded the difference was inherent in the patient selection dictated by an autopsy study. The Mayo Clinic and other centers are responsible for a number of similar studies which are summarized in Table 6.1.

The mere presence of an aneurysm proved to be a poor predictor of its behavior (142). Review of the data suggested size as a factor in aneurysmal rupture and this has been repeatedly confirmed (259). From a number of series (137), the risk of rupture of a small aneurysm (<5 cm) averaged 9% (range 0 to 18%); an intermediate-sized lesion (4.5 to 10 cm) had ruptured in 37% of evaluable cases (range 20 to 60%); and a large aneurysm (>7 cm) had ruptured in 76% of cases (range 70 to 95%). It is important in reviewing these papers to note the means by which the size of the aneurysm was estimated, as clinical evaluation can result in a different measurement than radiographic or sonographic evaluation (18, 31, 58).

The third consideration in assessing the risk of rupture was the presence of symptoms, as noted by Flanigan *et al.* (115) and Gliedman *et al.* (133). In their series from Kings County Hospital and in their review of the previous publications, they found survival was considerably less in

Table 6.1
Survival of Patients with Unresected Aortic Aneurysms

Series	No. of Patients	Aneurysms Ruptured (%)	Percent after Years of Survival				
			1 yr	2 yr	3 yr	4 yr	5 yr
Barratt-Boyes, 1957 (20)	51	52	53				13
Blakemore and Voorhees, 1954 (40)	131		38	12		8	13
Estes, 1950 (111)	102	63	67	58	49	27	19
Foster *et al.*, 1969 (117)	57	33					18
Gliedman *et al.*, 1957 (133)	68		20		13		8
Kampmeier, 1936 (173)	57		13		2		
Schatz *et al.*, 1962 (258)	119	44	88		53		36
Szilagyi *et al.*, 1966 (288)	223	35	54		32		17
Wolffe and Colcher, 1966 (308)	33						30
Wright *et al.*, 1956 (312)	68		60		16		4
Summary	909	45	49		27		17.5

symptomatic patients than when the aneurysm was diagnosed incidentally in an asymptomatic patient. The final factor in assessing prognosis in a patient with an aneurysm is the presence of associated atherosclerotic cardiac, vascular, or cerebrovascular disease (123). Gliedman *et al.* (133) concluded that although only 49% of their patients died of aneurysmal rupture, another 47% died of associated atherosclerotic conditions.

The major step in defining the mortality of aneurysmal disease was the analysis of the large series of Szilagyi (285) and Szilagyi *et al.* (288). Not only did these papers clarify the disease process, they compared the mortality and morbidity of surgical correction in carefully matched patients. When standardized for age, cardiac status, blood pressure, and renal function, the five-year survival was calculated as 48% if the aneurysm was less than 6 cm, and 6% if it was greater than 6 cm.

CLINICAL FEATURES

Clinical presentation of the patient with an abdominal aortic aneurysm has changed as physician awareness has increased. Since aneurysmal changes of the abdominal aorta are only one manifestation of the atherosclerotic process (229, 230), the patient may be referred to a physician because of other cardiovascular complaints (83, 259). Twenty-five percent of these patients have an old myocardial infarction (157), angina pectoris, or congestive heart failure (87). Over 40% have systemic hypertension (15 to 100% in collected series) (124, 147) and nearly 50% have both. Significant occlusive disease of the lower extremities, reported in 27% by DeBakey *et al.* (87) and in 35% by Haimovici (150), may prompt patient referral. Associated aneurysmal disease of the thoracic aorta, femoral, or popliteal arteries may also become symptomatic prior to complaints arising from the abdominal aortic aneurysm (58).

While Eastcott (101), in a collected personal series of 100 patients, found pain a presenting factor in 72% (see Table 6.2), more recent series report over 60% of the patients are completely asymptomatic (137). Where there is a complaint, the most common patient observation is not pain but awareness of an abdominal pulsation (170). This is usually

Table 6.2
Typical Presenting Clinical Features of 100 Consecutive Patients with Abdominal Aortic Aneurysms

Clinical Features		No. of Patients
Pain		63
Abdominal	(21)	
Leg	(11)	
Back	(31)	
Asymptomatic and discovered by physician		19
Asymptomatic and discovered by patient		10
Genitourinary symptoms		5
Gastrointestinal symptoms		3

reported to be infraumbilical and varies in significance from merely disquieting to interfering with bedtime reading. This is not uncommonly first noticed during a febrile episode or when the patient is taking a hot bath—times when the peripheral vascular resistance is decreased and the cardiac output increased. The physician must be especially aware in this clinical setting, as tortuosity of the aorta and abdominal neoplasms displacing the aorta and major arteries must be considered and ruled out.

The symptoms ascribed to aneurysms that may rupture into the free abdominal cavity or present as aortocaval, -enteric, and -ureteral fistulas are described in the section "Special Problems," along with their surgical management. Symptoms of the unruptured aneurysm are caused by 1) compression of adjacent organs, vascular or neural structures; 2) the inflammatory reaction which frequently accompanies the aneurysm (136); and 3) changes within the aorta caused by intramural thrombus (74).

Gastrointestinal manifestations may be caused by angulation and displacement of the 2nd and 3rd portions of the duodenum. There may be insufficiency of the inferior mesenteric artery (IMA) as its origin is compromised by the expanding aneurysmal sac, if the superior mesenteric artery (SMA) or the maginal artery of Drummond is compromised as well. Constipation or an irritable bowel syndrome may develop, although the mechanism is not clear. Weight loss is described in 20% of patients (272).

Genitourinary tract symptoms have been reported and one paper describes a series of patients whose complaints were attributed to their inguinal herniae (216). This is apparently secondary to irritation by an expanding aneurysmal sac of the genitofemoral nerve as it passes down the anterior surface of the psoas muscle. Compression of the left renal artery or vein may result in renal ischemia and/or hypertension (7). The ureter may be obstructed, causing left-sided renal pain or colic (76). Pressure on the testicular vessels may result in a varicocoele. A large sac may affect the genitofemoral nerve and produce inguinal hernia-like pain. Leg swelling may result from obstruction of the left common iliac vein.

Neurologic complaints include lumbosacral pain from inflammatory involvement of the vertebral fascia, varying in severity from slight, to excruciating, to the point of patient suicide (272). Spinal root compression by the expanding sac may cause sciatic pain, sensory loss, quadriceps paralysis, and foot drop. These neurologic effects also include various degrees of bladder dysfunction. Sexual disturbances— impaired or painful orgasms—have been attributed to changes in the sympathetic trunk and presacral plexus related to the aneurysmal periarteritis (304).

DIAGNOSIS

Physical Examination

Despite computers and sophisticated laboratory analyses, the surgeon's hands are among the most important diagnostic tools in identifying an abdominal aortic aneurysm (47, 195). Any pulsatile mass is significant, especially if it extends below the patient's umbilicus (Fig. 6.1). The pulsations of the abdominal aneurysm are classically described as pushing the examiner's fingers apart rather than merely anteriorly. Note must be made of the proximal extent of the aneurysm. If the examiner is unable to place his hand between the mass and the xiphoid, there may be suprarenal extension of the aneurysm. By correcting for the thickness of the anterior abdominal wall, the examiner can rather accurately size the aneurysm. The Hertzer and Beven review of comparative techniques (158) found that physical examination usually overestimated the true size of the aneurysm by 1 cm, but the examiner was within 1 cm of the true diameter in 58% of cases.

Physical examination is difficult in emaciated and obese patients. Very thin patients will tend to have an easily palpable aorta and a normal or tortuous vessel may seem to be widened. The obese patient's overlying abdominal wall fat makes examination difficult. Further confusion in the diagnosis can result from spinal deformities in the patient; a normal vessel will seem more prominent in front of a lordotic spine. A tense abdominal wall may make a valid examination nearly impossible.

Routine Radiography

The simplest and most common tests suggesting a diagnosis of an aneurysm are radiographs of the abdomen, anteroposterior and cross-table lateral films. Since 55 to 58% of aneurysms are calcified (137), this radiopacity can be readily seen. With large, uncalcified aneurysms, a soft

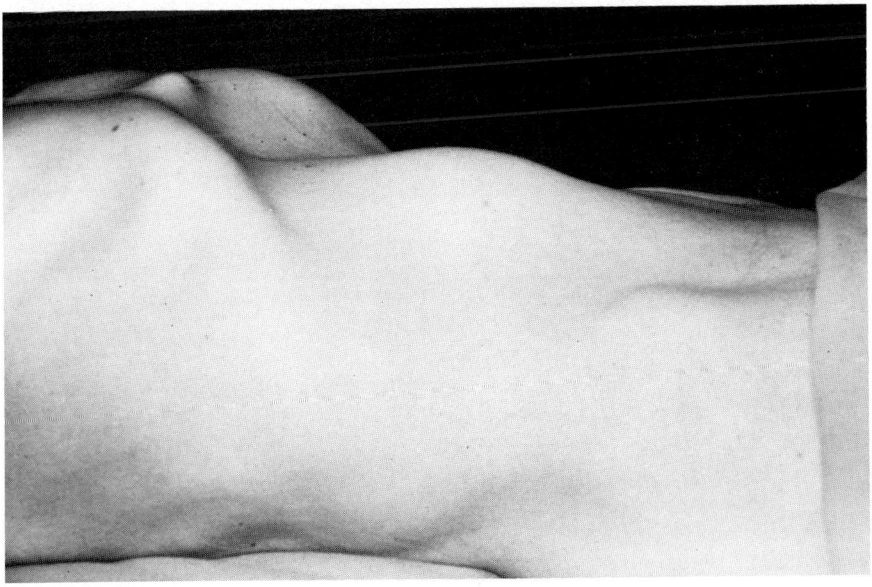

Figure 6.1. Patient presented with a pulsatile abdominal mass.

tissue mass may be discernible. Large aneurysms may also displace other organs and cause abnormal gas patterns. Hertzer and Beven (158) found that the size derived from the lateral abdominal radiograph was within 1 cm of the true size in 72% of patients. The overall diagnostic accuracy of routine radiography is estimated at 88%. Although an upper gastrointestinal (GI) series, barium enema, or intravenous pylogram (IVP) may be performed to clarify these, other methods have proven more reliable.

A radiograph of the chest should also be obtained. Widening of the mediastinum may be an indication either of a thoracoabdominal aneurysm or suprarenal extension of an abdominal aneurysm. DeBakey and Cooley (86) and DeBakey *et al.* (87) demonstrated a concomitant aneurysm of the thoracic aorta in 4% of patients with abdominal aortic aneurysms.

Ultrasonography

B-mode ultrasonography has become an easy means of confirming and measuring abdominal aortic aneurysms (228) (Figs. 6.2 and 6.3). Leopold *et al.* (197) reviewed a series of 38 patients with suspected aneurysms; they reported 26 aneurysms to be present—25 were confirmed by other techniques. Of the 12 cases reported as negative, all were, in fact, negative. The single false-positive result proved to be a lymphoma. Their overall accuracy was 97.4%, but technical interpretation at other centers is

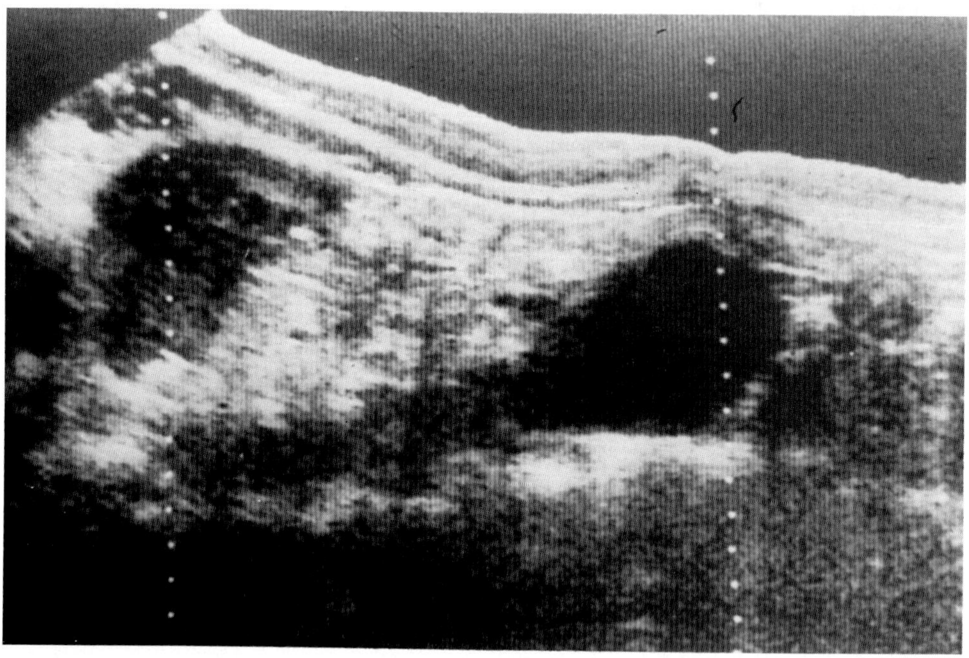

Figure 6.2. Ultrasound demonstration of cross-section of abdominal aortic aneurysm.

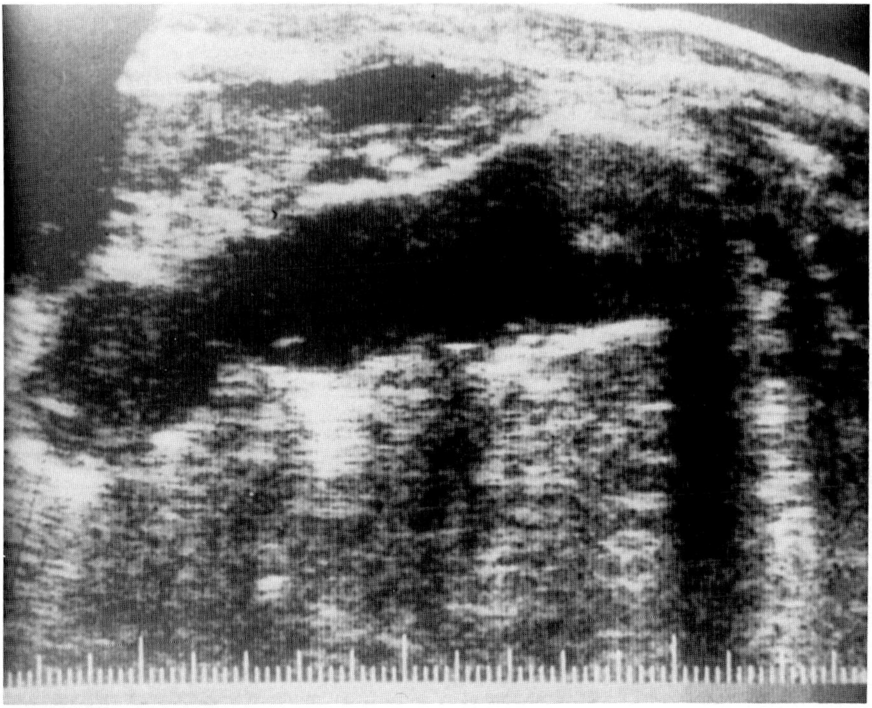

Figure 6.3. Lateral view of an abdominal aortic aneurysm demonstrated by B-mode ultrasonography.

probably not this good and detection rates are, therefore, likely to be lower. Sizing can be easily done in the A-mode with similar accuracy. The Hertzer and Beven study (158) found ultrasonography the most reliable technique, with the measured size being within 1 cm of the aneurysm's true size in 92% of cases.

Computerized Axial Tomography Scan

The computerized axial tomography (CAT) scan (242) has been considered of greater accuracy than ultrasound techniques (Fig. 6.4). As in much of clinical surgery, the choice between these two modalities is one of cost to patient and radiologist experience. Ultrasonography is inexpensive, but requires a competent technician and an experienced radiologist. The CAT scan is more expensive, but is very forgiving of technician inexperience. It can be performed on the obese patient, is not adversely affected by overlying gas patterns, and requires virtually no patient preparation. While the CAT scan will match ultrasonography in the diagnosis and sizing, it may prove better in documenting proximal extension with regard to the renal arteries and in describing associated iliac artery aneurysms where ultrasonography is especially weak. Use of

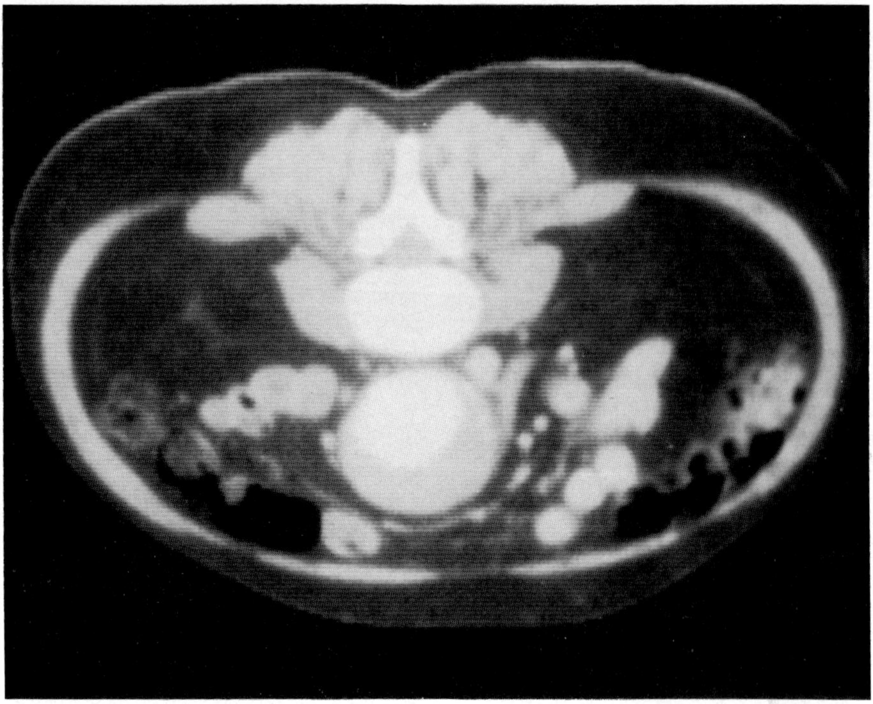

Figure 6.4. CAT scan cross-section view which demonstrates the abdominal aortic aneurysm surrounded by clot anterior to the vertebral column.

intravenous contrast material adds further information to the conventional CAT scan.

Aortography

Aortography, in the evaluation of the unruptured abdominal aortic aneurysm, is still a matter of some controversy (Fig. 6.5). Aortography is not valid in screening patients for the presence of an aneurysm because it can only show the arterial lumen. Since the lumen may be filled with clot, it is difficult to evaluate the size of the aneurysm. Both ultrasonography and the other radiographic procedures discussed earlier are simpler, more accurate, less expensive, and are associated with less patient morbidity. The benefits of aortography lie in defining the anatomic extent of disease and the presence of additional aneurysmal or occlusive disease (170). The controversy that exists is over whether this additional information justified aortography in all patients. Aortography can demonstrate significant associated disease (Table 6.3).

Supported by similar data, routine preoperative aortography is supported by Bauer *et al.* (24), Cyr *et al.* (77), Foster (116), Johnson and Nabseth (169), Kahn and Callow (172), Kwaan *et al.* (182), and Robicsek

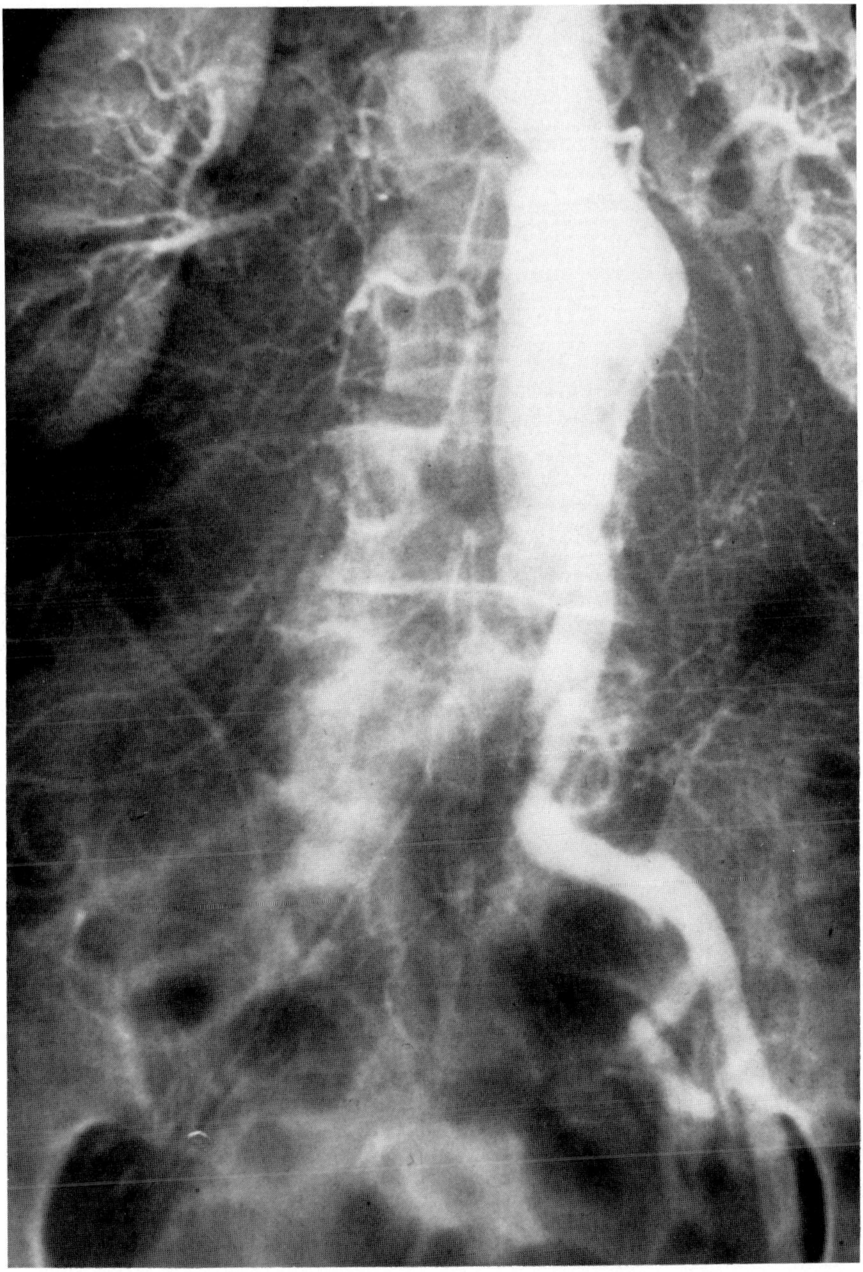

Figure 6.5. Aortogram demonstrating an abdominal aortic aneurysm and occlusion of right common iliac artery.

Table 6.3
Results of Aortography in Patients with Abdominal Aortic Aneurysms

Series	Renal Lesions (%)	Other Aneurysms (%)	Occlusive Disease (%)
Bauer *et al.*, 1978 (24)	32		49
Brewster *et al.*, 1975 (49)	39	56	
Kwaan *et al.*, 1977 (182)	6	33	77

et al. (254). There are, however, other surgeons who do not feel the routine study offers significant advantages—a group which includes Danielson and Payne (80), Gaspar (127), Ochsner and DeCamp (230), and Rob and Williams (252). Their contention is that the majority of the data gleaned from aortography would be discovered by the surgeon at the operating table and any changes in his operative plan may then be decided upon. Danielson and Payne (80) felt that " . . . consistent successful surgical results could be obtained without pre-operative aortograms." Similarly, in 1977, Gaspar (127), in his commentary of Kwaan's paper, could only find two of his own patients who would have benefited from routine aortography. Thompson *et al.* (292) reserve aortography " . . . for those cases in which the diagnosis is questionable, there is associated occlusive disease or there may be problems with the renal arteries." We regard the question of aortography as one of judgment, favoring routine aortography where it is readily available and can be obtained at low morbidity. The current techniques are not those of 20 or 30 years ago and many of the objections to angiography are no longer valid. Moreover, surgery for abdominal aortic aneurysms is not for the casual, occasional vascular surgeon; rather, it requires the combined efforts and talents of appropriate, preoperative, and intraoperative evaluation and expertise.

The information gained from aortography adds to that of physical examination. Femoral and popliteal aneurysms can be detected clinically and repaired at the time of operation (127), but the aortogram more clearly defines their extent.

Our experience also indicates that the information found from aortography adds to that which would be discovered during operation. Although suprarenal extension may have been suggested by preoperative physical examination and is obvious in the operating room, the surgeon armed with this knowledge beforehand can better plan his operation according to the risks of his patient. Abnormal renal vasculature will be found during routine dissection of the aneurysm, but awareness of this beforehand may preserve aberrant vessels before they are divided.

What changes in the operating plan are dictated by aortography? Knowledge of suprarenal extension of the aneurysm allows the surgeon to prepare by increasing the availability of cross-matched blood, or preparing chilled renal perfusates before aortic cross-clamping (49). Similarly, associated renovascular disease may not be readily visible at the operating table and there would be no way to determine which patients would benefit from renal artery reconstruction. In most patients, renal artery occlusive disease may be managed by percutaneous angioplasty in the angiography suite, with a low incidence of re-stenosis. Finally, the aortogram may demonstrate that a poor-risk patient has such extensive vascular disease so as to contraindicate operation. Aortography was an important factor in making this decision in seven of the Brewster *et al.* (49) patients.

Those who do not favor routine aortography do accept specific indications for its use. Indications for aortography include: hypertension (49), intestinal angina (49, 127), associated occlusive disease (49), where there is a question of suprarenal extension (49, 314), a non-calcified aneurysm (49), or a high-pitched epigastric bruit suggestive of visceral artery disease (49).

Aortography is not without complications, although their incidence can be reduced. In reported series, the mortality of aortography ranges from 0.06 to 1.7% (8, 49, 182, 189, 190, 211, 219, 278). Complications may be due to mechanical factors resulting from the manipulation of percutaneous needles, catheters, or guide wires. The jet stream of contrast during pressure injection can damage the aorta or cause the catheter tip to whip around and cause damage. The tip may even break off and embolize. Other mechanical complications include thrombosis, local bleeding and hematoma at the puncture site, perforation or dissection of the vessel, dislodgment of an atheromatous plaque with distal embolization, subintimal injection of contrast, infection at the puncture site, and late development of a false aneurysm at the site of puncture. Other complications may result from the contrast material, either as hypersensitivity to the iodinated dyes or to the effects on the kidneys and central nervous system of the volume of dye injected. Pyogenic reactions may occur. Electrical shock during angiography has also been reported. The frequency of serious complications ranges from 2.4 to 3.0%; the frequency of minor complications from 0.5 to 2.1% (Table 6.4).

This is not the place for a lengthy description of arteriographic techniques for which the reader is referred elsewhere (see Table 6.4). There are a number of points which should be enumerated, however. Aortog-

Table 6.4
Complications of Aortography

Series	Complication Rate (%)		Death (%)	No. of Patients
	Minor	Major		
Abrams, 1971 (8)			1.70	1,706
Brewster *et al.*, 1975 (49)	2.1			190
Kwaan *et al.*, 1977 (182)				132
Lang, 1963 (189)	0.7	3.0	0.06	11,302
McAfee, 1957 (209)	0.74		0.28	13,207
Molnar and Paul, 1972 (220)	0.5	2.1		1,762
Steinberg and Stein, 1965 (278)				225

raphy is commonly performed using the standard Seldinger catheter technique. The femoral vessels are preferred, as other vessels are associated with increased complication rates although the transbrachial or transaxillary approach are acceptable alternatives. Translumbar aortography is an older technique which may be utilized when the patient has significant associated occlusive disease. Major improvements in morbidity can be achieved by attention to the patient before radiography. All patients should have a BUN and creatinine determined beforehand. A serum creatinine over 3 mg/dl, or a clearance below 20 ml/min, are relative contraindications for aortography. The patient should be well hydrated before the procedure. If there is coexistent cerebrovascular disease, proper planning with the radiologist can result in a split dye technique—providing visualization of the arch, four vessels, and the distal aorta for minimal dye exposure. Finally, the patient should be adequately premedicated prior to transportation to the angiography suite.

Because the flow is reportedly slower in the area of the aneurysm, somewhat longer cassette intervals are recommended (278). Radiographs are obtained as proximal as the renal arteries and as far distally as there is suspected associated vascular disease. Lateral radiographs are obtained to visualize the origins of the celiac vessels.

After the aortogram, compression of the puncture site is maintained for 15 to 20 minutes. The status of the distal artery tree is examined in the angiography suite and subsequently. Pressure dressings are maintained for 8 hours with the patient kept in bed for at least that time. Although some question has recently been raised regarding puncture-associated hematoma and subsequent infection, there is no indication for antibiotics as part of the angiographic preparation.

Radionuclide Angiography

Bergan and Yao (27) and Bergan *et al.* (28) described a technique of noninvasive angiography. Technetium-99m-tagged albumin is injected intravenously and the patient's abdomen scanned with a standard γ-camera technique. The labeled albumin adheres to the intraluminal thrombus and thus demonstrates the aneurysm. As such, the technique provides data similar and complementary to contrast aortography. Twenty-eight patients with confirmed abdominal aortic aneurysms were studied. There were two false-negative studies and another false-positive examination. The authors themselves place limitations on this technique. It cannot be relied upon to demonstrate the size of an aortic aneurysm.

OPERATION

Having described the natural history of abdominal aortic aneurysms, there are obvious operative indications for their resection. The risk of aneurysmal rupture balanced against the risks of elective operation (128) supports resection once the aneurysm is greater than 5 cm in diameter (204). Smaller aneurysms which have been shown to be enlarging (usually by ultrasonography) should be resected. Finally, the symptomatic patient who may have an expanding aneurysm is another surgical candidate. Prudent management does not include "emergency" operations for these patients. In a recent series (167) where "urgent" and "emergent" management were compared, the latter produced an increase in operative mortality for non-ruptured aneurysms without any improvement in the mortality of patients with ruptured aneurysms.

The elective operation for repair of an abdominal aortic aneurysm demands an optimal preoperative status (275). Cardiac, pulmonary, renal, and metabolic problems must be treated appropriately (67, 268). Prophylactic antibiotics are usually begun one to two hours prior to surgery, or in the operating suite itself. Because of broad-spectrum coverage, which includes both staphylococci and the more common gram-negative bacteria, a cephalosporin is usually selected. A mechanical bowel preparation is recommended, especially for patients with large aneurysms. EKG monitoring is begun in the operating room prior to induction of anesthesia. Aortic surgery under general endotracheal anesthesia remains the technique of choice. After induction, a Foley catheter and a nasogastric tube are placed. An arterial line for monitoring both blood pressure and acid-base status is strongly recommended. Whereas the older literature suggested central venous pressure monitoring as a guide to fluid management, the more prudent approach today calls for placement of a Swan-Ganz catheter. The patient's volume status can be better maintained by following the pulmonary artery wedge pressure, resulting in increased hemodynamic stability during anesthetic induction and aortic clamping (144, 306).

Although Dubost selected the retroperitoneal approach to aneurysmectomy, the majority of surgeons today prefer the transabdominal approach. The left chest is prepped, along with the abdomen, to allow aortic cross-clamping above the diaphragm, if necessary. The field is extended to below both knees in the event of distal artherosclerotic disease or embolism. Lahey (intestinal) bags are placed on the feet to allow the operating surgeon to evaluate the distal circulation without difficulty. The towels are secured to the patient with sutures and a Vi-drape is placed over the field to prevent the towels from slipping off the table. A xiphoid-to-pubis incision is made (Fig. 6.6). After the abdominal cavity is entered, a thorough examination is performed with attention to the presence of an occult malignancy. Most authorities would agree on treating the malignancy first, deferring the vascular procedure. The recent report by Swanson *et al.* (284) has caused us to question this management. They demonstrated a high rate of aneurysmal rupture in the postoperative period, presumably secondary to induced collagenase. If the malignancy is not unresectable and there is no urgent indication for an intestinal operation, such as bleeding or obstruction, we might first resect the aneurysm. Peritoneal soilage from inadvertent bowel injury, or the discovery of an unsuspected abscess, mitigates against further aneurysmal surgery. The presence of asymptomatic cholelithiasis poses a peculiar problem for the surgeon. Because of the significant risk

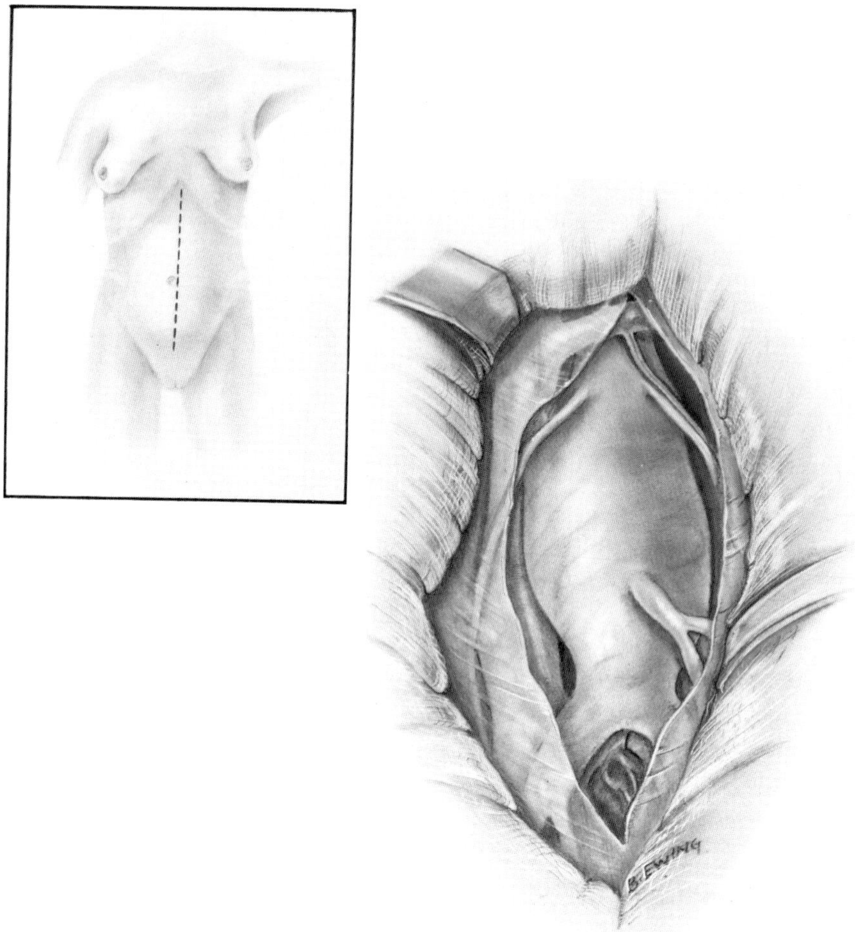

Figure 6.6. Abdominal aortic aneurysm with the inferior mesenteric artery (IMA). The upper left diagram demonstrates the midline incision.

of postoperative cholecystitis if the gall bladder is not removed, we recommend cholecystectomy at the conclusion of the vascular procedure after the peritoneum is closed over the aortic graft (only if the vascular procedure has gone well). To combat the transient bacteremia associated with this procedure, the prophylactic antibiotic regimen may require supplementation.

After the abdominal exploration, a self-retaining retractor is placed and the small bowel retracted to the patient's right. Although some surgeons recommend a bowel bag to avoid dessication of the bowel, we find this cumbersome and prefer protecting the bowel with moist Mickulicz pads and gentle handling. The transverse colon is retracted superiorly and the retroperitoneum is entered through a vertical incision over the sac and to the left of the small bowel mesentery. This dissection is carried cephalad beyond the aneurysm, up to the level of the left renal vein. Care is taken to avoid injury to the blood supply of the duodenum.

Vascular control of the aorta should first be obtained by cautious mobilization of the aorta proximally (Figs. 6.7 and 6.8). The vessel is dissected to the adventitia so that a vascular clamp may be placed securely. It is not necessary to strip down the posterior wall to make it thinner. The surgeon must make a decision as to whether the distal aorta is sufficiently free of disease to allow a simple tube graft—this is the preferred prosthesis and is more common with operations on earlier or smaller aneurysms. A suitable point below the aneurysm and proximal to the aortic bifurcation may be chosen. The more usual condition, however, requires the use of a Y-graft and vascular control of the iliac arteries must be effected. Anatomically, this area is somewhat treacherous because of the adjacent uterus, as well as the sometimes adherent iliac veins. Distal control may be achieved at the level of the iliac arteries or distal aorta, even if the graft must be anastomosed to the femoral arteries.

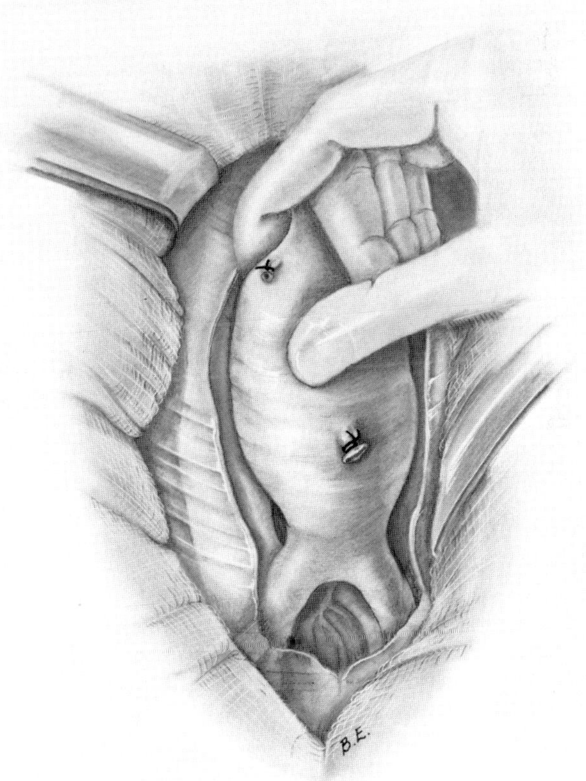

Figure 6.7. Attempt at proximal control, going around the "neck" of the aneurysm.

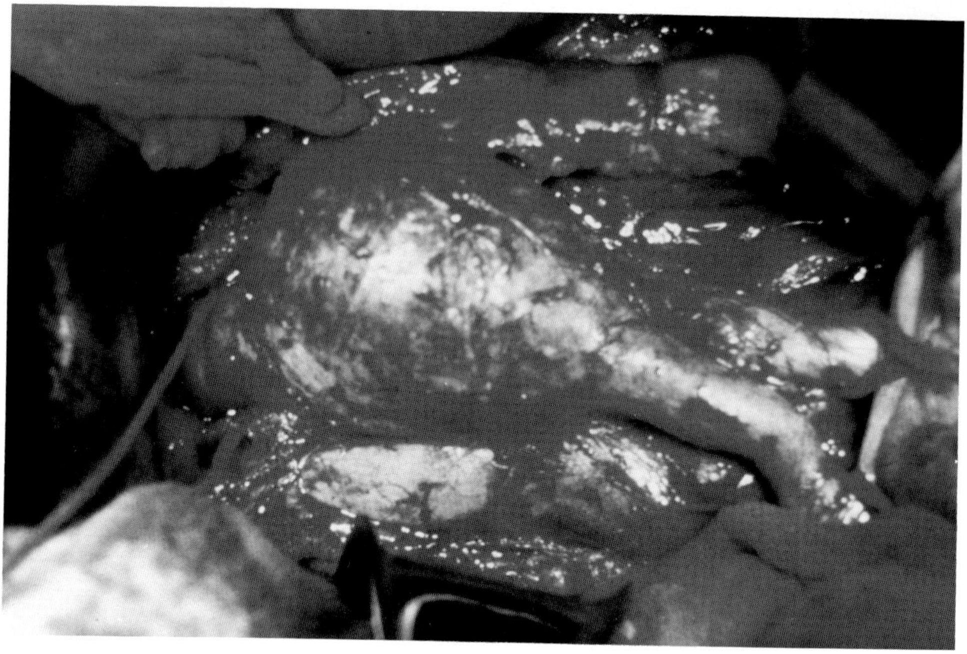

Figure 6.8. Tape is passed about the "neck" of the aneurysm.

Having assessed the patient's vascular anatomy, a decision is made regarding the specific graft material and size (275). The most common prostheses are knitted or woven Dacron. The former is characterized by a larger pore size in the fabric and must be pre-clotted prior to its use. This restriction is not placed on the woven fabric which is, of necessity, the material of choice for a ruptured aneurysm. It is also recommended for older patients and in those who cannot tolerate excessive blood loss or physiologic manipulation at the head of the table. PTFE grafts which do not require pre-clotting are now available in both straight tube and Y-grafts. The size of graft selected should minimize any difference between the graft diameter and the proximal aorta and the distal vessel. Turbulence and sludging will occur if the graft diameter is too large. If the aorta is ectatic and its diameter too large, anterior or posterior V's may be excised and the graft sutured to this reduced circumference.

If a porous, knitted fabric has been selected, it is pre-clotted by a variation of the method of Sauvage. Before heparinization, 30 ml of blood is withdrawn from an available blood vessel and irrigated through the graft. Care must be taken to assure the whole graft is exposed to the blood so that fibrin is deposited in all the interstices.

The patient is then prepared for aortic cross-clamping. Even though the clamps are applied below the renal arteries, the kidneys are vulnerable to ischemic damage. Preservation of optimal renal function is achieved by maintaining a high plasma volume load and inducing a brisk diuresis with mannitol. The second consideration at this point is anticoagulation to prevent distal thrombosis during the period of clamping. Heparin is injected intravenously at a dose of 3,500 to 5,000 units for the average-sized patient. At least five minutes should pass before the clamps are applied to allow the anticoagulation to become effective. The distal vessels are clamped first to avoid distal embolization (165, 276), as we have found this procedure does not significantly increase intramural pressure in the aneurysm; however, the proximal clamp is applied nearly simultaneously. Some authors believe that distal clamping results in renal emboli through turbulence of the intra-aortic debris.

The anterior sac of the aneurysm is then opened sharply and thrombus and debris removed (Figs. 6.9 and 6.10). It may be difficult, and even unnecessary, to transect the whole aorta and the back wall may be left intact, decreasing the chance of lumbar vein damage. A sample of the saccular thrombus should be sent for aerobic and anaerobic bacterial culture, especially if the patient was febrile or complained of tenderness over the sac. Bleeding will be encountered from the lumbosacral vessels and, perhaps, from the IMA as well. It is safer to control this bleeding within the aneurysmal sac—this can usually be accomplished with non-absorbable 0-0 suture (Fig. 6.11). If there is too much calcification of the

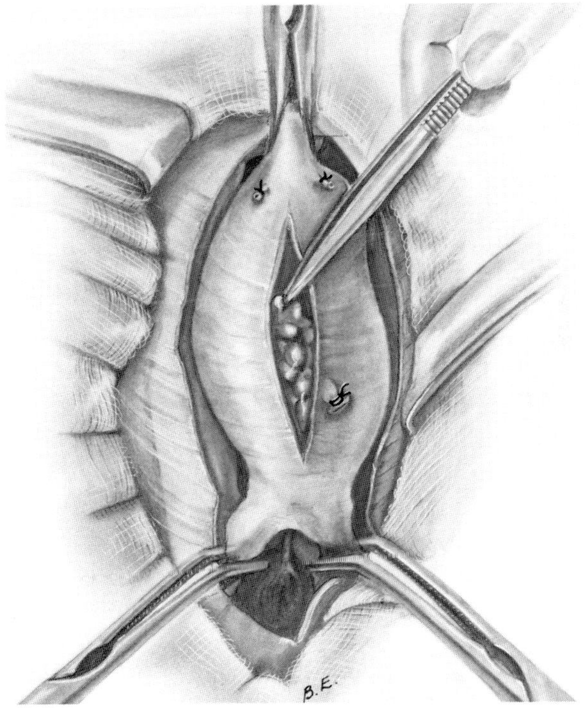

Figure 6.9. Opening into the aneurysm—debris noted in the lumen. Proximal and distal control is seen.

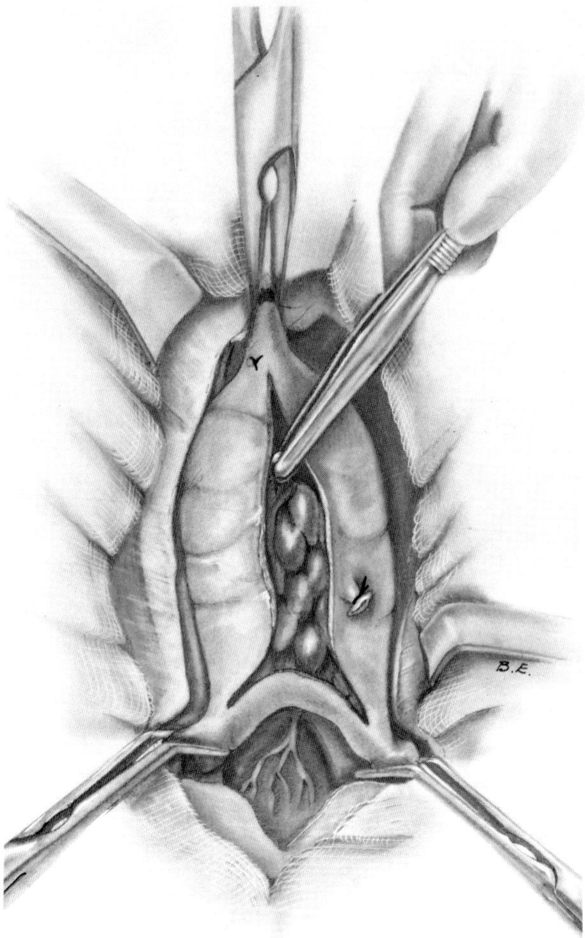

Figure 6.10. Because the aneurysm may extend into the iliac vessels, the incision must go there as well.

posterior wall, both these vessels and the mid-sacral artery may be controlled by placing hemo-clips from the left underside of the sac. The proximal aorta is then transected to allow for an end-to-end anastomosis to the graft (Figs. 6.12 to 6.14). The proximal end of the graft is cut so as to place the bifurcation high. Forgetting to shorten the proximal end of the graft will result in a "baggy-pants" bowing or arching of the graft, inviting turbulence, thrombosis, or aortoenteric fistula. An additional cuff of Dacron may be brought up around the proximal graft to serve as

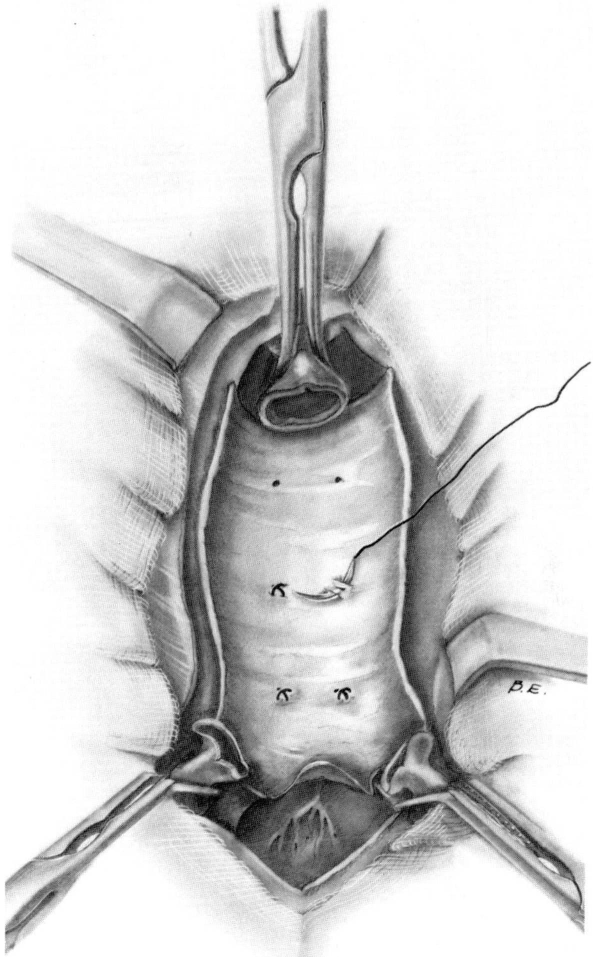

Figure 6.11. Lumelar arteries are controlled from inside the lumen. The ends of the aneurysm are fashioned into "cuffs."

buttressing, especially if the aortic wall appears dangerously thin (Figs. 6.15 and 6.16).

The suture of choice is a 3-0 or 4-0 synthetic material placed in a simple running fashion. The suture line may be begun either posteriorly or equilaterally. Monofilament material combines good tensile strength with minimal tissue reactivity—it slides well, but this quality requires that seven knots be tied for it to seat properly. The sutures should be deeply placed in the aortic wall at least 5 mm from the transected edge.

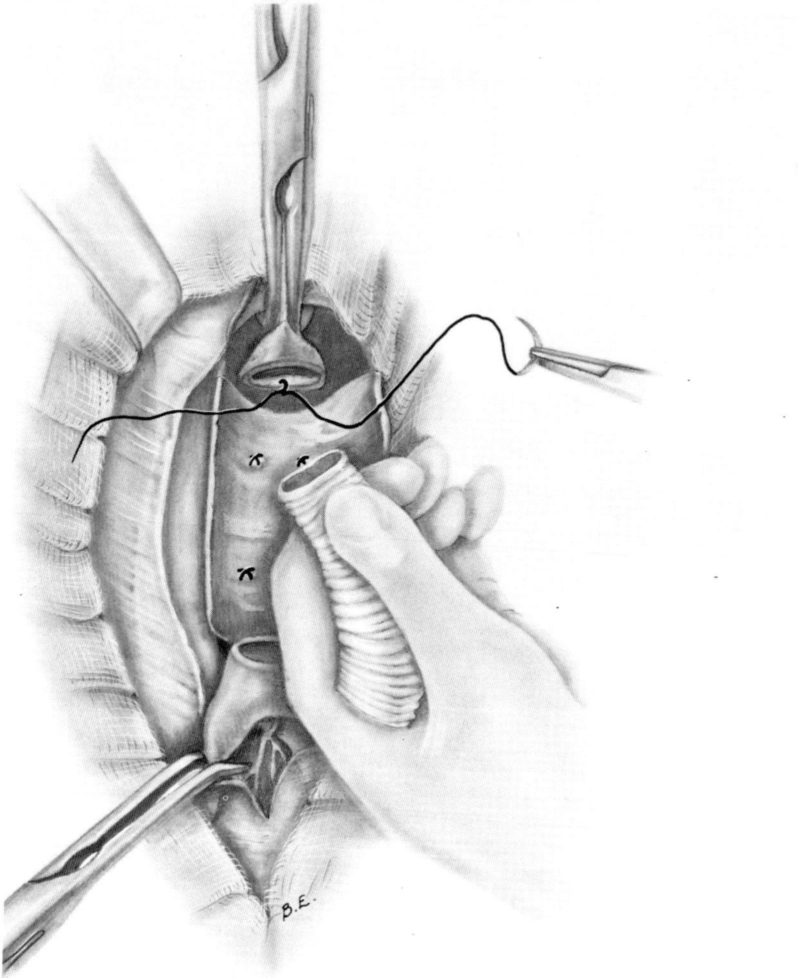

Figure 6.12. Proximal end-to-end anastomosis is started with a double-ended needle on the posterior aspect.

If the aorta is very attenuated at the level of the anastomosis, this suture line may be supported by mattress sutures placed over Teflon pledgets. Attention is then directed towards the distal anastomosis. The same suture and technique is used on the distal anastomosis in a tube graft. If a Y-graft is employed, 4-0 or 5-0 suture is usually employed with the iliac or femoral artery anastomosis (Figs. 6.16 and 6.17). If the patient had unilateral limb ischemia or claudication, the less-compromised limb should be re-perfused first, as its collaterals are not as well developed

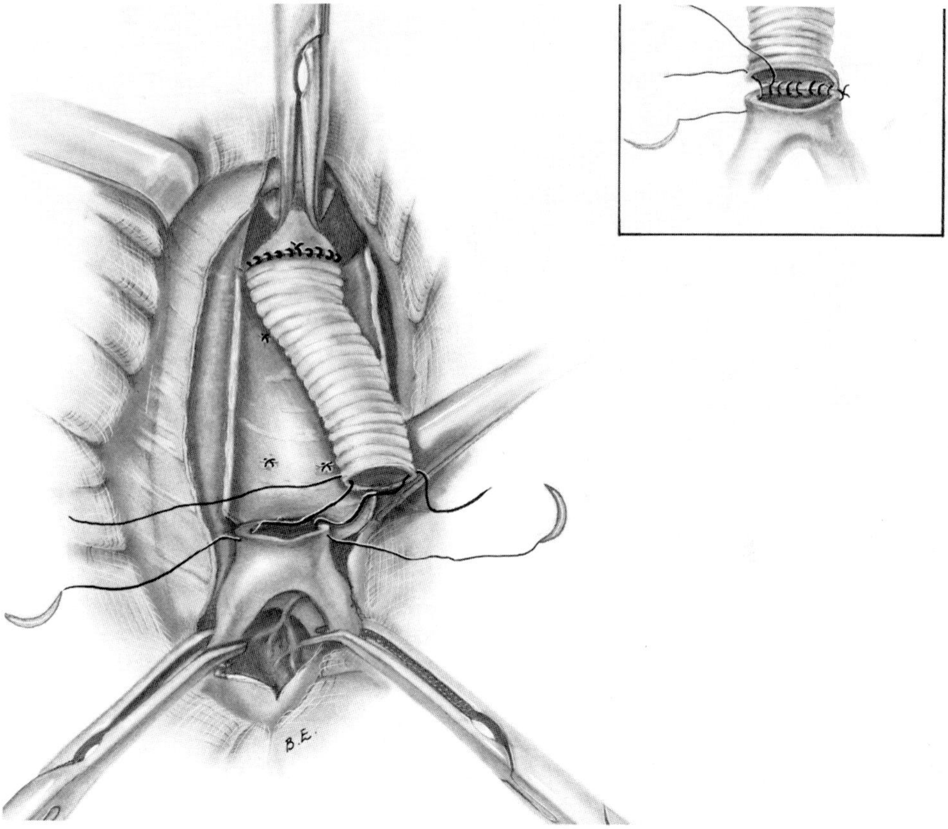

Figure 6.13. Distal end-to-end anastomosis is completed using another technique, sutures begun at the sides. Each suture is run over and over half-way.

and ischemia could result in ischemic myositis. Prior to completion of this distal anastomosis of the Y-graft, the distal vascular clamp is released to flush back any clot or debris. The aortic clamp is then released and quickly reapplied to flush the graft as well. When the anastomoses are completed, many anesthesiologists infuse sodium bicarbonate to compensate for the metabolic acidosis as the ischemic limb is re-perfused. Bleeding is controlled with additional sutures as indicated. The vascular clamps are now moved down to the unconnected limb of the Y-graft, which should be anastomosed to the contralateral iliac artery in the same manner. If the common femoral artery is selected, adequate tunnels are developed to the groin and end-to-side anastomoses are made, with back- and fore-flush before completion.

Anticoagulation is continued during the aneurysmal resection. Since the half-life of heparin is about 90 minutes, many surgeons use sequential, additional half doses of heparin every 60 to 90 minutes. A tube graft

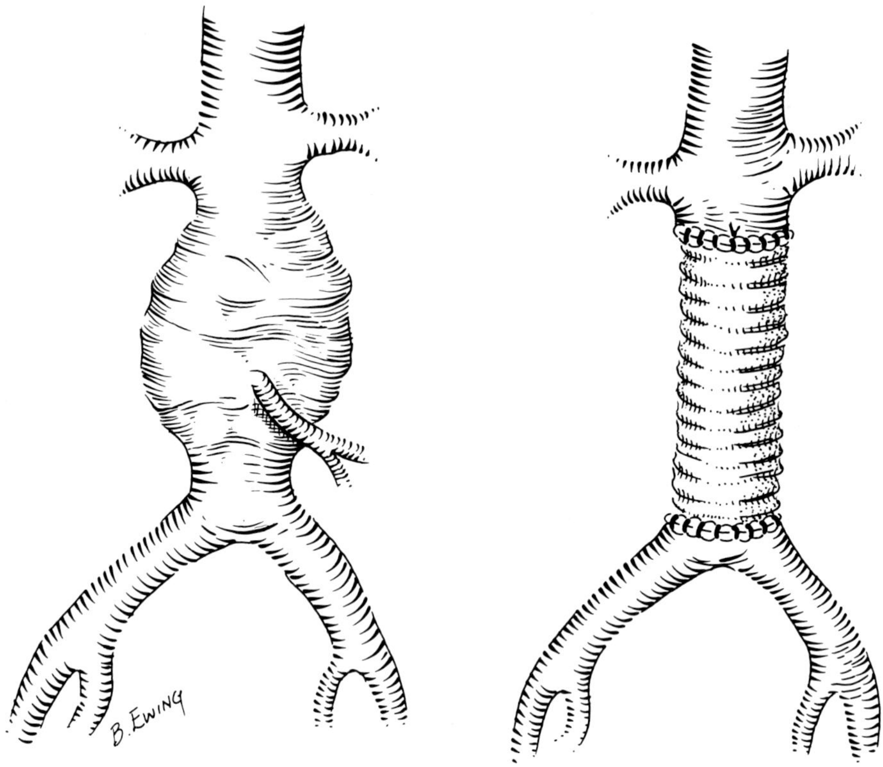

Figure 6.14. Completed tubular-type graft anastomosis.

should be completed within this time frame and further heparin should not be required. If a graft cuff was previously developed, it is now placed over the proximal anastomosis as additional support for hemostasis. Thanks to an efficient collateral network arising from the SMA *via* the marginal artery of Drummond, the IMA can usually be sacrificed. It is noteworthy that the IMA is often occluded in aneurysmal disease. If there is good backflow through the IMA, this collateral network is most probably intact. If there is question of ischemia of the left colon, the artery must be reanastomosed into the graft. The techniques of this procedure are discussed in the section entitled "Postoperative Complications: Ischemic Colitis."

With the prosthesis in place, the surgeon must inspect the blood flow to make certain a more distal reconstruction is not required (290). Doppler ultrasound is a useful tool in this regard, although clinical estimation of strongly palpable pulses should be appreciated—the Lahey bags placed on the feet facilitate this. A Fogarty catheter is sometimes used prior to the closure of the distal anastomoses to assure that no thrombus or debris have embolized downstream. Angiography following

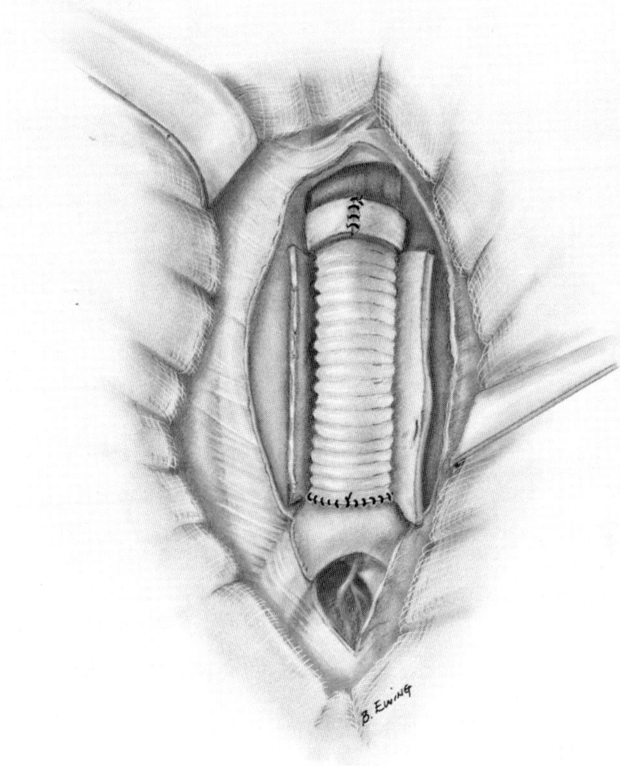

Figure 6.15. Note the use of the graft as a cuff at the proximal anastomosis.

aneurysmal surgery is reserved for problem cases. The final consideration before closure of the abdomen is reversal of the anticoagulation. If the operation has proceeded expeditiously and the patient has received no additional heparin after the first dose, no reversal is usually required. In longer, more complex cases, however, the activated clotting time may be used as a guideline to determine the dose of protamine necessary to re-establish normal clotting. At the end of 60 minutes, a dose of protamine equalling the dose of heparin should suffice. Protamine must be infused slowly because it is a potent vasodilator. Coagulation studies should be obtained again in the recovery room.

The authors are divided on the question of closing the remains of the aneurysmal sac around the prosthesis (Fig. 6.18). Although this adds another tissue layer between the bowel and the graft, it may trap a postoperative hematoma and does not absolutely prevent aortoenteric fistulas. The retroperitoneum is carefully closed over the graft for the same reason. The abdomen is irrigated copiously to remove as much

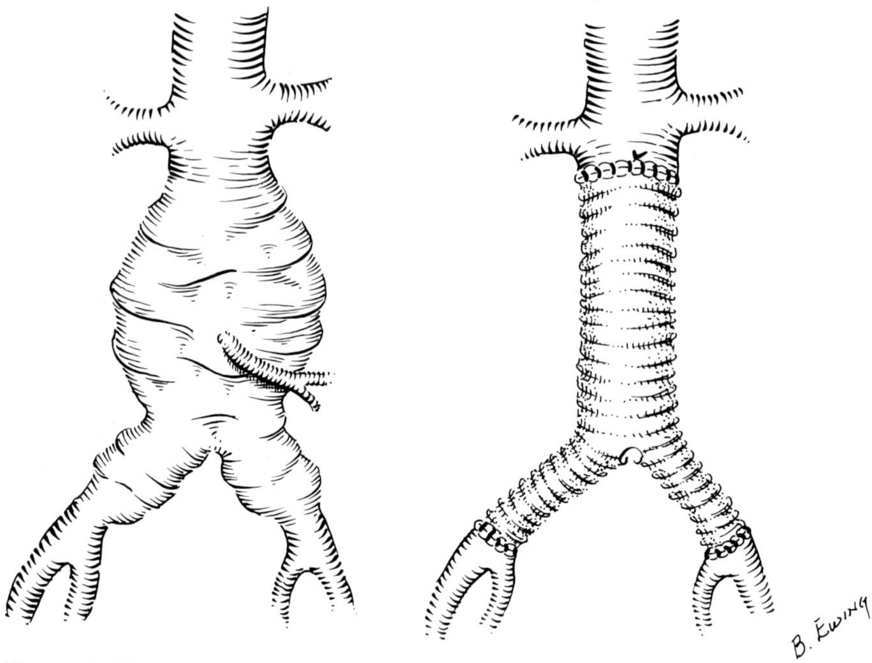

Figure 6.16. A bifurcation graft is sometimes required when the aneurysms extend into the iliac vessels.

extravasated blood and debris as practical. The remainder of the abdominal closure is the same as in any laparotomy.

Experience has shown that postoperative continuation of antibiotics for about 48 hours is prudent. The patient's nasogastric tube should remain in place until any ileus resolves. Cardiopulmonary and renal function should be carefully monitored and frequent, systematic observations of the peripheral circulation recorded. Intraoperative fluid therapy may necessitate prolonged tracheal intubation and the authors do not extubate their patients the night of operation. The value of the Swan-Ganz catheter intra- and postoperatively cannot be overemphasized. Intra-arterial lines may be maintained as long as frequent blood gas collection and pressure monitoring are necessary. However, expeditious removal of all lines is advised to avoid avenues for bacteremia. Ambulation is begun when the patient is hemodynamically stable.

SPECIAL PROBLEMS

Fortunately, most abdominal aortic aneurysms may be managed by elective resection and graft replacement. Complicated presentations are of two types—those which reflect the patient's pre-existing abnormal anatomy (horseshoe kidneys, etc.) and those which occur consequent to the aneurysm's natural history (rupture into adjacent structures, rupture into the free abdominal cavity, and thrombosis) (232).

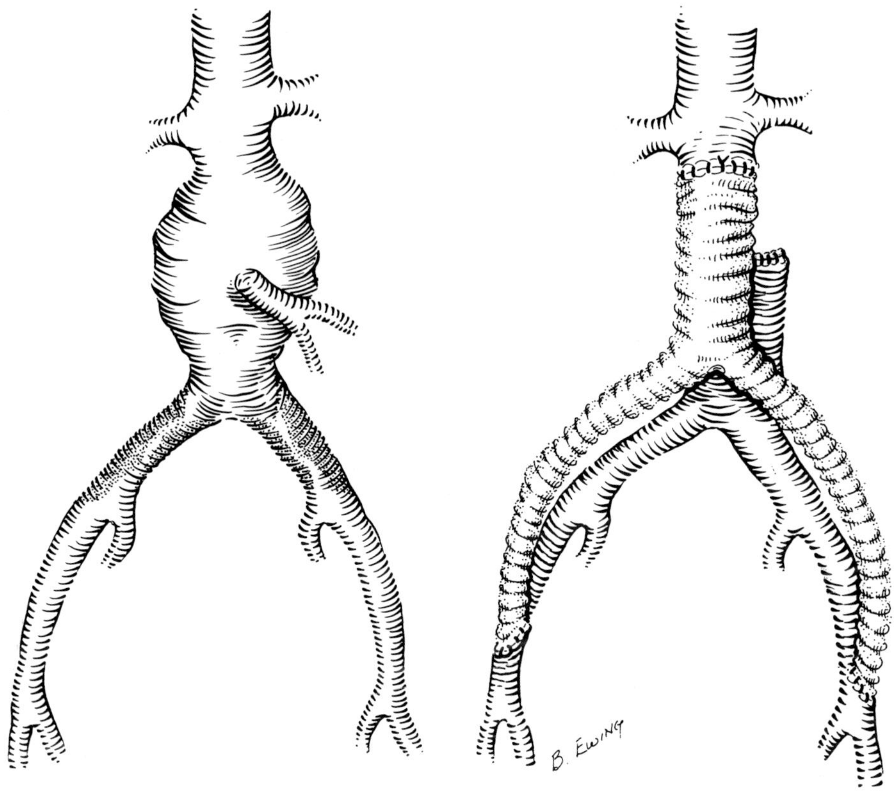

Figure 6.17. When combined aneurysmal and stenotic disease occur in synchrony, an aortobifemoral graft may be required.

Ruptured Aortic Aneurysms

Surely the most dramatic presentation of an abdominal aortic aneurysm is its rupture into the retroperitoneal space. Although aneurysms may leak slowly into the retroperitoneum, the patient usually describes no previous symptoms. The patient may describe severe back and/or abdominal pain, or may have collapsed because of pain or hypovolemic shock before arriving at the hospital. The patient's prognosis depends upon his status at presentation (286), the speed with which the diagnosis can be made, and the efficiency of resuscitation. Although autotransfusion has been credited with increasing survival after aneurysmal rupture, the mortality rate continues between 40 and 65% (203, 205, 221, 263, 265, 315).

Resuscitation must be started prior to coming to definitive operation. Aggressive fluid therapy must be begun through large-bore intravenous catheters. A Swan-Ganz catheter and arterial line are even more necessary than in the patient undergoing elective operation. MAST trousers may be employed for the patient in shock to support the central vascular

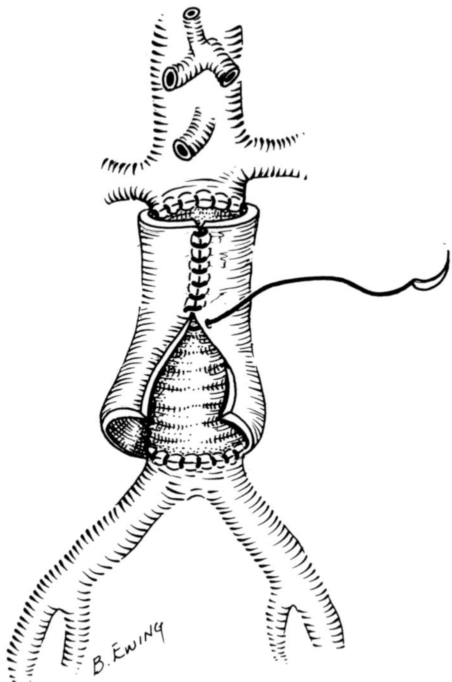

Figure 6.18. Aneurysmal walls may be used to wrap the graft to decrease the incidence of aortoenteric fistula.

bed. Autotransfusion equipment is prepared, if available. The operation must never be delayed, however, by placement of arterial and Swan-Ganz catheters. Control of hemorrhage is essential.

The operative procedure begins with proximal aortic control. This is usually achieved initially just below the diaphragm, with the aortic clamp being advanced caudally as the level of the aneurysm is demonstrated. Attempts should be made to clamp below the renal arteries, if this is compatible with the site of the aneurysm. The aorta may be compressed digitally against the vertebral bodies as the level of the bleeding is established. Alternatively, compression may be achieved with an aortic compressor (Fig. 6.19), or with a Foley balloon catheter (Fig. 6.20) advanced proximally through the site of rupture and inflated. Distal control of the distal aorta or iliac vessels is achieved in the usual fashion. Working within the aneurysm, control of the sacral and lumbar arteries must be quickly effected. The procedure at this point is identical to that of the elective aneurysmectomy.

Primary Aortoenteric Fistula

The patient with an aortoenteric fistula presents most commonly with massive upper gastrointestinal bleeding, although melena and hematochezia may have been reported beforehand. There may even have been a

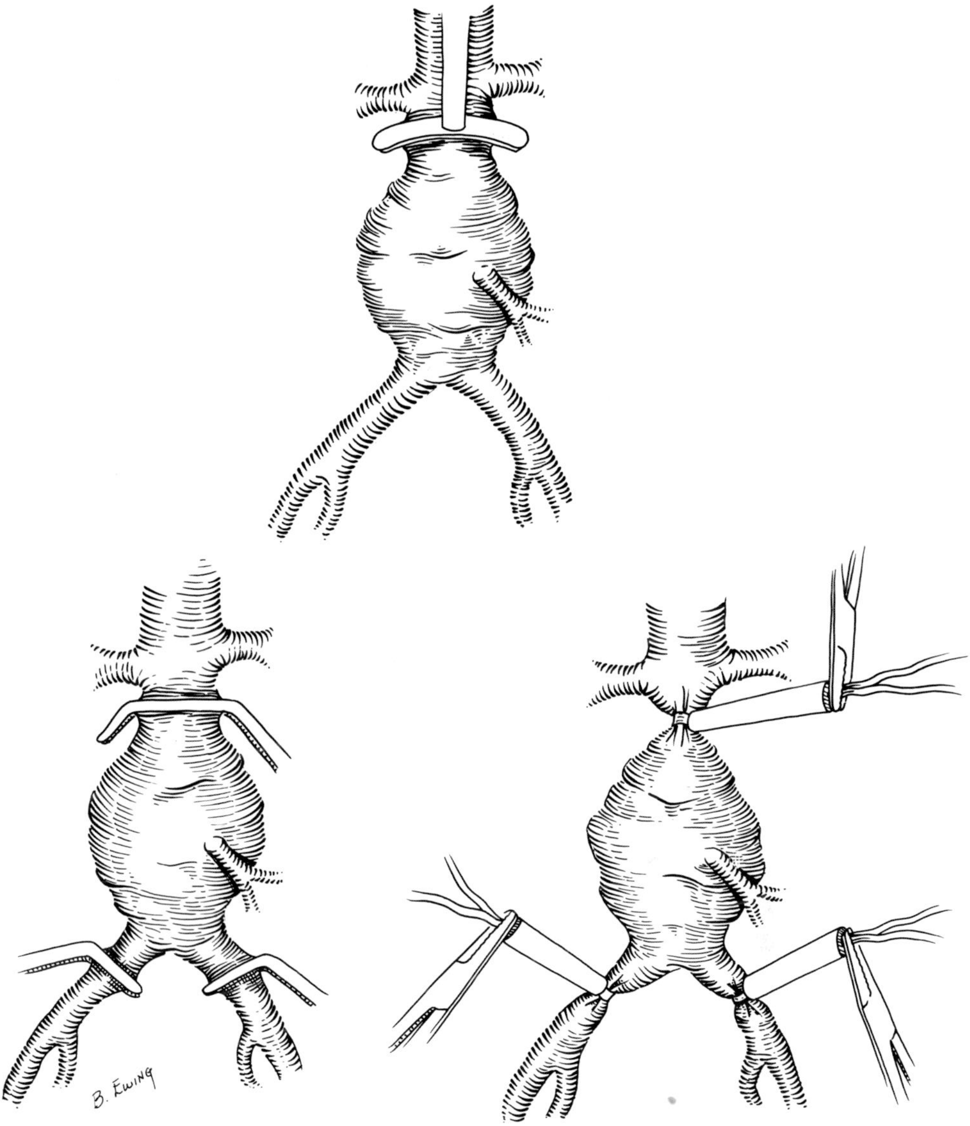

Figure 6.19. Use of an aortic compressor.

dramatic, though brief, "herald bleed" preceding the massive hemorrhage. There is nothing especially distinctive about this hemorrhage to lead the clinician to the correct diagnosis. History of an abdominal aortic aneurysm, or history or clinical demonstration of a pulsatile abdominal mass, are usually sufficient clues, if sought for.

The anatomic proximity of the duodenum to the aneurysm makes this

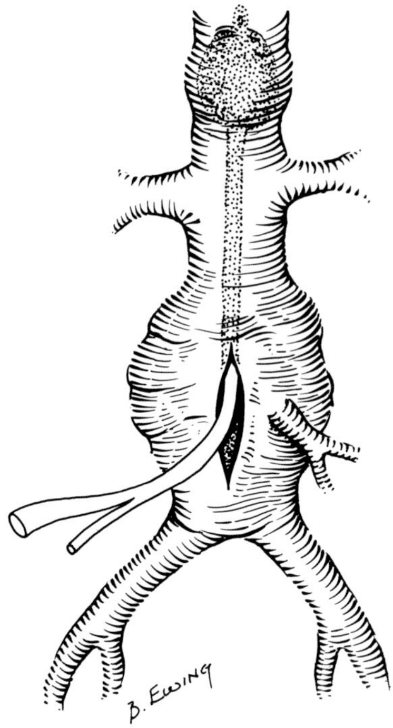

Figure 6.20. Use of a Foley balloon catheter to stem the tide of hemorrhage in a ruptured abdominal aortic aneurysm. In the elective operation, it may provide temporary proximal aortic control to operate on the renal arteries.

the most common site of the fistula. Rupture into the jejunum is less common and colonic fistulas are very rare. The etiology of the primary fistula is probably different from that of the secondary fistula (postaortic grafting) and reflects the adherence of the bowel to the inflammatory reaction around the aneurysm.

The initial maneuver in the operating room is proximal and distal control of the aorta. A careful search should be made for the enteric fistula. If the surrounding tissue is clearly viable, the point of fistulization may be closed primarily after debridement. If the surrounding tissue appears ischemic, the bowel must be resected to good viable tissue. Omentum, or adjacent bowel serosa, may be placed around the bowel defect to buttress the closure. Cultures, thorough debridement, and irrigation are a necessity.

Though infection probably does not contribute to the fistulization, therapy must be directed against it in the postoperative period. We do not place intra-abdominal catheters for continuous irrigation of antibiotic solutions, but rely instead on prolonged parenteral therapy with the appropriate broad-spectrum antibiotics. The re-establishment of vascular continuity is *via* an extra-anatomic approach. The aorta is secured to the vertebral fascia with monofilament synthetic sutures after debridement and closure.

Aortocaval Fistula

Patients will commonly present with an abdominal bruit, widened pulse pressure, venous hypertension, edema, arterial insufficiency of the lower extremity, hematuria, and congestive heart failure (48). The successful repair of an aortocaval fistula was reported by DeBakey *et al.* (87) in 1964. The Reckless *et al.* (248) review of the literature identified 71 cases up to 1972 with an operative mortality of 25%.

Operative management must avoid embolization of thrombus either distally to the legs or caudally through the vena cava to the lungs. Proximal and distal vascular control are achieved first. We then perform the operation in the usual fashion and close the defect in the vena cava through the aneurysmal sac (98).

Horseshoe Kidney

Clinical presentation of the patient with an associated horseshoe kidney is generally unremarkable, although the patient may have had previous urinary tract infections. The preoperative diagnosis is usually made from the IVP and because this radiographic procedure may be the only means of making this diagnosis, a routine IVP is strongly recommended if one has not performed an aortogram (112). If any anomalous structure is demonstrated on the urogram, aortography is necessary to define the vascular anatomy. It is important to remember, however, that neither procedure is infallible. Preoperative evaluation of all patients includes demonstration of a negative urinalysis and culture.

Horseshoe and pelvic kidneys are not rare (34, 153, 188); the incidence of horseshoe kidneys being 1:400 and of pelvic kidneys, 1:1000. The number of reported cases of associated aortic aneurysms, though, is less than 50 (34, 65). Their significance to the vascular surgeon stems less from their urinary status than from their associated vascular anomalies. In Bietz and Merendino's report (34) of 34 cases of associated horseshoe kidney, 16 patients had associated anomalous arterial supply to the kidney and six had a separate blood supply to the isthmus.

After demonstrating the horseshoe kidney in the operating room, the surgeon must delineate all of the renal artery supply without damaging these vessels in the process (188). If the aneurysm can be resected without compromising the blood supply of the isthmus, this should be done and the aortic graft tunneled behind it. A thinned fibrous isthmus may be resected with impunity. If there is a separate arterial supply, a larger isthmus may be resected. Care must be taken to excise all ischemic parenchymal tissue. There is a risk of bacteruria in these patients and, if the isthmus is incised or divided, the patient's antibiotic therapy should include a drug directed against gram-negative organisms. This therapy should be continued longer than the usual perioperative period.

Abnormal Renal Arteries

An attempt should be made to preserve all major anomalous renal arteries (73). If these arise out of the aneurysm itself, they should be excised with a button of parent aorta to facilitate reimplantation into the graft. If there are a large number of such aberrant vessels, the surgeon may frequently be unable to perform an aneurysmectomy without autotransplantation of the kidney (74). Ureteral pathology may be associated, as well, with abdominal aneurysms (156).

Associated Venous Anomalies

Aberrant venous anatomy compromises resection of abdominal aortic aneurysms as much as does abnormal artery anatomy (168, 188, 283). Double or left-sided inferior vena cava have a reported incidence of 3 and 0.5%, respectively. The vena cava may overlap the aneurysm, or the aneurysm may be obscured by a very short right renal vein which is difficult to retract (148). This abnormal anatomy should be recognized prior to placement of aortic clamps. Certainly one, though not both, renal veins may be sacrificed in the repair of an abdominal aneurysm (45).

Rarely, the left renal vein may occur in a retroaortic position, either as the sole venous drainage of the left kidney or in association with a normally placed vessel. Injury to this vein requires division of the aorta to effect successful repair, although the vein can be sacrificed if necessary. This aberrant left renal vein may also be the site of a fistula to the aneurysm—this presentation is virtually identical to that of an aortocaval fistula. Technical vissisitudes may require the placement of clamps near the diaphragmatic hiatus for proximal control with resultant damage to the cisterna chyli and the sequellae of chylous ascites (44, 215).

Mycotic Aneurysm

See Chapter 8.

Thrombosed Distal Aorta

The intramural thrombus within the aneurysm may propagate to the point of complete aortic occlusion. Depending upon the rate of this occurrence and the presence of collateral channels, the patient may present with signs and symptoms of claudication or with frank ischemia of the distal extremity.

Operation of the former patient is relatively straightforward with resection of the aneurysm, graft replacement, and embolectomy. The patient with a non-pulsatile thrombosed aneurysm may require only an extra-anatomic approach as the repair. The postoperative status of the distal extremity dictates its management. Mortality of this presentation rises with the vascular compromise initially seen. In some patients, massive distal embolism has been reported just prior to aneurysmal rupture (26, 99).

COMPLICATIONS

Excessive bleeding and graft thrombosis are significant causes of operative mortality and morbidity. These complications usually occur during or shortly after operation and are associated with errors in surgical technique or management, although occasionally bleeding may be secondary to a graft defect. Pseudoaneurysms, on the other hand, are usually late events, occurring many years after surgery; but often they too may be ascribed to errors in surgical technique.

Hemorrhage

Venous bleeding, the most common source of severe intraoperative blood loss, can arise from normal structures or anomalous veins which are injured during the aneurysmorrhaphy, such as veins damaged by retractor trauma. The lateral branches of the left renal vein may be injured in placing the proximal aortic clamp. This injury can be avoided by clearing the aneurysmal sac from below and mobilizing the vein carefully. As this is done, excessive tension must be avoided which could rip the left gonadal vein. The intense inflammatory component, frequently found around aortic aneurysms, may make the vena cava tightly adherent to the aneurysmal sac. Javid's modification of aneurysmorrhaphy, wherein the wall is left *in situ*, will avoid a caval tear. Adherence of the iliac veins is another problem which can be managed by careful technique.

The major common source of arterial bleeding is from the lumbar arteries. As discussed in the section on "Operation," these can usually be managed by ligation from within the sac; if this is not possible, bleeding could be controlled with hemo-clips. The iliac artery may be the source of intra-operative hemorrhage with large aneurysms, but this is usually easily obviated by control of the common femoral artery.

Errors in anticoagulant management constitute a third source of intraoperative hemorrhage. Thrombocytopenia secondary to platelet antibodies to heparin has been reported, but is an uncommon finding. For reasons not well understood, some patients, especially post-menopausal females, are unusually sensitive to heparin and will have prolonged partial thromboplastin times, although the half-life of heparin usually is only 60 to 90 minutes. Severe hemorrhage is managed with fresh frozen plasma or small doses of protamine sulfate.

Thrombosis

The formation of thrombus within the graft occurs secondary to exposure to a thrombogenic surface, or is due to turbulence and sludging. Graft materials currently in use are inherently non-thrombogenic. Healing of the prosthesis is characterized by formation of a neointima and ingrowth of endothelial cells except for the PTFE graft. Exposed suture material, however, can be a source of thrombosis, as has been proven using silk sutures in experimental animals. Injury to the vessel wall during suturing may expose thrombogenic surfaces which stimulate clot formation and graft thrombosis.

The major error is suture technique, which results in thrombosis secondary to production of turbulence and sludging within the vessel. Crimping of the native vessel wall, or tenting up of atheromatous plaque, may impede the normal laminar blood flow. Mismatching the size of the graft and the native vessel can cause the same result. The rate at which the blood flows through a graft of large diameter is not sufficient to prevent platelets from aggregating at the graft surface. This process is self-limiting and ceases when the active channel equals the diameter of the aorta above.

Pseudoaneurysm

Early failure at the graft-vessel interface is usually associated with suture disruption and commonly results in exsanguinating hemorrhage (177, 224, 250, 291). Late failures result in the formation of pseudoaneurysms.

The relatively high incidence of pseudoaneurysmal formation in the early days of vascular surgery was attributed to the silk sutures commonly employed. Silk is a highly reactive substance and loses nearly all of its tensile strength within a year of implantation. The next suture material introduced to correct this was polyethylene, but soon this material was seen to be associated with the formation of false aneurysms. Polypropylene has been in use for many years and has been associated with few aneurysms; this material causes little tissue reaction and persists, apparently undegraded, for years. But despite the Starr *et al.* (277) contention that the suture material was the cause of pseudoaneurysmal formation, the problem did not disappear with the introduction of newer suture material.

Graft material may contribute to the formation of false aneurysms. Textile grafts undergo a dilatation of 15 to 20% after implantation (104). Dacron grafts lose tensile strength early (104), although Teflon grafts do not. These changes put additional stress on the suture line. Further stress occurs because of the non-distensibility of the prosthesis during arterial pulsation, which results in impedance mismatching (302). In his recent review, Gayliss (128) was able to assign a cause for 25 of 28 pseudoaneurysms, determining them usually to be secondary to suture failure.

Infections

See Chapter 8.

Renal Insufficiency

INCIDENCE

Acute renal failure (ARF) is one of the three most common complications following abdominal aortic aneurysm resection (the two others being myocardial infarction and postoperative bleeding) (246). The current incidence in elective resections is reported as averaging 3 to 4%, as seen in Table 6.5. The picture is more serious with ruptured aneurysms, with the incidence of renal failure ranging from 8 to 46% (Table 6.6) (17, 59, 81, 93, 124, 159, 178, 212, 266, 274, 313).

These statistics, however, reflect only part of the problem of acute renal failure. Once this condition has developed, the mortality rate ranges from 40 to 90% in most series. Although the mortality rate is less with elective aneurysmal resections than with surgery for ruptured aneurysms, it is still significant (Tables 6.7 and 6.8).

In both elective and emergent cases, renal failure is the major source of postoperative mortality. In the Abbott (2) and Abbott *et al.* (4) studies, the mortality rate in patients with ruptured aneurysms who developed

Table 6.5
Incidence of Acute Renal Failure (ARF) Following Elective Abdominal Aortic Aneurysm Resection

Author	No. of Patients	No. with ARF	Incidence (%)
Gardner *et al.*, 1970 (124)	56	1	2
Hicks *et al.*, 1975 (159)	225	9	4
King and Evans, 1975 (178)	78	3	4
McCombs and Roberts, 1979 (212)	368	9	3
Stokes and Butcher, 1973 (280)	87	2	2
Thompson *et al.*, 1975 (292)	108	9	8
Volpetti *et al.*, 1976 (298)	585	25	4
Summary	1,507	58	3

Table 6.6
Incidence of Acute Renal Failure (ARF) Following Operation for Ruptured Aneurysms

Author	No. of Patients	No. with ARF	Incidence (%)
Baird *et al.*, 1978 (17)	50	16	32
Chawla *et al.*, 1975 (59)	43	14	33
Darling, 1970 (81)	60	13	22
DiGiovanni *et al.*, 1975 (93)	78	28	36
Gardner *et al.*, 1970 (124)	24	2	8
Hicks *et al.*, 1975 (159)	56	10	18
King and Evans, 1975 (178)	18	6	33
McCombs and Roberts, 1979 (212)	38	8	21
Sink *et al.*, 1976 (266)	28	13	46
Yashar *et al.*, 1972 (313)	32	6	19
Summary	427	116	27

Table 6.7
Mortality Rate from Acute Renal Failure (ARF) in Elective Aneurysmectomy

Author	No. of Patients	No. with ARF	No. Died	Mortality Rate (%)
David *et al.*, 1974 (84)	69	9	8	89
Hicks *et al.*, 1975 (159)	225	9	4	44
Luft *et al.*, 1975 (200)	12	12	5	42
Thompson *et al.*, 1975 (292)	108	9	0	0
Volpetti *et al.*, 1976 (298)	585	25	12	48
Summary	999	64	29	45

Table 6.8
Mortality Rate from Acute Renal Failure (ARF) in Ruptured Aneurysmectomy

Author	No. of Patients	No. with ARF	No. Died	Mortality Rate (%)
Abbott *et al.*, 1975 (3)	32	32	28	88
Chawla *et al.*, 1975 (59)	43	14	8	57
DiGiovanni *et al.*, 1975 (93)	78	28	15	54
Hicks *et al.*, 1975 (159)	56	10	7	70
Luft *et al.*, 1975 (200)	16	16	12	75
Sink *et al.*, 1976 (266)	28	13	9	69
Tilney *et al.*, 1973 (295)	18	18	17	95
Summary	271	131	96	73

ARF was 88%, but the mortality was only 25% in those who had ARF but not a ruptured aneurysm.

CLINICAL PICTURE

It is not necessary to describe the generally well-known physiologic consequences of renal failure. It is, however, constructive to review these consequences in the particular type of patient under discussion. Water and sodium accumulation exacerbate any pre-existing cardiac failure and render these patients more likely to require additional ventilatory support. Electrolyte disturbances, especially accumulation of potassium and hydrogen ions are not well tolerated by hearts already suffering from coronary artery disease. These patients are frequently elderly and in poor nutritional health and cannot tolerate the unavoidable protein depletion of conventional therapy. Defects in wound healing are common in patients with ARF. Lastly, the renal failure patient's immune dysfunction may lead to sepsis and consequent graft infection.

PATHOPHYSIOLOGY

Techniques are necessary to avoid renal failure and improve the prognosis once ARF has supervened. In analyzing the problem, there are three points of etiologic consideration: global, mechanical, and local factors. Hypovolemic hypotension and cardiac depression from acidosis or hypoxemia are examples of global events which may lead to decreased renal perfusion. Mechanical factors include the placement of vascular clamps, proximal extension of the aneurysm, and condition of the renal arteries. Events occurring within the renal parenchyma in response to surgical manipulation constitute local factors in the development of ARF.

The importance of thorough preoperative evaluation of cardiac and renal status cannot be overstated and the elective operation should be performed only after these systems have been optimized. All patients should have a creatinine clearance calculated and a preoperative IVP performed if aortography was deferred. Aortography will have elucidated renal artery disease, especially suprarenal extension of the aneurysm. The operating surgeon must sometimes choose between the mortality of the "unoperated" aortic aneurysm and the possible mortality from renal failure in patients with significant pre-existing chronic renal failure. We believe a serum creatinine over 3.5 mg/100 ml, or a creatinine clearance less than 25 ml/min, are relative contraindications to elective aneurysmorrhaphy.

Intraoperatively, blood pressure, cardiac function, and fluid balance must be carefully monitored. EKG monitoring and maintenance of urine output are routine operative measures. Use of a Swan-Ganz catheter is strongly advised. An arterial line measures blood pressure and allows for drawing arterial blood gases. Blood lost should be replaced at a rate sufficient to maintain an effective hematocrit, either by the infusion of banked blood or by autotransfusion. The use of the "G-suit" or "antishock trousers" has been suggested as part of the management in ruptured aortic aneurysms, although the exact mechanism of its benefit is unclear (2).

The patient is at greatest risk of hypotension when the aortic clamp is released to allow perfusion of one limb of the graft because of 1) decreased vascular resistance of the ischemic tissue; 2) release of accumulated lactic acid; and 3) increase in potassium. The solution to this so-called "declamping shock" is similarly twofold. First, the clamps should be removed slowly, offering some resistance to rapid limb re-perfusion as the patient receives increased intravenous fluids. Second, acidosis is prevented by bolus therapy with sodium bicarbonate prior to unclamping. If sequential intraoperative pH monitoring and correction are performed, this bolus is not necessary.

Anomalies of the patient's renal vascular tree have been partly discussed previously. Brewster *et al.* (46) reported a large number of unexpected renal artery abnormalities in his patients. The management of the horseshoe kidney is a difficult, but fortunately rare, problem. More common, though, is extension of the aneurysm to the level of at least one of the renal arteries, necessitating that the proximal aortic clamp be placed above this vessel. Abbott (2) advocated infusion of a chilled perfusate to increase the kidney's tolerance to ischemia, but we have not utilized it; instead, if warm ischemia time is expected to exceed 45 minutes, we cool the kidney externally by application of chilled Ringer's lactate in lap pads. Aberrant renal arteries should be preserved. Renal arteries arising from aneurysmal portions of the aorta may be anastomosed into the aortic graft, cutting out a button of the original aorta and, thus, having a greater circle to sew with less chance of stenosis.

Our understanding of ARF has increased dramatically in the last few years. A segmental renal circulation has been demonstrated, with the cortical blood supply being the largest and most important component (6). Prolonged renal ischemia leads to a decreased cortical flow on reperfusion and this maintenance of hypoperfusion after unclamping seems to be the final pathway of ARF. Experimental data have shown this phenomenon to be caused by the renin-angiotensin system (29).

Although one cannot suppress the renin system, Thompson *et al.* (293)

showed that solute loading (high salt solutions such as lactated Ringer's or normal saline) could blunt this response. It has also been demonstrated that mannitol, given prior to and during aortic clamping, causes a redistribution of blood which preserves cortical circulation (5, 21, 22). Moreover, some investigators have shown that mannitol completely abolishes the "no-reflow" phenomenon (118). The clinical usefulness of mannitol during aortic cross-clamping has, nevertheless, been a subject of controversy (63). Prophylactic diuresis with ethacrynic acid or furosemide has also been given for the prevention of postoperative renal failure (274). Recently, low-dose dopamine has been shown to prevent post-ischemic ARF if given prior to renal artery clamping. Clinically, we combine Thompson's regimen of large solute infusions with 12.5 g of intravenous mannitol given prior to aortic clamping.

MANAGEMENT

Once the patient manifests the clinical or laboratory signs of renal failure, his subsequent postoperative management must include avoidance of fluid overload and consideration of his kidney's progressive inability to metabolize or excrete drugs (131, 132). Although ARF is a reversible condition, severe cases should be managed with early hemodialysis. Nutritional therapy has been advocated on the basis of experimental and clinical studies.

Ischemic Colitis

Ischemic colitis following abdominal aortic reconstruction is a major, although infrequent, cause of postoperative morbidity and mortality. As with many of the other complications of abdominal aortic aneurysm surgery, it represents an area where current knowledge aims at both prevention and treatment.

INCIDENCE

The absolute incidence of ischemic colitis in a large number of reported cases ranges from 0.2 to 10% (30, 32, 36, 71, 110, 149, 166, 169, 218, 235, 240, 251, 253, 270, 316). This number, however, is not very meaningful. Older studies are almost always retrospective and include only those cases with grossly manifest disease. The more recent series are largely prospective and reflect diagnoses made with colonoscopy which may not be clinically significant. This 6% incidence applies to both elective aneurysmal resection and aortic reconstruction for aortoiliac occlusive disease (110, 149). The incidence rises dramatically in some series of patients with ruptured aneurysms to as much as 60% (149). The mortality associated with ischemic colitis has been reported to be as high as 90% (33, 71, 110, 169, 210, 235, 253, 270, 316). Although small bowel ischemia can also occur, it is a rare condition.

PATHOLOGY

Boley *et al.* (42) described three forms of ischemia which represent points on a continuum and reflect the anatomic and prognostic status of the condition. Type I is described as reversible transient ischemic colitis, with a reported incidence of 20% of published cases. It is probably more frequent and not published. The ischemia extends only into the mucosa and, by definition, is transient, mild, and reversible. The mucosa becomes friable and there may be submucosal edema and hemorrhage. The bacterial barrier breaks down as the mucosa is sloughed. Healing takes place in days to weeks and there are usually no adverse sequelae. Type II involves both the mucosa and muscularis, reflects more severe ischemia, and may result in healing with fibrosis, scarring, and stricture. The most severe condition is type III which represents transmural ischemia and may result in frank gangrene with perforation and patient death. This last type is reported in 60% of published cases of ischemic colitis.

PATHOPHYSIOLOGY

The anatomic basis of this complication is most commonly an interruption of the arterial blood supply to the left colon. The descending and sigmoid colon blood supply is usually derived from the IMA. Superiorly, the IMA anastomoses with the SMA which supplies the right and transverse colon through its ileocolic, right colic, and middle colic arteries *via* the marginal artery of Drummond. Inferiorly, it anastomoses with the internal iliac artery *via* the hemorrhoidal plexus (the superior hemorrhoidal artery being a branch of the IMA and the middle and inferior hemorrhoidal arteries being derived from the hypogastric artery). An anatomic danger point, known as Griffiths' point (32, 130, 143), marks the site along the splenic flexure where the SMA and IMA systems are joined. It is absent in 5% of patients and these patients are immediately in danger following IMA ligation. The marginal artery may also be incomplete along the sigmoid colon, a condition observed in as many as 20% of individuals (279).

Another important connection between the SMA and IMA systems is the wandering or meandering mesenteric artery (226); it arises from the SMA close to its origin and joins the IMA also close to its origin. This artery is distinct from the marginal artery and apparently has few, if any, branches coursing directly to the colon. It is found in about two-thirds of normal individuals and can be seen on routine aortography in 27% of patients with abdominal aortic aneurysms (110). The wandering mesenteric artery allows flow in both directions and may be the principle blood supply of the small bowel if the SMA is occluded at its origin; in which case, the IMA is the progenitor of the primary vascular supply to the GI tract.

Errors in handling the IMA are the cause of most of the cases of ischemic colitis (30, 32, 33, 36, 56, 71, 130, 149, 169, 210, 227, 235, 237, 240, 253, 270, 316). Ischemic colitis may be consequent to the ligation of a vessel which should have been spared, or by the incorrect placement of ligatures which compromise retrograde flow from the left colic, sigmoid, or hemorrhoidal arteries. Rarely, ischemic colitis may be secondary to the interruption of important arterial collaterals, or caused by mesenteric compression by the hematoma of a ruptured aneurysm—by direct colon trauma secondary to retractor placement or by prolonged hypotension and hypoperfusion.

DIAGNOSIS

The most frequent sign of clinically significant ischemic colitis is diarrhea, sometimes bloody, and occurring usually 24 to 48 hours after operation (30, 33, 169, 210, 235, 240, 270, 316). The diarrhea may occur as late as 14 days afterwards. Although the bloody character of the stool is dramatic and should alert the physician to this diagnosis, its prognostic significance is unclear (33, 235).

Other signs and symptoms of the conditions may be difficult to separate from the expected complaints of the postoperative patient. There may be abdominal pain which is commonly left-sided and ranges from mild to severe. The progression to peritonitis may be marked by leukocytosis, hypotension, oliguria, and acidosis.

Gastrograffin, or low-pressure "thin" barium contrast studies, have been employed in the acute postoperative period. The characteristic "thumb-printing" sign establishes the diagnosis. Alternatively, procto-sigmoidoscopy and flexible colonoscopy have been recommended (30, 57, 109, 149, 210, 316), but we favor the contrast studies. Although we commonly employ sigmoidoscopy, we recognize it is limited in that most disease occurs higher than 25 cm. Air insufflation during colonoscopy carries with it a risk of perforation. When colonoscopy is performed, it should be done within 48 hours of the onset of symptoms. Since the colitis is essentially left-sided, the colonoscope need not be advanced beyond 40 cm (150). The finding of edema and diffuse hemorrhage suggests early or mild colitis. Pseudomembranes and ulcerations are consistent with more advanced disease. Finally, a yellowish-green, non-contractile surface is diagnostic of frank gangrene. Once colitis has been demonstrated, there is no point in advancing the instrument beyond the disease.

PREVENTION

Considering the variable incidence of this complication and its high mortality, attempts have been made to define a high-risk population. This high-risk group includes patients with: 1) symptoms of visceral ischemia; 2) a ruptured aortic aneurysm; 3) a patent IMA; 4) IMA-to-SMA flow in the meandering mesenteric artery; 5) zero intraoperative Doppler flow in the colic arteries; 6) IMA stump pressure <40 mm Hg; and 7) occluded and/or stenosed hypogastric arteries.

Preoperative aortography may provide valuable information (36, 49, 109, 110, 169, 254). The patency of the IMA can be easily discovered by examining a lateral film, as can the presence of a wandering mesenteric artery and, usually, the direction of flow within it. Similarly, the adequacy of the inferior collateralization *via* the hypogastric artery may be discovered. Measurement of IMA stump pressures, as well as fluoroscopic and Doppler evaluations of the left colon circulation, may compensate for the unreliability of the clinical parameters of the colon, arterial pulsations, and peristalsis (36, 52, 110, 174, 225, 235, 240). Their use is recommended only in cases where there is a question of bowel viability. The patient with a thrombosed IMA, or preoperative demonstration of SMA-to-IMA flow in the meandering mesenteric artery, is probably not a candidate for sophisticated, esoteric examinations, as he will not have ischemic problems postoperatively.

The use of a sterile Doppler probe to assess adequacy of the arterial circulation of the colon was championed by Hobson *et al.* (160), who demonstrated in a 1976 study that patients with good flow failed to develop ischemic colitis (161). In a subsequent study, they found 6 patients of 59 with an abdominal aortic aneurysm in whom compression of the IMA produced a marked diminution of Doppler signal (161). All patients had preservation of the IMA, either by reimplantation into the graft or construction of an end-to-side proximal anastomosis, and none developed clinical evidence of ischemic colitis.

A technique has been developed for measuring IMA stump pressure (109). The divided stump is cannulated with an 18-gauge Teflon catheter and attached to a pressure transducer in the usual fashion. The pressure is measured simultaneously with the systemic blood pressure. Two measurements are produced—a stump pressure and a stump/systemic ratio. Patients in this series were followed with colonoscopic examination. Only one developed ischemic colitis and he had both a stump pressure less than 40 mm Hg and a stump/systemic ratio <0.4. If either of these techniques demonstrate a bowel dependent upon the IMA, it must be preserved.

Mechanical cleansing of the large bowel (with or without appropriate antibiosis) may reduce the incidence of postoperative colitis (30, 32, 36, 270, 316), as the presence of bacteria increases the risk of infection in ischemic tissues. We employ this cleansing in the event there is an unanticipated bowel injury. Bowel distension is prevented during the operation because the increased wall tension consequent to dilatation increases vascular resistance in the bowel.

The other major means for the prevention of ischemic colitis are technical. Care must be taken to ligate the IMA (if it needs ligation) close to the aneurysmal sac before it divides into left colic and sigmoid branches (108) (Fig. 6.21). A tie placed too far distal will effectively ligate both of these branches. Care must also be taken here to prevent debris from entering the colonic vasculature and producing the bowel equivalent of "trash foot" (210, 270). Gentle retraction, especially of the sigmoid colon, is the rule. Hypotension and hypoperfusion must, of course, be avoided. Finally, the graft itself must be chosen and anastomosed in a fashion to preserve either IMA flow (if present) or adequate hypogastric flow (30, 109, 192, 270). Compromised colonic arterial flow may demand a distal end-to-side anastomosis, depending upon the patient's anatomy.

The most common technique for IMA reimplantation calls for its excision, along with a button of the original aorta—a technique which

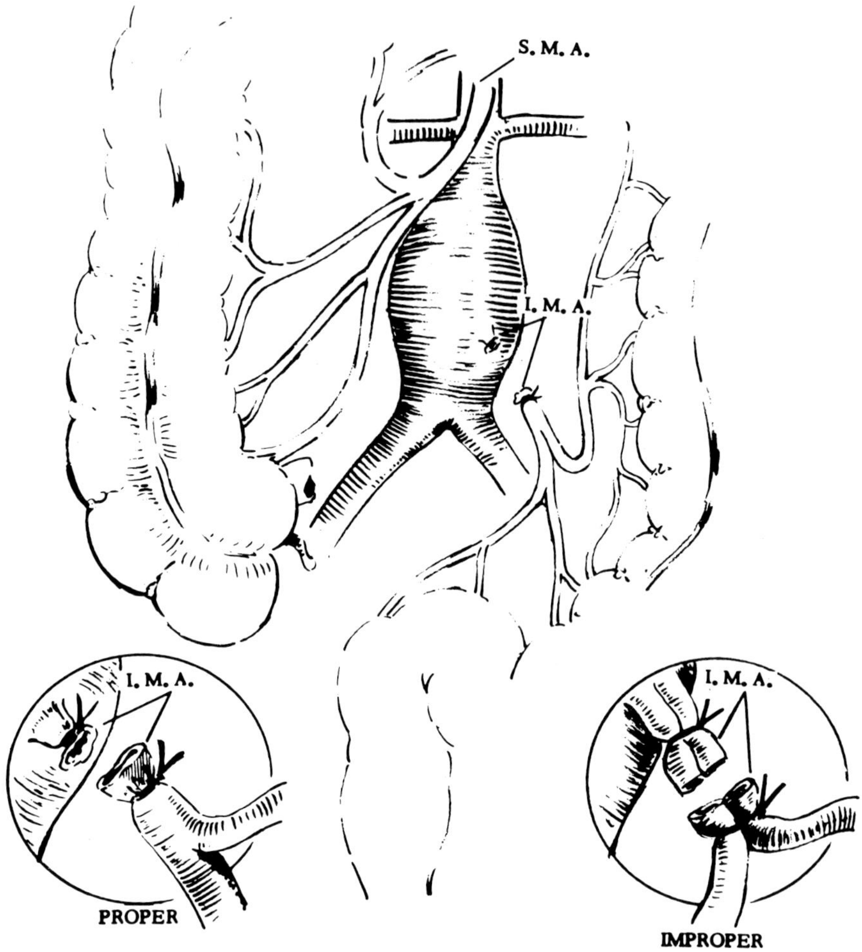

Figure 6.21. Inferior mesenteric artery branches into the left colic artery (LCA) and superior sigmoidal artery (SSA). Ligation of the IMA close to the aorta will preserve collateral circulation between LCA and SSA. Improper ligation of IMA will obliterate this collateral circulation. [Reproduced with permission from Johnson and Nabseth (169).]

can be traced back to Alexis Carrel (56) (Fig. 6.22). If a button was not taken, or if the arterial orifice is small, the vessel may be spatulated and sutured to the prosthesis either directly or *via* a short interposition vein graft (66, 108).

TREATMENT

Once colon ischemia has been diagnosed, the patient must be monitored closely or operated upon. Serial colonoscopic examinations, though not often practical, are indicated until there is definite evidence of

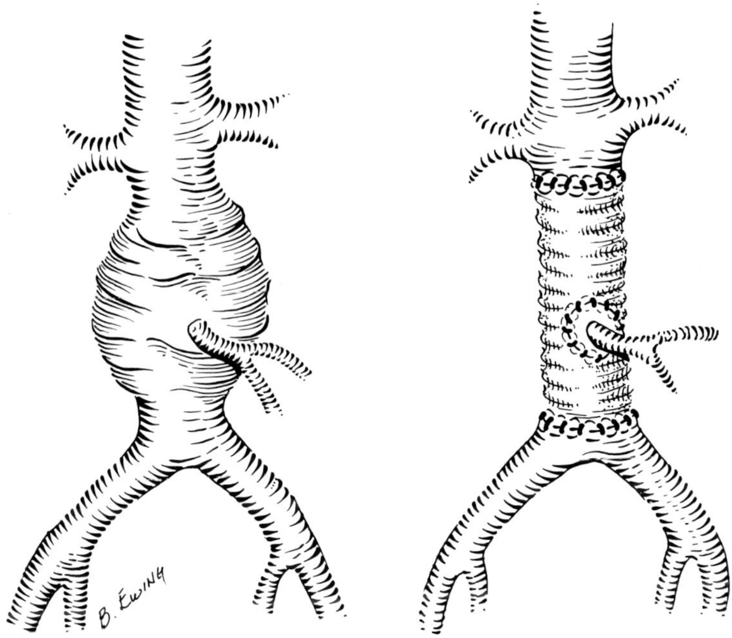

Figure 6.22. Technique of revascularization of the inferior mesenteric artery by direct reimplantation into the aortic prosthesis. Note cuff of aorta retained on IMA patch.

improvement. Although reversible lesions will improve in seven to ten days (42, 110), the patient will require careful support during this time if he is to survive. Of especial importance is maintenance of fluid and electrolytes, continued bowel decompression, and broad-spectrum antibiotics aimed at colonic organisms. Operative intervention is necessary if the patient is not improving, or if the ischemic picture progresses beyond two weeks. Signs and symptoms which should point toward emergency operation include fever, lower left quadrant pain, increasing leukocytosis, or the demonstration of a palpable mass. The goal of reoperation is the removal of necrotic and non-viable bowel and is best achieved by segmental colectomy and either a double-barreled colostomy or a Hartmann procedure and end-colostomy. Any abscess is drained. Rectal necrosis requires proctectomy and perineal drainage. The latter is a rare event occurring when collaterals *via* the hypogastric are obliterated through disease or iatrogenically.

Secondary Aortoenteric Fistulas

Postoperative aortoenteric fistulas are uncommon causes of gastrointestinal bleeding (50, 53, 60, 61, 64, 70, 79, 85, 89, 106, 126, 164, 181, 198, 248, 260, 262, 307); moreover, they exhibit few distinguishing characteristics which separate them from other more common causes. The incidence has been reported as high as 10% in one series (95), but more commonly in the range of 1 to 4% (121). When the cause of bleeding is not properly recognized, the mortality of this condition is 100%.

The first reported case of postoperative fistula to a homograft was made in 1952 by Lord Brock (50), followed shortly by Claytor's report of fistulization to a prosthetic graft (60), and by Heberer's first successful repair (155).

PATHOGENESIS

The third portion of the duodenum is the most commonly involved portion of the bowel in the aortoenteric fistula (85, 105, 126, 248, 294). Mechanical injury and infection contribute to the development of the fistula, although the relative roles of each are obscure (61, 89, 106, 126, 181). The duodenum is vulnerable to injury during mobilization of a large aneurysm, especially as it may have been adherent to the aneurysm consequent to the periarteritis of the condition. The majority of cultures taken during operation for repair of a fistula will grow out of enteric organisms, suggesting the previous presence of enteric spillage. The canine model of Busuttil *et al.* (53) strongly implicated infection as the causative agent, though their model has not been universally accepted (180).

Several technical points bear on the pathogenesis of the fistula. Inadequate reperitonealization is an important factor in some patients (89, 106, 126), resulting in an adherent loop of bowel, with the pulsatile force in the aorta probably transmitted to the bowel wall. Fistulas have also been seen in association with false aneurysms developing at the suture line of a prosthetic graft (180). Prosthetic material itself generates an inflammatory response. Modern graft material is readily incorporated with less reactivity.

There are two types of fistulas (89)—those which occur at the suture line and those which arise at some distance and then extend to involve the suture line. In the former, which constitutes the majority of reported cases, there is a small communication between the aortic suture line and the bowel. This connection is intermittently occluded by thrombus, with recurrent bleeding episodes until the hole enlarges beyond the capacity of the hemostatic mechanisms. In the less common condition, or paraprosthetic fistula (89, 233), there is bleeding from the traumatized bowel, but no fistula until the process extends to involve the suture line.

CLINICAL PRESENTATION

The degree of gastrointestinal bleeding runs the gamut from melena to hematemesis, and to hematochezia. As would be expected from the above pathophysiology, many patients will have an initial "herald bleed" which stops with reconstruction of the thrombin plug (61, 85, 89, 106, 126, 181, 198). Unless there is surgical intervention, this condition will progress to massive bleeding when local hemostatic mechanisms fail. Some patients will be diagnosed when the bleeding is still occult and the patient presents with unexplained anemia and guaiac-positive stools.

DIAGNOSIS

Aortoenteric fistulas do not lend themselves to very successful diagnosis. A number of techniques have been employed with variable success. Though their diagnostic accuracy in combination approaches 50% (106), individual tests are closer to 15 to 30% (219, 273). Fiberoptic endoscopy is a commonly employed technique in all cases of upper gastrointestinal bleeding (19, 181, 219, 233). Findings of gastritis, or of a bleeding duodenal ulcer, establish a non-fistula diagnosis. Classic findings of the fistula include arterial bleeding, a pulsatile structure in the wall or lumen, a suture line, or a bile-stained prosthesis (19). The endoscopist should be experienced and explore the duodenum to at least its third portion. Endoscopy in a readied operating suite is recommended to decrease delay in commencing operation.

Aortography is the next recommended procedure if the diagnosis has not been made (85, 125, 126, 181, 222, 296). Suggestive findings include frank extravasation of dye, a kinked prosthetic graft (121), the presence of a false aneurysm, or dye within the gastrointestinal tract. A lateral radiograph is a necessity.

Gastrointestinal contrast studies should follow the above investigations, if indicated (85, 89, 95, 114, 181). These studies may demonstrate the so-called "coiled spring" sign (contrast material coating the outside of the graft) or demonstrate an extramural sinus, bowel wall defect, or partial bowel obstruction (114, 314, 315). An aortocolonic fistula may be diagnosed on barium enema (25, 79).

In their review of aortoenteric fistulas, Rosenthal *et al.* (255) put great store in the value of blood cultures. All seven of their patients were febrile on presentation and six had positive cultures for enteric bacteria. In fact, these cultures were almost the only positive findings in these patients.

TREATMENT

Management is surgical and urgent. As soon as possible, the patient should be started on appropriate antibiotics which are modified as sensitivities are obtained on positive blood cultures. In the absence of such demonstration, prophylactic antibiotics to sensitive enteric organisms should be started. The operation has three distinct goals: 1) elimination of all infected graft material (105, 181); 2) repair or resection of involved bowel; and 3) restoration of arterial circulation. The surgeon may first perform an extra-anatomic bypass (such as an axillobifemoral), closing the new incisions before approaching the aortoenteric fistula, or he may deal with the fistula first (especially in emergent circumstances) (Fig. 6.23). In this second case, care must be taken to re-prep and drape the patient to avoid contaminating the new prostheses. Small bowel repairs may be buttressed by another loop of bowel or by omentum. An extra-anatomic graft is employed, with rigorous attention directed towards non-contamination. With prompt recognition and appropriate management, survival has been reported in as many as 70% of cases (180).

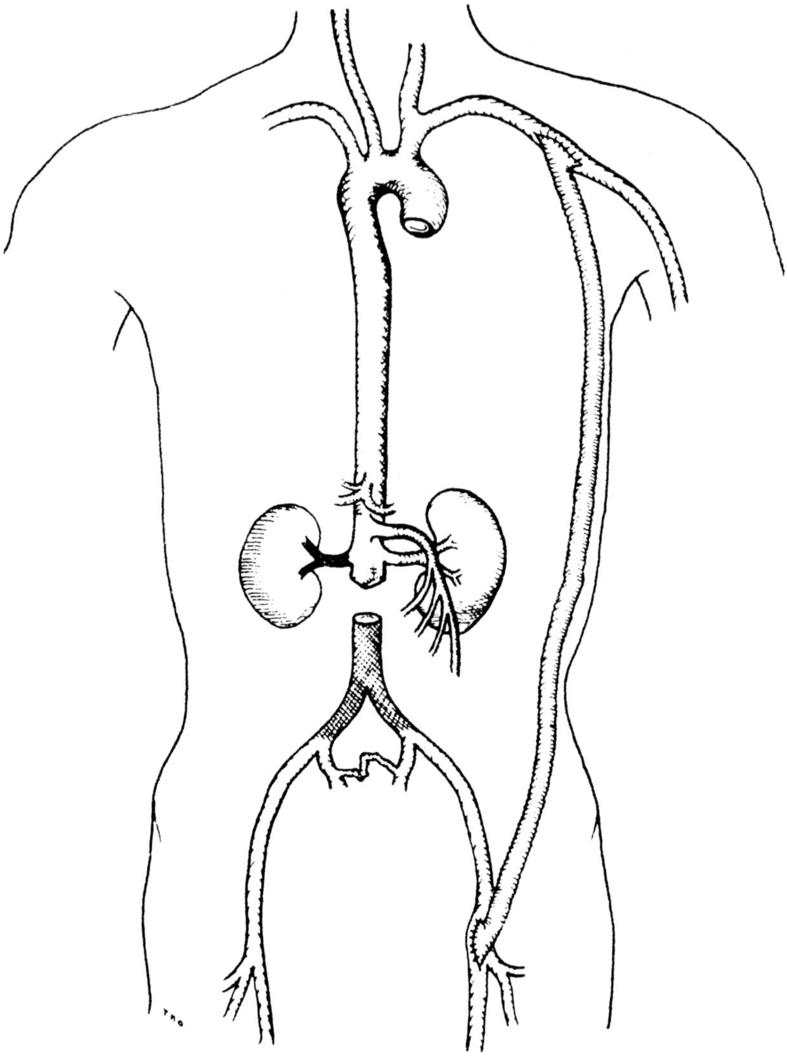

Figure 6.23. Diagram of the technique of axillofemoral graft. The graft is funneled between the axillary and femoral incisions and is sutured end-to-side of the first portion of the axillary artery and to the common femoral artery.

Neurologic Complications

Neurologic deficits caused by spinal cord ischemia may be devastating, but are fortunately rare. These have been encountered mostly in thoracic, but lessin abdominal aortic aneurysmorrhaphy and in aortic reconstruction for aortoiliac occlusive disease. The deficits range from transient sensory deficits to permanent paraplegia.

INCIDENCE

Fewer than 40 patients with neurologic changes following abdominal aortic aneurysm surgery have been reported in the literature (11, 23, 68, 72, 102, 107, 113, 129, 134, 135, 138, 145, 146, 152, 162, 196, 215, 217, 238, 249, 261, 262, 267, 269, 287, 317). A representative incidence figure (0.43%) comes from the Elliot *et al.* (107) experience at the Henry Ford Hospital in Detroit (Table 6.9).

CLINICAL PICTURE

Patients with cord ischemia manifest a variety of sensory and motor deficits. The largest number suffer from complete sensory and motor loss, most commonly beginning in the area from T-10 to L-2 and extending caudally. The next most common pattern includes partial sensory and motor loss (usually with preservation of vibratory and proprioception, these being posterior column modalities). Nearly half of these patients die and there is frequently postmortem evidence of ischemia, infarction, or cord softening. The prognosis is better in the absence of established paraplegia (see Table 6.10), with nearly all surviving patients manifesting partial or full recovery.

PATHOPHYSIOLOGY

Spinal cord ischemia may be due to hypotension or to more specific causes. Direct causes include: interruption of the cord blood supply, either by occlusion during the aneurysectomy or by exclusion of those vessels from the reconstruction; embolization with debris to those vessels (37, 249, 267); production of a "steal" phenomenon; or spinal anesthesia (183). The first is probably the most common etiology.

Numerous investigators have contributed to our knowledge of this anatomy, notably the postmortem studies of Adamkiewicz (9, 10) and Kadyi (171), and a recent number of angiographic studies (90–92, 94,

Table 6.9
Neurologic Deficits in Patients with Aortic Aneurysms (107)

Surgical Lesion	No. of Cases	Neurologic Deficit	
		No.	%
Unruptured aneurysms	1,602	3	0.19
Ruptured aneurysm	259	5	1.90
Total	1,861	8	0.43

Table 6.10
Consequences of Neurologic Impairment (107, 261)*

Deficit	No. of Patients	Recovery			Dead
		None	Partial	Full	
Paraplegia	21	3	2	1	15
Paraparesis	19	1	10	5	3

* Includes patients with cord ischemia after reconstruction for aortoiliac occlusive disease.

119, 120, 193, 282). Proximally, the blood supply is derived from the vertebral, the ascending cervical, deep cervical, intercostal, and lumbar arteries. Extensive collateralization between these exists in the cervical and sacral cords (with the additional contribution of the internal iliac and middle sacral vessels). The thoracic cord, however, is marked by a relative paucity of these collateral channels and is at greatest risk of ischemic injury (107, 176, 301).

Proceeding distally, the cord is supplied by three, long, vascular channels, one anterior and two posterior, which run along the surface of the cord and send off penetrating branches. The anterior spinal artery (tractus arteriosus of Kadyi) is a single channel which courses in the medial longitudinal fissure, beginning cranially at the union of the two anterior spinal branches of the vertebral arteries and ending caudally in the filum terminale. The posterior spinal arteries (tractus arteriosus posterior of Kadyi) are paired channels running in the posterolateral sulcus down to the conus medullaris. Each begins as the continuation of the posterior spinal branch of the corresponding vertebral artery. Microscopically, the anterior vessel supplies the anterior two-thirds of the cord, while the posterior columns and horns are supplied by the posterior spinal artery (214).

In addition, these channels receive additional blood from three to ten radicular branches arising from the ascending cervical, costocervical, intercostal, and lumbar arteries. Each lumbar artery divides into an anterior branch, essentially to muscle and skin, and a posterior branch from which arises a lateral spinal artery (191). The lateral spinal arteries have variable importance to the cord and may only supply the nerve root. Those radicular arteries which enter the cord divide, ascending and descending, to join the anterior and posterior spinal arteries. These anastomoses are the anatomic bases of border areas (Grinzonnen), especially susceptible to ischemic damage (318). These radicular vessels are not consistent, the clean segmental anatomy of the embryo being replaced by subsequent atrophy and disappearance. Where the aorta courses to the left of the spine, the radicular branches tend to originate from the left of the paired intercostal and lumbar vessels.

The largest of the radicular arteries (only 1.0 to 1.8 cm in diameter) (299) originates from the posterior muscular branch of an inferior intercostal or a superior lumbar artery. This vessel is referred to as the arteria radicularis magma, the great radicular artery, or the artery of Adamkiewicz. In the earliest studies, namely those of Adamkiewicz (9, 10) and Kadyi (171), this artery is described as arising anywhere from the intercostal of T-9 to the third lumbar artery (9, 10, 171). Suh and Alexander (282) placed its origin even wider, namely from T-8 to L-4. The origin, however, of modern angiography has again narrowed the domain of this vessel, which is now most commonly arising from the left T-9 intercostal, but may be derived as early as T-8 or as low as L-1 (92, 96). In one recent series, it is found between T-9 and T-12 in 75% of cases (94). The vessel follows the nerve roots of T-5 to T-8 in 15% of cases and roots of L-1 or L-2 in another 10% (297). If the artery of

Adamkiewicz arises high, there is frequently an anterior radicular artery in the infrarenal lumbar area (297). The artery enters the cord after passing through the intervertebral foramen and courses in a caudal direction, making a hairpin curve (97).

The precariousness and variable anatomy of the spinal cord's blood supply and the poor collateralization explain the cases of ischemic injury. By injection techniques, Tanon (289) demonstrated the lumbar arteries could be the principle blood supply of the cord. It has been demonstrated in monkeys that occlusion of the major radicular artery is followed by ischemic softening of the spinal cord (238). Clinically, the artery of Adamkiewicz may be jeopardized when the proximal aortic clamp is placed above the vessel's origin—this would occur under normal circumstances if the origin were low (the vascular clamp usually placed about L-1), or if the clamp had to be placed high (at the diaphragmatic level, for instance, in the management of a ruptured aneurysm). A clamp between the diaphragm and celiac arteries would interrupt nearly all of the blood supply to the lower cord. The cord does, however, usually tolerate this clamping for 10 to 15 minutes, and reportedly for as long as 20 minutes at normal body temperature (107). Interruption of the lumbar arteries has also been reported as the proximate cause of cord ischemia. Finally, hypotension and low-perfusion states probably prevent maintenance of any collateral flow, possibly explaining the greater incidence of this complication in patients with ruptured aneurysms.

PREVENTION

Surgery of the thoracic aorta is associated with nearly 20 times the incidence of cord ischemia as surgery of the abdominal aorta. A number of experimental and technical suggestions have been advanced for its avoidance (21, 92, 96, 97, 102, 179, 301, 305, 306, 314). In the majority of abdominal aortic aneurysm patients, however, no obvious, single cause is usually demonstrable. Neurologic deficits can be prevented by 1) avoiding hypotension, 2) minimizing the time the aorta is cross-clamped above the celiac axis, 3) maintaining adequate anticoagulation, and 4) protecting against distal embolization into the spinal vessels (107). We do not recommend extensive angiographic localization of the relevant spinal vessels during preoperative arteriography, but if an extra large lumbar artery is noted on that arteriogram, it is preserved during the operation. Furthermore, we do not meticulously dissect the lumbar vessels in an attempt to demonstrate the radicular branches arising from them.

TREATMENT

There is no specific treatment for these neurologic sequelae once they have occurred. An immediate neurologic consultation should be obtained and the patient critically reassessed. Any obvious volume deficits should be rapidly corrected, as should any associated hypotension. The neurologic changes may be transient, but in the face of permanent disability, appropriate rehabilitation should be begun as early as practical.

SUMMARY

The vascular surgeon of today stands on the shoulders of giants. Within our lifetimes we have seen the syphilitic aortic aneurysm almost disappear from clinical practice, but have seen the toll of atherosclerosis. We have watched the development of a definitive reconstructive operation with low mortality, but continue to be plagued by the ruptured aneurysm. We can return the patient with an abdominal aortic aneurysm to a normal lifestyle, but cannot deal effectively with his associated degenerative diseases.

The improvements in therapy of the next generation will come with the prevention of postoperative complications, but we will share that field with biochemists, physiologists, and engineers. These will include improvements in graft materials which resist infection and better maintain their vascular integrity, improvements in diagnosis and follow up of vascular disease, and improvements in managing postoperative morbidity. Until the day when abdominal aortic aneurysms no longer occur, we will continue to apply the techniques described and strive for even better results than those reported.

References

1. Abbott, O. A. Clinical experience with the application of polythene cellophane upon aneurysms of the thoracic vessels. *J. Thorac. Surg. 18:* 435–461, 1949.
2. Abbott, W. M. Renal failure complicating vascular surgery. In *Complications of Vascular Surgery*, edited by V. M. Bernhard and J. B. Towne, pp. 363–377. Grune & Stratton, New York, 1980.
3. Abbott, W. M., Abel, R. M., Beck, O. H., Jr., and Fisher, J. E. Renal failure after ruptured aneurysm. *Arch. Surg. 110:* 1110–1112, 1975.
4. Abbott, W. M., Abel, R. M., and Fischer, J. E. Treatment of acute renal insufficiency after aorto-iliac surgery. *Arch. Surg. 103:* 590–594, 1971.
5. Abbott, W. M., and Austen, W. G. The reversal of renal cortical ischemia during aortic occlusion by Mannitol. *J. Surg. Res. 16:* 482–489, 1974.
6. Abbott, W. M., Cooper, J. D., and Austen, W. G. The effect of aortic clamping and declamping on renal blood flow distribution. *J. Surg. Res. 14:* 385–392, 1973.
7. Abrahams, D. G., and Parry, E. H. O. Hypertension due to renal artery stenosis caused by abdominal aortic aneurysm. *Circulation 26:* 104–107, 1962.
8. Abrams, H. L. The hazards of thoracic aortography. In *Angiography*, edited by H. L. Adams, ed. 2, p. 295. Little, Brown and Co., Boston, 1971.
9. Adamkiewicz, A. Die blutgefasse des menschliechen ruckenmarkes. I. Theil die gefasse der ruckenmarkssubstanz. *Sitz. Akad. Wiss. Wien Math. Nature Klass. 84:* 469–473, 1882.
10. Adamkiewicz, A. Die blutgefasse des menschlichen ruckenmarkes. II. Theil die gefasse der ruckenmarksoberflache. *Sitz. Akad. Wiss. Wien Math. Nature Klass. 85:* 101–106, 1882.
11. Adams, H. D., and VanGetruyden, H. Neurologic complications of aortic surgery. *Ann. Surg. 144:* 574–610, 1956.
12. Alexander, J., and Byron, F. X. Aortectomy for thoracic aneurysm. *J.A.M.A. 126:* 1139–1145, 1944.
13. Altman, P., and Voorhees, A. B., Jr. Aneurysm of the aorta treated by wiring: case report of a 38-year survival. *Ann. Surg. 184:* 738–742, 1976.
14. Babcock, W. W. *A Textbook of Surgery*, p. 404. W. B. Saunders, Philadelphia, 1928.
15. Bahnson, H. T. Considerations in the excision of aortic aneurysms. *Ann. Surg. 138:* 377–386, 1953.

16. Bahnson, H. T. Definitive treatment of saccular aneurysms of the aorta with excision of sac and aortic suture. *Surg. Gynecol. Obstet. 96:* 383–401, 1953.
17. Baird, R. J., Gurry, J. F., Kallam, J. F., and Wilson, D. R. Abdominal aortic aneurysms. Recent experience with 210 patients. *Can. Med. Assoc. J. 118:* 1229–1235, 1978.
18. Baker, A. G., Roberts, B., Berkowitz, H., and Barker, C. F. Risk of excision of abdominal aortic aneurysm. *Surgery 68:* 1129–1134, 1970.
19. Baker, M. S., Fisher, J. H., van der Reis, L., and Baker, B. H. The endoscopic diagnosis of an aortoduodenal fistula. *Arch. Surg. 111:* 304–306, 1976.
20. Barratt-Boyes, B. D. Symptomatology and prognosis of abdominal aortic aneurysm. *Lancet 2:* 716–720, 1957.
21. Barry, K. G., Cohen, A., Knochel, J. P., Whelan, T. J., Jr, Beisel, W. R., Vargas, C. A., and LeBlanc, P. C. Mannitol infusion. II. The prevention of acute functional renal failure during resection of aneurysm of the abdominal aorta. *N. Engl. J. Med. 264:* 967–971, 1961.
22. Barry, K. G., Cohen, A., and LeBlanc, P. Mannitolization. I. The prevention and therapy of oliguria associated with cross-clamping of abdominal aorta. *Surgery 50:* 335–340, 1961.
23. Bates, T. Paraplegia following resection of abdominal aortic aneurysm. *Br. J. Surg. 58:* 913–916, 1971.
24. Bauer, G. M., Porter, J. M., Eidemiller, L. R., Rosch, J., and Keller, F. The role of arteriography in abdominal aortic aneurysm. *Am. J. Surg. 136:* 184–189, 1978.
25. Beach, P. M., and Risley, T. S. Aorticosigmoid fistulization following aortic resection. *Arch. Surg. 92:* 805–807, 1966.
26. Bell, J. W. Acute thrombosis of the subrenal abdominal aorta. *Arch. Surg. 95:* 681–684, 1967.
27. Bergan, J. J., and Yao, J. S. T. Modern management of abdominal aortic aneurysms. *Surg. Clin. North. Am. 54:* 175–193, 1974.
28. Bergan, J. J., Yao, J. S. T., Henkin, R. E., and Quinn, J. L., III. Radionuclide aortography in detection of arterial aneurysms. *Arch. Surg. 109:* 80–83, 1974.
29. Berkowitz, H. D., and Shetty, S. Renin release and renal cortical ischemia following aortic cross clamping. *Arch. Surg. 109:* 612–617, 1974.
30. Bernatz, P. E. Necrosis of the colon following resection for abdominal aortic aneurysms. *Arch. Surg. 81:* 373–378, 1960.
31. Bernstein, E. F., Fisher, J. C., and Varco, R. L. Is excision the optimum treatment for all abdominal aortic aneurysms? *Surgery 61:* 83–93, 1967.
32. Bernstein, W. C., and Bernstein, E. F. Ischemic ulcerative colitis following inferior mesenteric arterial ligation. *Dis. Colon Rectum 6:* 54–61, 1963.
33. Bicks, R. O., Bale, G. F., Howard, H., and McBurney, R. F. Acute and delayed colon ischemia after aorta aneurysm surgery. *Arch. Intern. Med. 122:* 249–253, 1968.
34. Bietz, D. S., and Merendino, K. A. Abdominal aneurysm and horseshoe kidney: a review. *Ann. Surg. 181:* 333–341, 1975.
35. Bigger, I. A. The surgical treatment of aneurysm of the abdominal aorta. Review of the literature and report of two cases, one apparently successful. *Ann. Surg. 112:* 879–894, 1940.
36. Birnbaum, W., Rudy, L., and Wylie, E. J. Colonic and rectal ischemia following abdominal aneurysmectomy. *Dis. Colon. Rectum 7:* 293–302, 1964.
37. Blaisdell, F. W., and Cooley, D. A. The mechanism of paraplegia after temporary thoracic aortic occlusion and its relationship to spinal fluid pressure. *Surgery 51:* 351–355, 1962.
38. Blakemore, A. H., and King, G. B. Electrothermic coagulation of aortic aneurysms. *J.A.M.A. 111:* 1821–1827, 1938.
39. Blakemore, A. H., and Voorhees, A. B., Jr. Aneurysm of the aorta: review of 365 cases. *Angiology 5:* 209–231, 1954.
40. Blakemore, A. H., and Voorhees, A. B., Jr. The use of tubes constructed from Vinyon "N" cloth in bridging arterial defects—experimental and clinical. *Ann. Surg. 140:* 324–334, 1954.
41. Blum, L. Ruptured aneurysm of abdominal aorta. *N.Y. State J. Med. 68:* 2061–2066, 1968.

42. Boley, S. J., Brandt, L. J., and Veith, F. J. Ischemic disorders of the intestines. *Curr. Probl. Surg. 15(4):* 1–85, 1978.
43. Borrie, J., and Griffin, S. G. Twenty-seven cases of syphilitic aneurysms of the thoracic aorta and its branches. *Thorax 5:* 293–324, 1950.
44. Bradham, R. R., Gregorie, H. B., and Wilson, R. Chylous ascites following resection of abdominal aortic aneurysm. *Am. J. Surg. 36:* 238–240, 1970.
45. Brener, B. J., Darling, R. C., Frederich, P. L., and Linton, R. R. Major venous anomalies complicating abdominal aortic surgery. *Arch. Surg. 108:* 159–165, 1974.
46. Brewster, D. C., Buth, J., Darling, R. C., and Austin, W. G. Combined aortic and renal artery reconstruction. *Am. J. Surg. 131:* 457–463, 1976.
47. Brewster, D. C., Darling, C., Raines, J., Sarno, R., O'Donnell, T. F., Ezpeleta, M., and Athanasoulis, C. Assessment of abdominal aortic aneurysm size. *Circulation 56(2):* 164–169, 1977.
48. Brewster, D. C., Ottinger, L., and Darling, R. C. Hematuria as a sign of aorto-caval fistula. *Ann. Surg. 186:* 766–771, 1977.
49. Brewster, D. C., Retana, A., Waltman, A. C., and Darling, R. C. Angiography in the management of aneurysms of the abdominal aorta. Its value and safety. *N. Engl. J. Med. 292:* 822–825, 1975.
50. Brock, R. C. Aortic homografting: A report of 6 successful cases. *Guy's Hosp. Rep. 102:* 204–228, 1953.
51. Brock, R. C. *The Life and Work of Astley Cooper*, p. 56. E. & S. Livingstone, Edinburgh, 1952.
52. Bussemaker, J. B., and Lindeman, J. Comparison of methods to determine viability of small intestine. *Ann. Surg. 176:* 97–101, 1972.
53. Busuttil, R. W., Rees, W., Baker, J. D., and Wilson, S. E. Pathogenesis of aortoduodenal fistula. Experimental and clinical correlates. *Surgery 85:* 1–13, 1979.
54. Carrel, A. Permanent intubation of thoracic aorta. *J. Exp. Med. 16:* 17–24, 1912.
55. Carrel, A. Results of permanent intubation of the thoracic aorta. *Surg. Gynecol. Obstet. 15:* 245–248, 1912.
56. Carrel, A. Technique and remote results of vascular anastomoses. *Surg. Gynecol. Obstet. 14:* 246–254, 1912.
57. Carter, R., Vannix, R., Hinshaw, D. B., and Stafford, C. E. Inferior mesenteric vascular occlusion: sigmoidoscopic diagnosis. *Surgery 46:* 845–846, 1959.
58. Chang F., Smith, J., Rahbar, A., and Farha, G. Abdominal aortic aneurysm—a comparative analysis of surgical treatment of symptomatic and asymptomatic patients. *Am. J. Surg. 136:* 705–708, 1978.
59. Chawla, S. K., Najafi, H., Ing, T. S., Dye, W. S., Javid, H., Hunter, J. A., Goldin, M. D., and Serry, C. Acute renal failure complicating ruptured abdominal aortic aneurysm. *Arch. Surg. 110:* 521–526, 1975.
60. Claytor, H., Birch, L., Cardwell, E. S., and Zimmerman, S. L. Suture-line rupture of a nylon aortic bifurcation graft into the small bowel. *Arch. Surg. 73:* 947–950, 1956.
61. Cohn, R., and Angell, W. W. Late complications from plastic replacement of aortic abdominal aneurysms. *Arch. Surg. 97:* 696–698, 1968.
62. Coleman, C. C., Jr, Deterling, R. A., Jr., and Parshley, M. S. Some long-term observations on aortic homografts. *Surgery 37:* 64–79, 1955.
63. Collard, M., Guey, A., Meary, M. F., Claveyrolas, P., Minh, V. T., Lyonnet, D., and Pinot, A. Distribution du debit sanguin renal dans l'insuffiance renale aigue, ou le probleme de la mesure du debit renal en clinique. *Lyon Med. 238:* 505–512, 1977.
64. Conn, J. H., Hardy, J. D., Chevez, C. M., and Fain, W. R. Infected arterial grafts: experience in 22 cases with emphasis on unusual bacteria and techniques. *Ann. Surg. 171:* 704–714, 1970.
65. Connelly, T. L., McKinnon, W., Smith, R. B., III, and Perdue, G. D. Abdominal aortic surgery and horseshoe kidney. Report of 6 cases and a review. *Arch. Surg. 115:* 1459–1463, 1980.
66. Connolly, J. E., and Kwaan, J. H. M. Prophylactic revascularization of the gut. *Ann. Surg. 190:* 514–522, 1979.
67. Cooley, D. A., and DeBakey, M. E. Surgical considerations of intrathoracic aneurysms of the aorta and great vessels. *Ann. Surg. 135:* 660–680, 1952.

68. Coupland, G. A. E., and Reeve, T. S. Paraplegia: a complication of excision of abdominal aortic aneurysm. *Surgery 64:* 878–881, 1968.
69. Crane, C. Atheriosclerotic aneurysm of the abdominal aorta. Some pathologic and clinical correlations. *N. Engl. J. Med. 253:* 954–958, 1955.
70. Crawford, E. S., DeBakey, M. E., Morris, G. C., Jr., and Garrett, E. Evaluation of late failures after reconstructive operations for occlusive lesions of the aorta and iliac, femoral, and popliteal arteries. *Surgery 47:* 79–104, 1960.
71. Crawford, E. S. Thoraco-abdominal and abominal aortic aneurysms involving renal, superior mesenteric, and celiac arteries. *Ann. Surg. 179:* 763–772, 1974.
72. Crawford, E. S., Fenstermacher, J. M., Richardson, W., and Sandiford, F. Reappraisal of adjuncts to avoid ischemia in the treatment of thoracic aortic aneurysms. *Surgery 67:* 182–196, 1970.
73. Crawford, E. S., Snyder, D. M., Cho, G. C., and Roehm, J. Progress in treatment of thoraco-abdominal and abdominal aortic aneurysms involving celiac, superior mesenteric and renal arteries. *Ann. Surg. 188:* 404–422, 1978.
74. Crisler, C., and Bahnson, H. T. Aneurysms of the aorta. *Curr. Probl. Surg.* December: 1–64, 1972.
75. Crisp, E. *Structure, Diseases, and Injuries of Blood Vessels.* J. Churchill, London, 1847.
76. Culp, O. S., and Bernatz, P. E. Urologic aspects of lesions in the abdominal aorta. *J. Urol. 86:* 189–195, 1961.
77. Cyr, R., Trudel, J., Rabbat, A. G., Trudel, S., Lafortune, M., and Lemire, G. Angiography: an essential diagnostic aid in asymptomatic aortic aneurysms. *Can. J. Surg. 20:* 57–59, 1977.
78. Dale, W. A. The beginnings of vascular surgery. *Surgery 76:* 849–866, 1974.
79. Dalinka, M. K., Gohel, V. K., Schaffer, B., and Hernberg, J. Gastrointestinal complications of aortic bypass surgery. *Clin. Radiol. 27:* 255–258, 1976.
80. Danielson, G. K., and Payne, W. S. Arteriography and abdominal aortic aneurysm. *JAMA 209:* 1366, 1969.
81. Darling, R. C. Ruptured arteriosclerotic abdominal aortic aneurysms. *Am. J. Surg. 119:* 397–401, 1970.
82. Darling, R. C., Messina, C., Brewster, D., and Ottinger, L. Autopsy study of unoperated abdominal aortic aneurysm. The case for early resection. *Circulation 56(2):* 161–164, 1977.
83. Dauchot, P. J., DePalma, R., Grum, D., and Zanella, J. Detection and prevention of cardiac dysfunction during aortic surgery. *J. Surg. Res. 26:* 574, 1979.
84. David, J. P., Marks, C., and Bonneval, M. A ten year institutional experience with ruptured abdominal aortic aneurysms. *Surg. Gynecol. Obstet. 138:* 591–594, 1974.
85. Dean, R. H., Allen, T. R., Foster, J. H., Mattingly, S., Clayson, K. R., and Edwards, W. H. Aortoduodenal fistula: an uncommon but correctable cause of upper gastrointestional bleeding. *Am. J. Surg. 44:* 37–43, 1978.
86. DeBakey, M. E., and Cooley, D. A. Surgical treatment of aneurysms of abdominal aorta by resection and restoration of continuity with homograft. *Surg. Gynecol. Obstet. 97:* 257–266, 1953.
87. DeBakey, M. E., Crawford, E. S., Cooley, D. A., Morris, G. O., Jr., Royster, T. S., and Abbott, W. P. Aneurysm of abdominal aorta: analysis of results of graft replacement therapy one to eleven years after operation. *Ann. Surg. 160:* 622–639, 1964.
88. Deterling, R. A., Jr., and Bhonslay, S. B. An evaluation of synthetic materials and fabrics suitable for blood vessel replacement. *Surgery 38:* 71–91, 1955.
89. DeWeese, M. S., and Fry, W. J. Small-bowel erosion following aortic resection. *JAMA 179:* 882–886, 1962.
90. Di Chiro, G. Unintentional spinal cord arteriography: a warning. *Radiology 112:* 231–233, 1974.
91. Di Chiro, G., and Doppman, J. L. Letter to the Editor. Paraplegia after resection of aneurysm. *N. Engl. J. Med. 281:* 799, 1969.
92. Di Chiro, G., and Wener, L. Angiography of the spinal cord. *J. Neurosurg. 39:* 1–29, 1973.
93. DiGiovanni, R., Nichols, G., Volpetti, G., Berkowitz, H., Barker, C., and Roberts, B. Twenty-one years' experience with ruptured abdominal aortic aneurysms. *Surg.*

Gynecol. Obstet. 141: 859–862, 1975.
94. Djindjian, R., and Faure, C. Accidents medullaires de l'aortographie. *J. Belge. Radiol. 50:* 207–211, 1967.
95. Donovan, T. J., and Bucknam, T. J. Aorto-enteric fistula. *Arch. Surg. 95:* 810–820, 1967.
96. Doppman, J. L., Di Chiro, G., and Morton, D. L. Arteriographic identification of spinal cord blood supply prior to aortic surgery. *J.A.M.A. 204:* 174–175, 1968.
97. Doppman, J. L., Di Chiro, G., and Ommaya, A. K. *Selective Arteriography of the Spinal Cord.* Warren H. Green, St. Louis, 1969.
98. Doty, D. B., Wright, C. B., Lamberth, W. C., Spoto, G., III, Garrett, M. V., and Cram, A. E. Aortocaval fistula associated with aneurysm of the abdominal aorta: current management techniques using autotransfusion techniques. *Surgery 84:* 250–252, 1978.
99. Drager, S., Riles, T., and Imparato, A. Management of acute aortic occlusion. *Am. J. Surg. 138:* 293–295, 1979.
100. Dubost, C., Allary, M., and Oeconomos, N. Resection of an aneurysm of the abdominal aorta. Reestablishment of the continuity by a preserved human arterial graft, with result after five months. *Arch. Surg. 64:* 405–408, 1952.
101. Eastcott, H. G. G. *Arterial Surgery,* ed. 2. J. B. Lippincott, Philadelphia, 1973.
102. Edmonston, H. T., and Gindin, R. A. Paraplegia as a complication of abdominal aortic resection. *Am. Surg. 36:* 383–386, 1970.
103. Edwards, W. B., and Tapp, J. S. Chemically treated Nylon tubes as arterial grafts. *Surgery 38:* 61–70, 1955.
104. Edwards, W. C., Snyder, R., Botzko, K., and Larkin, J. Dilation and durability changes in synthetic grafts of dacron and teflon. In *Complications of Vascular Surgery,* edited by V. M. Bernhard, and J. B. Towne. Grune & Stratton, New York, 1980.
105. Ehrenfeld, W. K., Lord, R. S. A., Stoney, R. J., and Wylie, E. J. Subcutaneous arterial bypass grafts in the management of fistulae between the bowel and plastic arterial prostheses. *Ann. Surg. 168:* 29–35, 1968.
106. Elliot, J. P., Jr., Smith, R. F., and Szilagyi, D. E. Aortoenteric and paraprosthetic-enteric fistulas. Problems of diagnosis and management. *Arch. Surg. 108:* 479–490, 1974.
107. Elliot, J. P., Jr., Szilagyi, D. E., Hageman, J. H., and Smith, R. F. Spinal cord damage secondary to surgery of the abdominal aorta. In *Complications in Vascular Surgery,* edited by B. M. Bernhard and J. B. Towne, pp. 407–426. Grune & Stratton, New York, 1980.
108. Ernst, C. B. Colon ischemia following abdominal aortic reconstruction. In *Complications of Vascular Surgery,* edited by V. M. Bernhard and J. B. Towne, pp. 379–406. Grune & Stratton, New York, 1980.
109. Ernst, C. B., Hagihara, P. F., Daugherty, M. E., and Griffen, W. O., Jr. Inferior mesenteric stump pressure: a reliable index for safe IMA ligation during abdominal aortic aneurysmectomy. *Ann. Surg. 187:* 641–646, 1978.
110. Ernst, C. B., Hagihara, P. F., Daugherty, J., Sachatello, C. R., and Griffen, W. D., Jr. Ischemic colitis incidence following abdominal aortic reconstruction: a prospective study. *Surgery 80:* 417–421, 1976.
111. Estes, J. E., Jr. Abdominal aortic aneurysm. A study of 102 cases. *Circulation 2:* 258–264, 1950.
112. Ezzet, F., Dorazio, R., and Herzberg, R. Horseshoe and pelvic kidneys associated with abdominal aortic aneurysm. *Am. J. Surg. 134:* 196–198, 1977.
113. Ferguson, L. R. J., Bergan, J. J., Conn, J., Jr., and Yao, J. S. T. Spinal ischemia following abdominal aortic surgery. *Ann. Surg. 181:* 267–272, 1975.
114. Ferris, E. J., Koltay, M. R., Koltay, O. P., and Sciammas, F. D. Abdominal aortic and iliac graft fistulae: unusual roentgenographic findings. *Am. J. Roentgenol. 94:* 416, 1965.
115. Flanigan, D. P., Quinn, T., and Kraft, R. O. Selective management of high risk patients with abdominal aortic aneurysm. *Surg. Gynecol. Obstet. 150:* 171–176, 1980.
116. Foster, J. H. Arteriography: cornerstone of vascular surgery. *Arch. Surg. 109:* 605–611, 1974.

117. Foster, J. H., Bolasny, B. L., Gobbel, W. G., Jr., and Scott, W. H. Comparative study of elective resection and expectant treatment of abdominal aortic aneurysms. *Surg. Gynecol. Obstet. 129:* 1–9, 1969.
118. Franklin, W. A., Ganote, C. E., and Jennings, R. B. Blood reflow after renal ischemia. Effects of hypertonic Mannitol on reflow and tubular necrosis after transient ischemia in the rat. *Arch. Pathol. 98:* 106–111, 1974.
119. Fried, L. C., Di Chiro, G., and Doppman, J. L. Ligation of major thoraco-lumbar spinal cord arteries in monkeys. *J. Neurosurg. 31:* 608–614, 1969.
120. Fried, L. C., Doppman, J. L., and Di Chiro, G. Direction of blood flow in the primate cervical spinal cord. *J Neurosurg. 33:* 325–330, 1970.
121. Fry, W. J., and Lindenauer, S. M. Infection complicating the use of plastic arterial implants. *Arch. Surg. 94:* 600–609, 1967.
122. Galen, J. *Observations on Aneurysm,* p. 3. translated by J. E. Erichsen. Syndenham Society, London, 1944.
123. Gardner, R. J., Gardner, N. L., Tarney, T. J., Warden, H. E., James E. C., and Watne, A. L. The surgical experience and a 1–16 year follow-up of 277 abdominal aortic aneurysms. *Am. J. Surg. 135:* 226–230, 1978.
124. Gardner, R. J., Lancaster, J. R., Tarney, T. J., Warren H. E., and Currie, R. A. Five year history of surgically treated abdominal aortic aneurysms. *Surg. Gynecol. Obstet. 130:* 981–987, 1970.
125. Gardner, T. J., Brawley, R. K., and Gott, V. L. Anastomotic false aneurysms. *Surgery 72:* 474–478, 1972.
126. Garret, H. E., Beall, A. C., Jr., Jordan, G. L., Jr., and DeBakey, M. E. Surgical considerations of massive gastrointestinal bleeding caused by aortoduodenal fistula. *Am. J. Surg. 105:* 6–12, 1963.
127. Gaspar, M. R. In discussion of Kwaan, J. H. M., Connolly, J. E., Vander Molen, R., and Conroy, R. The value of arteriography before abdominal aneurysmectomy. *Am. J. Surg. 134:* 108–114, 1977.
128. Gayliss, H. G. Pathogenesis of anastomotic aneurysms. *Surgery 90:* 509, 1981.
129. Gensler, S. W., and Hoffert, P. Paraparesis following resection of abdominal aortic aneurysm. *N.Y. State J. Med. 71:* 2093–2095, 1971.
130. Gibson, W. E., III, Pearce, C. W., and Creech, O., Jr. Infarction on the left hemicolon due to primary vascular occlusion. *Dis. Colon Rectum 12:* 323–326, 1969.
131. Giordano, C. Use of exogenous and endogenous urea for protein synthesis in normal and uremic subjects. *J. Lab. Clin. Med. 62:* 231–246, 1963.
132. Giovannetti, S., and Maggiore, Q. A low-nitrogen diet with proteins of high biological value for severe chronic uraemia. *Lancet 1:* 1000–1003, 1964.
133. Gliedman, M. L., Ayers, W. E., and Vestal, B. L. Aneurysms of the abdominal aorta and its branches. A study of untreated patients. *Ann. Surg. 146:* 207–214, 1957.
134. Golden, G. T., Sears, H. F., Wellons, H. A., and Muller, W. H., Jr. Paraplegia complicating resection of aneurysms of the infrarenal abdominal aorta. *Surgery 73:* 91–96, 1973.
135. Golden, G. T., Wellons, H. A., and Muller, W. H. Paraplegia after surgery for abdominal aortic aneurysms. *J.A.M.A. 233:* 768–769, 1975.
136. Goldstone, J., Malone, J. M., and Moore, W. S. Inflammatory aneurysms of the abdominal aorta. *Surgery 83:* 425–430, 1978.
137. Gore, I., and Hirst, A. E., Jr. Arteriosclerotic aneurysms of the abdominal aorta. *Prog. Cardiovasc. Dis. 16:* 113–150, 1973.
138. Grace, R. R., and Mattox, K. L. Anterior spinal artery syndrome following abdominal aortic aneurysmectomy. *Arch. Surg. 112:* 813–815, 1977.
139. Graham, L. M., Burkel, W. E., Ford, J. W., Vinter, D. W., and Stanley, J. C. Immediate seeding of enzymatically derived endothelium in Dacron vascular grafts. *Arch. Surg. 115:* 1285–1288, 1980.
140. Graham, L. M., Vinter, D. W., Ford, J. W., Burkel, W. E., and Stanley, J. C. Cultured autogenous endothelial cell seeding of prosthetic vascular grafts. *Surg. Forum 30:* 204–206, 1979.
141. Graham, L. M., Vinter, D. W., Ford, J. W., Rahm, R. H., Burkel, W. E., and Stanley,

J. C. Cultured autogenous endothelial cell seeding of prosthetic vascular grafts: early experimental studies with cultured autologous canine endothelium. *Arch. Surg. 115:* 929–933, 1980.
142. Gravgaard, E., Juul, S., Albrechtsen, O., and Mouritzen, C. Prognosis and treatment of abdominal aortic aneurysm. *Surg. Gynecol. Obstet. 151:* 777–780, 1980.
143. Griffiths, J. D. Surgical anatomy of the blood supply of the distal colon. *Ann. R. Coll. Surg. Engl. 19:* 241–256, 1956.
144. Grindlinger, G. A., Vegas, A. M., Manny, J., Bush, H. L., Mannick, J. A., and Hechtman, H. B. Volume loading and vasodilators in abdominal aortic aneurysmectomy. *Am. J. Surg. 139:* 480–486, 1980.
145. Gump, F. E. Letter to the Editor. Paraplegia after resection of aneurysm. *N. Engl. J. Med. 281:* 798, 1969.
146. Gump, F. E. Paraplegia following resection of infrarenal aortic aneurysms. *N.Y. State J. Med. 70:* 794–795, 1970.
147. Gwathmey, O., Adkins, P. C., and Blades, B. Emergency and elective treatment of abdominal aortic aneurysms. *Postgrad. Med. 25:* 677–684, 1959.
148. Hafner, C. D., Cranley, J. J., Krause, R. J., and Strasser, E. S. Acute abdominal aorto-vena caval fistula. *Vasc. Surg. 3:* 149–153, 1969.
149. Hagihara, P. F., Ernst, C. B., Griffin, W. O., Jr. Incidence of ischemic colitis following abdominal aortic reconstruction. *Surg. Gynecol. Obstet. 149:* 571–573, 1979.
150. Haimovici, H. H. (Ed.) *The Surgical Management of Vascular Disease.* J. B. Lippincott, Philadelphia, 1970.
151. Halpert, B., and Williams, R. K. Aneurysms of aorta. An analysis of 249 necropsies. *Arch. Pathol. 74:* 163–168, 1962.
152. Hara, M., and Lipin, R. J. Spinal cord injury following resection of abdominal aortic aneurysm. *Arch. Surg. 80:* 419–423, 1960.
153. Hardy, J. D., and Timmis, H. H. Abdominal aortic aneurysms: special problems. *Ann. Surg. 173:* 945–965, 1971.
154. Harrison, P. W., and Chandy, J. A subclavian aneurysm cured by cellophane fibrosis. *Ann. Surg. 118:* 478–481, 1943.
155. Heberer, G. Diagnosis and treatment of aneurysms of the abdominal aorta. *Ger. Med. Monthly 2:* 203–205, 1957.
156. Henry, L. G., and Bernhard, V. M. Ureteral pathology associated with aortic surgery: a report of three unusual cases. *Surgery 83:* 464–469, 1978.
157. Hertzer, N. R. Fatal myocardial infarction following abdominal aortic aneurysm resection. Three hundred forty-three patients followed 6–11 years postoperatively. *Ann. Surg. 192:* 667–673, 1980.
158. Hertzer, N. R., and Beven, E. G. Ultrasound aortic measurement and elective aneurysmectomy. *J.A.M.A. 240:* 1966–1968, 1978.
159. Hicks, G. L., Eastland, M. W., DeWeese, J. A., May, A. G., and Rob, C. G. Survival improvement following aortic aneurysm resection. *Ann. Surg. 181:* 863–869, 1975.
160. Hobson, R. W., II, Wright, C. B., O'Donnell, J. A., Jamil, Z., Lamberth, W. C., and Najem, Z. Determination of intestinal viability by Doppler ultrasound. *Arch. Surg. 114:* 165–168, 1979.
161. Hobson, R. W., II, Wright, C. B., Rich, N. M., and Collins, G. J., Jr. Assessment of colon ischemia during aortic surgery by Doppler ultrasound. *J. Surg. Res. 20:* 231–235, 1976.
162. Hogan, E. L., and Romanul, F. C. A. Spinal cord infarction occurring during insertion of aortic graft. *Neurology 16:* 67–74, 1966.
163. Hufnagel, C. A. Permanent intubation of the thoracic aorta. *Arch. Surg. 54:* 382–389, 1947.
164. Humphries, A. W., Young, D. P., deWolfe, V. G., and LeFeure, F. A. Complications of abdominal aortic surgery: I. Aorto-enteric fistula. *Arch. Surg. 86:* 43–50, 1963.
165. Imparato, A. M., Berman, I. R., Bracco, A., Kim, G. E., and Beaudet, R. Avoidance of shock and peripheral embolism during surgery of the abdominal aorta. *Surgery 73:* 68–73, 1973.
166. Javid, H., Julian, O. C., Dye, W. S., and Hunter, J. A. Complications of abdominal aortic grafts. *Arch. Surg. 85:* 650–652, 1962.

167. Johnson, G., Jr., McDevitt, N. B., Proctor, H. J., Mandel, S. R., and Peacock, J. B. Emergent or elective operation for symptomatic abdomonal aortic aneurysm. *Arch. Surg. 115:* 51–53, 1980.
168. Johnson, J., and Wood, M. Arteriovenous fistula secondary to rupture of atherosclerotic abdominal aortic aneurysm—5 cases. *Am. J. Surg. 136:* 171–175, 1978.
169. Johnson, W. C., and Nabseth, D. C. Visceral infarction following aortic surgery. *Am. Surg. 180:* 312–318, 1974.
170. Kadir, S., Athanasoulis, C. A., Brewster, D. C., and Moncure, A. C. Tender abdominal pulsatile abdominal mass. Abdominal aortic aneurysm or not? *Arch. Surg. 115:* 631–633, 1980.
171. Kadyi, H. Uber die blutgefasse des menschlichen Ruckenmarkes, nach einer im XV. Bande der Denschriften der Math Natur classe der Akademie der Wissenschaften in Krakau erschienin Monographie. Aus dem Polnishen ubersetzt vom Verfasser. Gubrynowicz and Schmidt, Lember, 1889.
172. Kahn, P. C., and Callow, A. D. Catheter arteriography in the evaluation of abdominal aortic aneurysms. *Am. J. Roentgenol. Rad. Ther. Nucl. Med. 98:* 879–887, 1966.
173. Kampmeier, R. H. Aneurysm of abdominal aorta: study of 73 cases. *Am. J. Med. Sci. 192:* 97–109, 1936.
174. Katz, S., Wahab, A., Murray, W., and Williams, L. F. New parameters of viability in ischemic bowel disease. *Am. J. Surg. 127:* 136–141, 1974.
175. Keen, W. W., and White, J. W. *An American Text-Book of Surgery*, ed. 2, pp. 225–248. W. B. Saunders, Philadelphia, 1897.
176. Killen, D. A., Edwards, R. B., and Adkins, R. B., Jr. Relation of the arterial pressure in the permanently bypassed descending thoracic aorta to the occurrence of spinal cord injury in the dog. *Surgery 59:* 534–539, 1966.
177. Kim, G. E., Imparato, A. M., Nathan, I., and Riles, T. S. Dilation of synthetic grafts and junctional aneurysms. *Arch. Surg. 114:* 1296–1303, 1979.
178. King, D. R., and Evans, W. E. Abdominal aortic aneurysm. *Vasc. Surg. 9:* 46, 1975.
179. Kinley, C. E., Paasche, P. E., MacDonald, A. S., and Marble, A. E. Stress at vascular anastomosis in relation to host artery: synthetic graft diameter. *Surgery 75:* 28–30, 1974.
180. Kleinman, L. H., and Bernhard, V. M. Aorto-enteric fistula: recognition and surgical management. In *Complications in Vascular Surgery*, edited by V. M. Bernhard and J. B. Towne. Grune & Stratton, New York, 1980.
181. Kleinman, L. H., Towne, J. B., and Bernhard, V. M. A diagnostic and therapeutic approach to aortoenteric fistulas: clinical experience with 20 patients. *Surgery 86:* 868–880, 1979.
182. Kwaan, J. H. M., Connolly, J. E., Molen, R. V., and Conroy, R. The value of arteriography before abdominal aneurysmectomy. *Am. J. Surg. 134:* 108–114, 1977.
183. Lake, P. A. Letter to the Editor. Paraplegia after resection of aneurysm. *N. Engl. J. Med. 281:* 798–799, 1969.
184. Lancisi, G. M. *De Aneurysmatibus*, revised and edited by W. C. Wright, p. 3. MacMillan, New York, 1952.
185. Lancisi, G. M. *De Aneurysmatibus*, revised and edited by W. C. Wright, p. 24. MacMillan, New York, 1952.
186. Lancisi, G. M. *De Aneurysmatibus*, revised and edited by W. C. Wright, p. 333. MacMillan, New York, 1952.
187. Lancisi, G. M. *De Aneurysmatibus*, revised and edited by W. C. Wright, p. 346. MacMillan, New York, 1952.
188. Landes, R., Trumbull, H., and Nicoloff, D. Abdominal aortic aneurysm with rupture into the inferior vena cava associated with horseshoe kidney. *Ann. Surg. 187:* 329–331, 1978.
189. Lang, E. K. A survey of the complications of percutaneous retrograde arteriography. Seldinger technic. *Radiology 81:* 257–263, 1963.
190. Lang, E. K. Complications of retrograde percutaneous arteriography. *J. Urol. 90:* 604–610, 1963.
191. Laufman, H., Berggren, R. E., Finley, T., and Anson, B. J. Anatomic studies of the lumbar arteries. *Ann. Surg. 152:* 621–634, 1960.

192. Launer, D. P., Miscall, B. G., and Beil, A. R., Jr. Colorectal infarction following resection of abdominal aortic aneurysms. *Dis. Colon Rectum 21:* 613–617, 1978.
193. Lazorthes, G., Poulhes, B. G., and Roulleau, J. La vascularisation arterielle de la moelle. Reserches anatomiques et applications a la pathologie medullaire et a la pathologie aortique. *Neur. Chir. 4:* 3–8, 1958.
194. Leather, R. P., Shah, D., Goldman, M., Rosenberg, M., and Karmody, A. M. Nonresective treatment of abdominal aortic aneurysms. Use of acute thrombosis and axillofemoral bypass. *Arch. Surg. 114:* 1402–1408, 1979.
195. Lee, K. R., Walls, W. J., Martin, N. L., and Templeton, A. W. A practical approach to the diagnosis of abdominal aortic aneurysms. *Surgery 78:* 195–201, 1975.
196. Lentin, M., and Salis, J. S. Paraplegia as a complication of infra-renal aneurysmorrhaphy. *Vasc. Surg. 6:* 224–226, 1972.
197. Leopold, G. R., Goldberger, L. E., and Bernstein, E. F. Ultrasonic detection and evaluation of abdominal aortic aneurysms. *Surgery 72:* 939–945, 1972.
198. Levy, M. J., Todd, D. B., Lillehei, C. W., and Varco, R. L. Aortico-intestinal fistulas following surgery of the aorta. *Surg. Gynecol. Obstet. 120:* 992–996, 1965.
199. Linton, R. B. Intrasaccular wiring of abdominal-arteriosclerotic aortic aneurysms by the "pack" method. *Angiology 2:* 485–498, 1951.
200. Luft, F. C., Hamburger, R. J., Dyek, J. K., Szwed, J. J., and Kleit, S. A. Acute renal failure following operation for aortic aneurysm. *Surg. Gynecol. Obstet. 141:* 374–378, 1975.
201. Mahorner, H. Historic and modern methods of treating aneurysms. *Surg. Gynecol. Obstet. 105(2):* 105–113, 1957.
202. Maniglia, R., and Gregory, J. E. Increasing incidence of arteriosclerotic aortic aneurysms. Analysis of six thousand autopsies. *Arch. Pathol. 54:* 298–305, 1952.
203. Mannick, J. A. Diagnosis of ruptured aneurysm of the abdominal aorta. *N. Engl. J. Med. 276:* 1305–1307, 1967.
204. Mannick, J. A. Surgical treatment of aneurysms of the abdominal and thoracic aorta. *Proc. Cardiovasc. Dis. 16:* 69–87, 1973.
205. Mannick, J. A., Brooks, J. W., Bosher, L. H., Jr., and Hume, D. M. Ruptured aneurysms of the abdominal aorta. A reappraisal. *N. Engl. J. Med. 271:* 915–920, 1964.
206. Matas, R. Aneurysm of the abdominal aorta at its bifurcation into the common iliac arteries. A pictorial supplement illustrating the history of Corinne D., previously reported as the first recorded instance of cure of an aneurysm of the abdominal aorta by ligation. *Ann. Surg. 112:* 909–922, 1940.
207. Matas, R. An operation for the radical cure of aneurysm based upon arteriorrhaphy. *Ann. Surg. 37:* 161–196, 1903.
208. Matas, R. *Surgery: Its Principles and Practice*, edited by W. W. Keen. W. B. Saunders, Philadelphia, 1921.
209. McAfee, J. G. Survey of complications of abdominal aortography. *Radiology 68:* 825–838, 1957.
210. McBurney, R. P., Howard, H., Bicks, R. O., and Rale, G. F. Ischemia and gangrene of the colon following abdominal aortic resection. *Am. Surg. 36:* 205–209, 1970.
211. McCombs, P. R., and DeLaurentis, D. A. Division of the left renal vein. Guidelines and consequences. *Am. J. Surg. 138:* 257–263, 1979.
212. McCombs, P. R., and Roberts, B. Acute renal failure following resection of abdominal aortic aneurysm. *Surg. Gynecol. Obstet. 148:* 175–178, 1979.
213. McGill, H. C., Jr. (Ed.) *Geographic Pathology of Atherosclerosis*, pp. 523–645. Williams & Wilkins, Baltimore, 1968.
214. Mehrez, I. O., Nabseth, D. C., Hogan, E. L., and Deterling, R. A., Jr. Paraplegia following resection of abdominal aortic aneurysms. *Ann. Surg. 156:* 890–898, 1962.
215. Meinke, A. H., III, Estes, N. C., and Ernst, C. B. Chylous ascites following abdominal aortic aneurysmectomy. Management with total parenteral hyperalimentation. *Ann. Surg. 190:* 631–663, 1979.
216. Merchant, R. F., Jr., Cafferata, H. T., and De Palma, R. G. Pitfalls in the diagnosis of abdominal aortic aneurysms. *Am. J. Surg. 142:* 756–758, 1981.

217. Michaels, L. Case report: spinal cord ischemia associated with repair of a ruptured abdominal aortic aneurysm. *Stroke 3:* 238–239, 1972.
218. Miller, R. E., and Knox, W. G. Colon ischemia following infrarenal aortic surgery: report of four cases. *Ann. Surg. 163:* 639–642, 1966.
219. Mir-Madjlessi, S. H., Sullivan, B. H., Jr., Farmer, R. G., and Beven, E. G. Endoscopic diagnosis of aortoduodenal fistula. *Gastrointest. Endosc. 19:* 187–188, 1973.
220. Molnar, W., and Paul, D. J. Complications of axillary arteriotomies. An analysis of 1,762 consecutive studies. *Radiology 104:* 269–276, 1972.
221. Moore, H. D. Diagnosis of rupture of abdominal aortic aneurysms. *Lancet 2:* 184–186, 1967.
222. Moore, H. D. Replacement of blood vessels by polythene tubes. *Surg. Gynecol. Obstet. 91:* 593–600, 1950.
223. Moore, W. S., Chvapil, M., Seiffert, G., and Keown, K. Development of an infection-resistant vascular prosthesis. *Arch. Surg. 116:* 1403–1407, 1981.
224. Moore, W. S., and Hall, A. D. Late suture failure in the pathogenesis of anastomotic false aneurysms. *Ann. Surg. 172:* 1064–1068, 1970.
225. Moossa, A. R., Skinner, D. B., Stark, V., and Hoffer, P. Assessment of bowel viability using 99m-Technetium-tagged albumin microspheres. *J. Surg. Res. 16:* 466–472, 1974.
226. Moskowitz, M., Zimmerman, H., and Felson, B. The meandering mesenteric artery of the colon. *Am. J. Roentgenol. 92:* 1088–1099, 1964.
227. Movius, H. J., II. Resection of abdominal arteriosclerotic aneurysm. *Am. J. Surg. 90:* 298–305, 1955.
228. Mulder, D. S., Winsberg, F., Cole, C. M., Blundell, P. E., and Scott, H. J. Ultrasonic "B" scanning of abdominal aortic aneurysms. *Ann. Thorac. Surg. 16:* 361–367, 1973.
229. Nemir, P., and Micozzi, M. Combined aneurysmal and occlusive arterial diease. *Circulation 56(2):* 169–170, 1977.
230. Ochsner, A., Jr., and DeCamp, P. T. Management of abdominal aorticoiliac aneurysms associated with occlusive arterial disease: a study of 31 operative cases. *South. Med. J. 53:* 732–735, 1960.
231. O'Donnell, T. F., Jr., Darling, R. C., and Linton, R. R. Is 80 years too old for aneurysmectomy? *Arch. Surg. 111:* 1250–1257, 1976.
232. Olcott, C., Holcroft, J., Stoney, R., and Wylie, E. Unusual problems of abdominal aortic aneurysms. *Am. J. Surg. 135:* 426–431, 1978.
233. O'Mara, C., and Imbembo, A. L. Paraprosthetic-enteric fistula. *Surgery 81:* 556–566, 1977.
234. Osler, W. Aneurysm of abdominal aorta. *Lancet 2:* 1089–1096, 1905.
235. Ottinger, L. W., Darling, R. C., Nathan, M. J., and Linton, R. R. Left colon ischemia complicating aorto-iliac reconstruction. *Arch. Surg. 105:* 841–846, 1972.
236. Page, I. H. The production of persistent arterial hypertension by cellophane perinephritis. *JAMA 113:* 2046–2048, 1939.
237. Papadopoulos, C. D., Mancini, H. W., and Marino, A. W. M., Jr. Ischemic necrosis of the colon following aortic aneurysmectomy. *J. Cardiovasc. Surg. 15:* 494–500, 1974.
238. Pasternak, B. M., Boyd, D. P., and Ellis, F. H. Spinal cord injury after procedures on the aorta. *Surg. Gynecol. Obstet. 135:* 29–34, 1972.
239. Pearse, H. E. Experimental studies on the gradual occlusion of large arteries. *Ann. Surg. 112:* 923–937, 1940.
240. Perdue, G. D., and Lowry, K. Arterial insufficiency to the colon following resection of abdominal aortic aneurysms. *Surg. Gynecol. Obstet. 115:* 39–44, 1962.
241. Pilcher, D. B., Davis, J. H., Ashikaga, T., Bookwater, J., Butsch, D. W., Chase, C. R., Ellman, B. R., Vacek, P. M., and Lord, C. F. Treatment of abdominal aortic aneurysm in an entire state over 7½ years. *Am. J. Surg. 139:* 487–494, 1980.
242. Pond, G. D., and Hillman, B. Evaluation of aneurysms by computed tomography. *Surgery 89:* 216–223, 1981.
243. Ponseti, I. V., and Baird, W. A. Scoliosis and dissecting aneurysm of the aorta in rats fed with Lathyrus odoratus seeds. *Am. J. Pathol. 28:* 1059–1078, 1952.
244. Poppe, J. K. Cellophane treatment of syphilitic aneurysms with report of results in six cases. *Am. Heart. J. 36:* 252–256, 1948.

245. Poppe, J. K., and de Oliveira, H. R. Treatment of syphilitic aneurysms by cellophane wrapping. *J. Thorac. Surg. 15:* 186–195, 1946.
246. Porter, J. M., McGregor, F., Jr., Acinapura, A. J., and Silver, D. Renal function following abdominal aortic aneurysmectomy. *Surg. Gynecol. Obstet. 123:* 819–825, 1966.
247. Power, D., and Colt, G. H. A case of aneurysm of the abdominal aorta treated by the introduction of silver wire. *Lancet 2:* 808–813, 1903.
248. Reckless, J. P. D., McColl, I., and Taylor, G. W. Aorto-caval fistulae. An uncommon complication of abdominal aortic aneurysms. *Br. J. Surg. 59:* 461–462, 1972.
249. Reich, M. P. Paraplegia following resection of an abdominal aortic aneurysm. *Vasc. Surg. 2:* 230–234, 1968.
250. Richardson, J. V., and McDowell, H. A. Anastomotic aneurysms following arterial grafting. A 10 year experience. *Ann. Surg. 184:* 179–182, 1976.
251. Rob, C., and Snyder, M. Chronic intestinal ischemia: a complication of surgery of the abdominal aorta. *Surgery 60:* 114–145, 1966.
252. Rob, C. G., and Williams, J. P. The diagnosis of aneurysms of the abdominal aorta (an analysis of 100 patients). *J. Cardiovasc. Surg. 2:* 55–59, 1961.
253. Robicsek, F. Discussion of Ottinger, L. W., Darling, R. C., and Nathan, M. J. Left colon ischemia complicating aorto-iliac reconstruction. *Arch. Surg. 105:* 841–846, 1972.
254. Robicsek, F., Daugherty, H. L., Mullen, D. C., Tam, W., and Scott, W. P. Value of angiography in the diagnosis of unruptured aneurysms of the abdominal aorta. *Ann. Thorac. Surg. 11:* 538–550, 1971.
255. Rosenthal, D., Deterling, R. A., Jr., O'Donnell, T. F., Jr., and Callow, A. D. Positive blood culture as an aid in the diagnosis of secondary aortoenteric fistula. *Arch. Surg. 114:* 1041–1044, 1979.
256. Ruffin, M. de G., Castleman, B., and White, P. D. P. Arteriosclerotic aneurysms and senile ectasia of thoracic aorta. *Am. Heart J. 22:* 458–468, 1941.
257. Scales, J. T. Tissue reactions to synthetic materials. *Proc. R. Soc. Med. 46:* 641–652, 1953.
258. Schatz, I. J., Fairbairn, J. F., II, and Juergens, J. L. Abdominal aortic aneurysms: a reappraisal. *Circulation 26:* 200–205, 1962.
259. Selle, J. G., Robicsek, F., Daugherty, H. K., and Cook, J. W. Thoracoabdominal aortic aneurysms. A review and current status. *Ann. Surg. 189:* 158–164, 1979.
260. Sheil, A. G. R., Reeve, T. S., Little, J. M., Coupland, G. A. E., and Lowenthal, J. Aorto-intestinal fistulas following operation on the abdominal aorta and iliac arteries. *Br. J. Surg. 56:* 840–843, 1969.
261. Sher, M. H., and Healy, E. H. Paraplegia following infrarenal aneurysmorrhaphy. *Vasc. Surg. 5:* 171–176, 1971.
262. Sheranian, L. O., Edwards, J. E., and Kirklin, J. W. Late results in 100 patients with abdominal aortic aneurysm treated by resectional placement of aortic homograft. *Surg. Gynecol. Obstet. 109:* 309–314, 1959.
263. Shumacker, H. B., Jr., Barnes, D. L., and King, H. Ruptured abdominal aortic aneurysms. *Ann. Surg. 177:* 772–779, 1973.
264. Shumacker, H. B., Jr., Harris, E. J., and Siderys, H. Pliable plastic tubes as aortic substitutes. *Surgery 37:* 80–93, 1955.
265. Shumacker, H. B., Jr., and King, H. The use of pliable plastic tubes as aortic substitutes in man. *Surg. Gynecol. Obstet. 99:* 287–294, 1954.
266. Sink, J. D., Myers, R. T., and James, P. M. Ruptured abdominal aortic aneurysms: review of 33 cases treated surgically and discussion of prognostic indicators. *Am. Surg. 42:* 303–307, 1976.
267. Skillman, J. J., Zervas, N. T., Weintraub, R. M., and Mayman, C. I. Paraplegia after resection of aneurysms of the abdominal aorta. *N. Engl. J. Med. 281:* 422–425, 1969.
268. Smith, P. K., Fuchs, J. C. A., and Sabiston, D. C., Jr. Surgical management of aortic abdominal aneurysms in patients with severe pulmonary insufficiency. *Surg. Gynecol. Obstet. 151:* 407–411, 1980.
269. Smith, R. A. Neurological complications of extraspinal arterial origin. *Am. Surg. 42:* 679–684, 1976.

270. Smith, R. F., and Szilagyi, D. E. Ischemia of the colon as a complication in the surgery of the abdominal aorta. *Arch. Surg. 80:* 806–821, 1960.
271. Sommerville, R. L., Allen, E. V., and Edwards, J. E. Bland and infected arteriosclerotic abdominal aortic aneurysms: a clinicopathologic study. *Medicine 38:* 207–221, 1959.
272. Sondheimmer, J. L., and Steinberg, I. Gastrointestinal manifestations of abdominal aortic aneurysms. *Am. J. Roentgenol. 92:* 1110–1122, 1964.
273. Spanos, P. K., Gilsdorf, R. B., Sako, Y., and Najarian, J. S. The management of infected abdominal grafts and graft-enteric fistulas. *Ann. Surg. 183:* 397–400, 1976.
274. Stahl, W. M., and Stone, A. M. Prophylactic diuresis with ethacrynic acid for prevention of postoperative renal failure. *Ann. Surg. 172:* 361–369, 1970.
275. Stallworth, J. M., and Ramirezf, A. A. A method of treatment of complicated aneurysms of the abdominal aorta. *Ann. Surg. 169:* 282–289, 1969.
276. Star, D., Lawrie, G., and Morris, G. Prevention of distal embolism during arterial reconstruction. *Am. J. Surg. 138:* 764–769, 1979.
277. Starr, D. S., Weatherford, S. C., Lawrie, G. M., and Morris, G. L., Jr. Suture material as a factor in the occurrence of anastomotic false aneurysms. An analysis of 26 cases. *Arch. Surg. 114:* 412–415, 1979.
278. Steinberg, I., and Stein, H. L. Visualization of abdominal aortic aneurysms. *Am. J. Roentgenol. 95:* 684–695, 1965.
279. Steward, J. A., and Rankin, F. W. Blood supply of the large intestine: its surgical considerations. *Arch. Surg. 26:* 843–891, 1933.
280. Stokes, J., and Butcher, H. R., Jr. Abdominal aortic aneurysms: factors influencing operative mortality and criteria of operability. *Arch. Surg. 107:* 297–302, 1973.
281. Strandness, D. E., and Sumner, D. S. *Hemodynamics for Surgeons.* Grune & Stratton, New York, 1975.
282. Suh, T. H., and Alexander, L. Vascular system of the human spinal cord. *Arch. Neurol. Psychiat. 41:* 569–659–677, 1939.
283. Suzuki, M., Collins, G., Bassinga, G., and Dilley, R. Aorto-left renal vein fistula—an unusual complication of abdominal aortic aneurysm. *Ann. Surg. 184:* 31–34, 1976.
284. Swanson, R. J., Littooy, F. J., Hunt, T. K., and Stoney, R. J. Laparatomy as a precipitating factor in the rupture of intra-abdominal aneurysms. *Arch. Surg. 115:* 299–304, 1980.
285. Szilagyi, D. E. Clinical fate of the patient with asymptomatic abdominal aortic aneurysm and unfit for surgical treatment. *Arch. Surg. 104:* 600–606, 1982.
286. Szilagyi, D. E., Elliott, J. P., and Smith, R. F. Ruptured abdominal aneurysms simulating sepsis. *Arch. Surg. 91:* 263–275, 1965.
287. Szilagyi, D. E., Hageman, J. H., Smith, R. F., and Elliot, J. P. Spinal cord damage in surgery of the abdominal aorta. *Surgery 83:* 38–56, 1978.
288. Szilagyi, D. E., Smith, R. F., DeRusso, F. J., Elliot, J. P., and Sherrin, F. W. Contribution of abdominal aortic aneurysmectomy to prolongation of life. *Ann. Surg. 164:* 678–699, 1966.
289. Tanon, L. Les arteres de la moelle dorsolombaire. Consideratuons anatomiques et cliniques. These de Paris, Vigot, Paris, 1908.
290. Tchirkow, G., and Bevin, E. G. Leg ischemia following surgery of abdominal aortic aneurysm. *Ann. Surg. 188:* 166–170, 1978.
291. Thompson, B. W., Read, R. C., and Campbell, G. S. Uninfected false aneurysms after arterial reconstruction with prosthetic grafts. *Am. J. Surg. 138:* 920–923, 1979.
292. Thompson, J. E., Hollier, L. E., Patman, R. D., and Persson, A. V. Surgical management of abdominal aortic aneurysms: factors influencing mortality and morbidity—a 20 year experience. *Ann. Surg. 181:* 654–661, 1975.
293. Thompson, J. E., Vollman, R. W., Austin, D. J., and Kartchner, M. M. Prevention of the hypotensive and renal complications of aortic surgery using balanced salt solution. Thirteen year experience with 670 cases. *Ann. Surg. 167:* 767–778, 1968.
294. Thompson, W. M., Johnsrude, I. S., Jackson, D., Okder, R., and Wechsler, A. Late complications of abdominal aortic reconstructive surgery: roentgen evaluation. *Ann. Surg. 185:* 326–334, 1977.
295. Tilney, N. L., Bailey, C. J., and Morgan, A. P. Sequential system failure after rupture of abdominal aortic aneurysm: an unsolved problem in postoperative care. *Ann. Surg.*

178: 117–122, 1973.
296. Tilson, M. D., and Dang, C. Generalized arteriomegaly. A possible predisposition to the formation of abdominal aortic aneurysms. *Arch. Surg. 116:* 1030–1032, 1981.
297. Turnbull, I. M. Blood supply of the spinal cord. In *Handbook of Clinical Neurology*, edited by P. J. Vinken and G. W. Bruyn, vol. 12, part II, chapter 18, pp. 478–491. American Elsevier, New York, 1972.
298. Volpetti, B., Bacher, C. J., Berkowitz, H., and Roberts, B. Twenty-two year review of elective resection of abdominal aortic aneurysm. *Surg. Gynecol. Obstet. 142:* 321–324, 1976.
299. Voorhees, A. B., Jr. Discussion of Moore, W. S., and Hall, A. D. Late suture failure in the pathogenesis of anastomotic false aneurysms. *Ann. Surg. 172:* 1064–1068, 1970.
300. Voorhees, A. B., Jr., Jaretzki, A. T., and Blakemore, A. H. The use of tubes constructed of Vinyon "N" cloth in bridging arterial defects—experimental and clinical. *Ann. Surg. 140:* 324–329, 1954.
301. Wakabayashi, A., and Connolly, J. E. Prevention of paraplegia associated with resection of extensive thoracic aneurysms. *Arch. Surg. 111:* 1186–1189, 1976.
302. Walden, R., L'Italien, G. J., Megerman, J., and Abbott, W. M. Matched elastic properties and successful arterial grafting. *Arch. Surg. 115:* 1166–1169, 1980.
303. Wangensteen, O. H., and Wangensteen, S. D. *The Rise of Surgery.* University of Minnesota Press, Minneapolis, 1978.
304. Weinstein, M. H., and Machleder, H. I. Sexual function after aorto-iliac surgery. *Ann. Surg. 181:* 787–790, 1975.
305. Welsh, P. A. Surgical treatment of multiple aortic aneurysms. *Geriatrics 24:* 69–71, 1969.
306. Whittemore, A. D., Clowes, A. W., Hechtman, H. B., and Mannick, J. A. Aortic aneurysm repair. Reduced operative mortality associated with maintenance of optimal cardiac performance. *Ann. Surg. 192:* 414–421, 1980.
307. Wierman, W. H., Straham, R. W., and Spencer, J. R. Small bowel erosion by synthetic aortic grafts. *Am. J. Surg. 112:* 791–797, 1962.
308. Wolffe, J. B., and Colcher, R. E. Diagnosis and conservative management of atherosclerotic aneurysms of the abdominal aorta. *Vasc. Dis. 3:* 49–57, 1966.
309. Wolinsky, H., and Glagov, S. A lamellar unit of aortic medial structure and function in mammals. *Circ. Res. 20:* 99–111, 1967.
310. Wolinsky, H., and Glagov, S. Comparison of abdominal and thoracic aortic medial structure in mammals. Deviation of man from the usual pattern. *Circ. Res. 25:* 677–686, 1969.
311. Wolinsky, H., and Glagov, S. Nature of species differences in the medial distribution of aortic vasa vasorum in mammals. *Circ. Res. 20:* 409–421, 1967.
312. Wright, I. S., Urdaneta, E., and Wright, B. Re-opening the case of the abdominal aortic aneurysm. *Circulation 13:* 754–768, 1956.
313. Yashar, J. J., Indeglia, R. A., and Yashar, J. Surgery for abdominal aortic aneurysms. *Am. J. Surg. 123:* 398–405, 1972.
314. Youmans, C. R., and Derrick, J. R. Gastrointestinal erosion after prosthetic arterial reconstructive surgery. *Am. J. Surg. 114:* 711–715, 1967.
315. Young, A., Sandberg, G., and Couch, N. Reduction of mortality of abdominal aortic aneurysm resection. *Am. J. Surg. 134:* 585–590, 1977.
316. Young, J. R., Humphries, A. W., DeWolf, V. G., and LeFeure, F. A. Complications of abdominal aortic surgery. Intestinal ischemia. *Arch. Surg. 86:* 51–59, 1963.
317. Zuber, W. F., Gaspar, M. R., and Rothschild, P. D. The anterior spinal artery syndrome—a complication of abdominal aortic surgery: report of five cases and review of the literature. *Ann. Surg. 172:* 909–915, 1970.
318. Zulch, K. J. Mangeldurchblutung an der grenzzone zweier gefassegebiete als ursache bisher ungklarter ruckenmarksschadigungen. *Dtsch. Z. Nervenheilkd. 172:* 81–89, 1954.

CHAPTER 7

Management of Femoral and Popliteal Aneurysms

EDWARD A. STEMMER, M.D.

Although peripheral artery aneurysms are only 5% as frequent as abdominal aortic aneurysms, 90% of these lesions occur in the femoral and popliteal areas (1); one-third develop in the femoral artery; while two-thirds occur in the popliteal space. In view of the ready accessibility of peripheral aneurysms to inspection and palpation, it is somewhat surprising to note that one-third of patients with femoral or popliteal aneurysms present because of some surgical emergency (e.g., rupture, thrombosis, infection, embolization, or gangrene) distal to the involved vessel (1).

The history of treatment of peripheral aneurysms dates at least to 170 A.D., when Galen described the lesions and emphasized their potential for life-threatening hemorrhage. Shortly thereafter, Antyllus described treating femoral aneurysms by ligation both above and below the sac. Although this technique frequently resulted in loss of limb from gangrene, it remained the standard of treatment for more than 1,000 years. Actual excision of the aneurysmal sac was performed by Philagrius following the reintroduction of Antyllus's procedure by Ambrose Pare in the 16th century, as reported in the review by Queral *et al.* (12). In 1785, John Hunter described ligation of the femoral artery some distance proximal to a popliteal aneurysm in a successful effort to preserve collaterals and reduce the frequency of amputation following ligation (4). In 1896, J. B. Murphy successfully restored direct arterial continuity by end-to-end anastomosis following resection of a pseudoaneurysm of the femoral artery (13). In 1902, Rudolph Matas (9) applied his technique of endoaneurysmorrhaphy to obliterate a popliteal aneurysm and restore continuity of flow. From 1902 to 1912, Carrel and Guthrie described many of the basic techniques of direct arterial repair. Goyanes, in 1906, and Lexer, in 1907, first employed veins as interposition grafts for the repair of peripheral aneurysms. Although the problems associated with distal ischemia following obliteration of peripheral aneurysms had been recognized from the outset (2, 4, 9, 10), it was not until 1935 that sympathectomy was employed by Bird (2) as an adjunct to endoaneurysmorrhaphy. The modern treatment of aneurysms began in 1951, when Dubost *et al.* (7) described the use of arterial homografts. The following year, Blakemore and Voorhees (3) employed textile grafts (Vinyon "N") in the treatment of aneurysmal disease.

ETIOLOGY

Femoral and popliteal aneurysms can develop as the result of arteriosclerotic disease, trauma, syphilis, or infection. While true aneurysms secondary to trauma or syphilis were relatively common in John Hunter's time, they are infrequently seen now. Similarly, primary mycotic aneurysms (a term coined by Sir William Osler in 1885) are uncommon (10). Some 90% of the true aneurysms of the femoral and popliteal arteries are arteriosclerotic in origin.

Modern medical and social habits, however, have resulted in significant changes in the types of femoral aneurysms that are seen. With the advent of retrograde angiography, cardiac catheterization, aortofemoral bypass grafting, balloon counterpulsation, and direct arterial puncture for monitoring, pseudoaneurysms of the femoral artery now outnumber the true femoral artery aneurysms. Often these pseudoaneurysms are septic as well. Figure 7.1 illustrates a mycotic pseudoaneurysm secondary to balloon counterpulsation employed to treat cardiogenic shock following myocardial infarction. The drug culture has also produced an increasing number of mycotic aneurysms and pseudoaneurysms as addicts purposely or inadvertently puncture their femoral arteries.

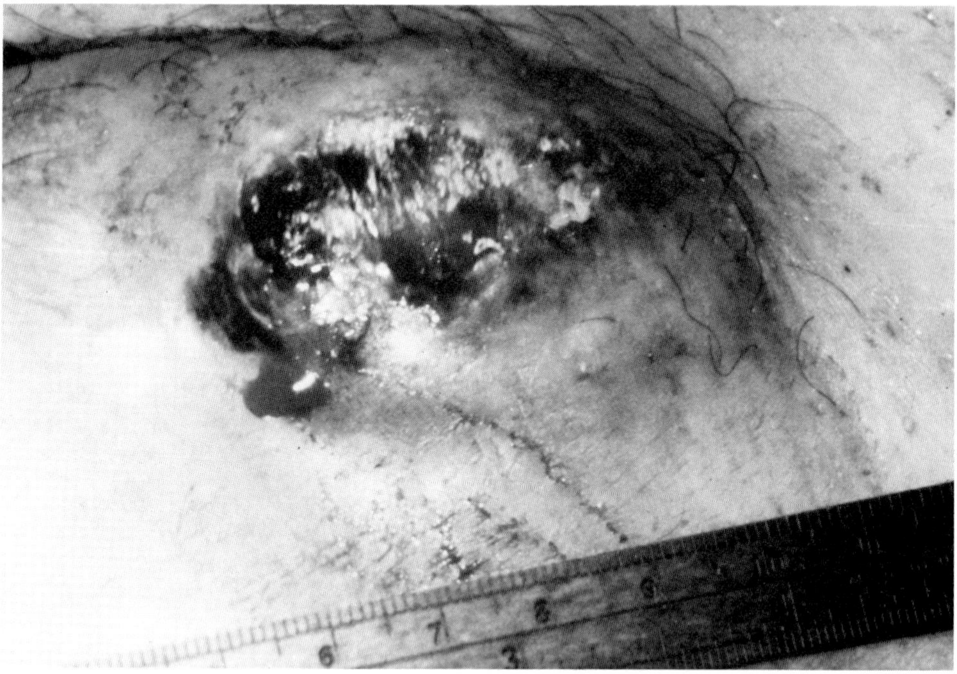

Figure 7.1. Infected femoral pseudoaneurysm secondary to prolonged intra-aortic balloon counterpulsation.

CLINICAL PRESENTATION AND COURSE

Most commonly, femoral aneurysms are discovered when a pulsatile mass is detected by the patient or by the physician on routine physical examination. Approximately one-third of patients with femoral aneurysms are asymptomatic; another one-third present with swelling, tenderness, and local pain (14). Somewhat surprisingly, the remaining one-third of the patients present with some type of surgical emergency, which underscores the treacherous nature of this entity (1). The incidence of thrombosis of a femoral aneurysm has been reported to be as high as 65% (14). Pappas *et al.* (11) reported a 16% incidence of amputation secondary to complications, while rupture of the aneurysm occurred in 5 to 15% of patients. Seventy to 95% of patients with a femoral aneurysm have aneurysms elsewhere, most often in the abdominal aorta. While infection is only infrequently associated with anastomotic pseudoaneurysms of the femoral artery, it is a frequent occurrence when the pseudoaneurysm occurs as a result of drug abuse. Somewhat uniquely, three infected pseudoaneurysms of the femoral artery have occurred in our hospital as a result of long-term intra-aortic balloon counterpulsation. Rupture of an infected pseudoaneurysm is inevitable unless prompt treatment is instituted.

Ninety to 100% of popliteal aneurysms occur in males, usually between the ages of 50 to 80 years. As with femoral aneurysms, the diagnosis of a popliteal aneurysm is usually made by palpation and inspection. The frequency with which the patient presents with complications of a popliteal aneurysm, however, is greater than is the case in patients with a femoral aneurysm. Chitwood *et al.* (4) reported that 15% of the patients in their series presented with thrombophlebitis, 27% with claudication, 15% with gangrene, and 19% with embolization. Barker (1) estimated that in his experience 10% of acute femoropopliteal occlusions were due to complications of popliteal aneurysms. Calcification of a popliteal aneurysm is commonly visible on X-ray of the extremity. These aneurysms are present bilaterally in from 30 to 50% of patients. Even when the popliteal aneurysm is initially asymptomatic, complications develop in 30 to 75% of untreated patients followed for one to eight years (5, 8, 15). Amputation is necessary in from 16 to 44% of untreated patients who develop a complication of their disease (6).

As Barker and others have stated, it is apparent that elective surgical repair of femoral and popliteal aneurysms is mandatory for all but the most debilitated patients. In the presence of an infected aneurysm or pseudoaneurysm, urgent treatment is necessary if rupture of the aneurysm is to be avoided.

OPERATIVE MANAGEMENT

Elective repair of true aneurysms in the femoropopliteal area is indicated primarily for prevention of the complications of the disease (as described earlier). Semi-elective repair of non-infected pseudoaneurysms is indicated to prevent the almost certain rupture of these lesions if operation is deferred. Urgent or even emergent repair of infected aneurysms or pseudoaneurysms is necessary to treat the septic process, as well as prevent rupture. As illustrated in Figure 7.1, these lesions commonly involve and erode the overlying skin. Except in the case of infected aneurysms, simple ligation, the standard of treatment until the late 19th century, has little place today. Resection or exclusion of the aneurysm with reconstruction of the arterial circulation is the appropriate treatment, with the possible exception of popliteal aneurysms in which the runoff vessels are occluded. In this latter situation, ligation of the aneurysm with concomitant lumbar sympathectomy, as advocated by Bird (2) in 1935, may preserve the patient's extremity. Except in emergent situations, angiography should be performed routinely to demonstrate the patency of distal vessels, as well as to delineate the extent of the aneurysm. Ultrasonography has a limited role in the diagnosis of femoral or popliteal aneurysms, since most are readily apparent on physical examination. On occasion, however, this technique may be valuable in distinguishing a puncture pseudoaneurysm from a hematoma early in the course of the disease. Ultrasonography may also aid in the diagnosis of a contralateral popliteal aneurysm in a patient known to have one such lesion.

A variety of graft materials may be employed; primarily, these consist of autogenous vein, Dacron, and expanded polytetrafluorethylene (Gore-Tex). Bovine heterografts have proven to be unacceptable substitutes, since they themselves are prone to aneurysmal dilatation (Fig. 7.2). Autogenous vein yields the best long-term results (particularly in the popliteal region); but, in the femoral area, the available vein may be of too small a caliber to match the common femoral artery.

True femoral aneurysms most often begin distal to the deep epigastric vessels and usually do not extend into the deep or superficial femoral arteries; they can usually be approached through a groin incision extending distally over Hunter's canal. Care should be taken to preserve the deep epigastric vessels, if possible, since they may be an essential part of the collateral circulation. After proximal and distal control are obtained, the aneurysm is opened and then excised. Vascular continuity is reestablished using a suitable graft. If a synthetic graft is employed, it is imperative that nonabsorbable synthetic sutures be employed, since silk sutures deteriorate with time, leading to the formation of anastomotic pseudoaneurysms. Should the femoral aneurysm extend proximally into the external iliac artery, control of this vessel can be readily obtained by an extraperitoneal approach above the inguinal ligament. Should the aneurysm extend into the deep or superficial femoral arteries, a bifurcation type of graft is employed. Prophylactic antibiotics are routinely employed for all vascular reconstructive procedures in the groin. Bypass grafting leaving the femoral aneurysm in continuity with the circulation is not indicated, since this procedure does not eliminate the potential complications of a femoral aneurysm.

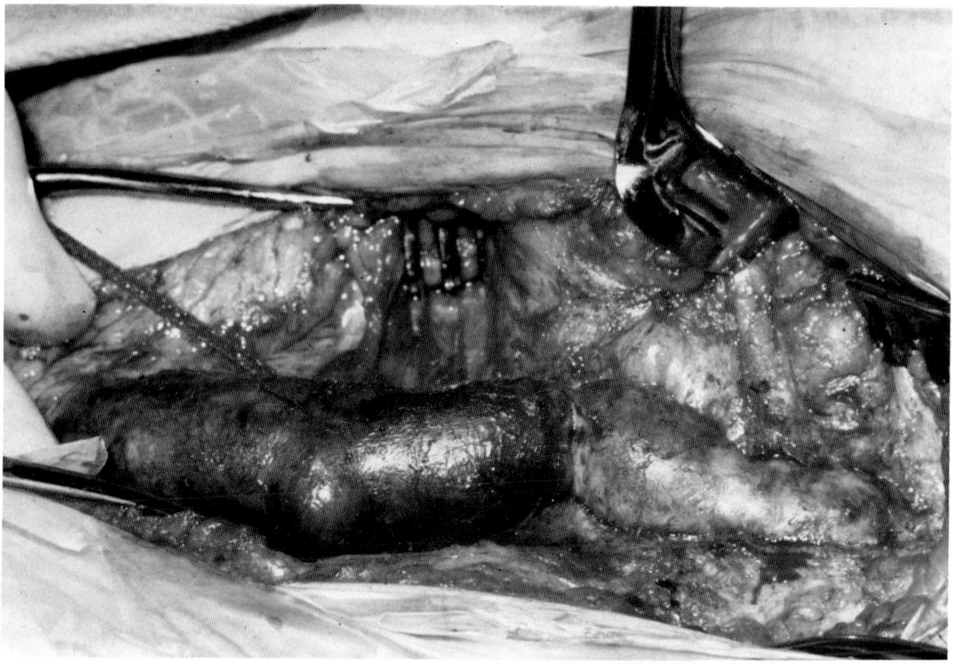

Figure 7.2. Aneurysmal dilatation of a bovine heterograft placed in the femoro-popliteal region.

Anastomotic pseudoaneurysms of the femoral artery are a complication of aortoiliac reconstruction utilizing synthetic grafts. While infection of the femoral suture line is not a frequent cause of these aneurysms, should infection occur, the formation of an anastomotic pseudoaneurysm is inevitable. Most often when these aneurysms are explored, the surgeon finds an intact suture in the synthetic graft which has retracted from the common femoral artery (Fig. 7.3). It is important to remember that scars contract in three dimensions; therefore, the femoral limbs of the synthetic graft should not be stretched tightly at the time of the distal anastomosis. The rule, of course, is to suture without tension. Suturing of the cloth limb to an endarterectomized segment of the common femoral artery will significantly increase the incidence of this complication.

Repair of an anastomotic pseudoaneurysm of the common femoral artery is much like that of a true aneurysm, with two important exceptions. Isolation of the feeding vessels must also include control of the limb of the synthetic graft. In addition, tissue reaction in the area may make control of the deep femoral artery difficult, dangerous, or impossible. In any event, once inflow and outflow vessels are controlled (Fig. 7.4), the aneurysm is opened and the inevitable clot evacuated (Fig. 7.5). If control of the profunda femoris artery has not been achieved, it may

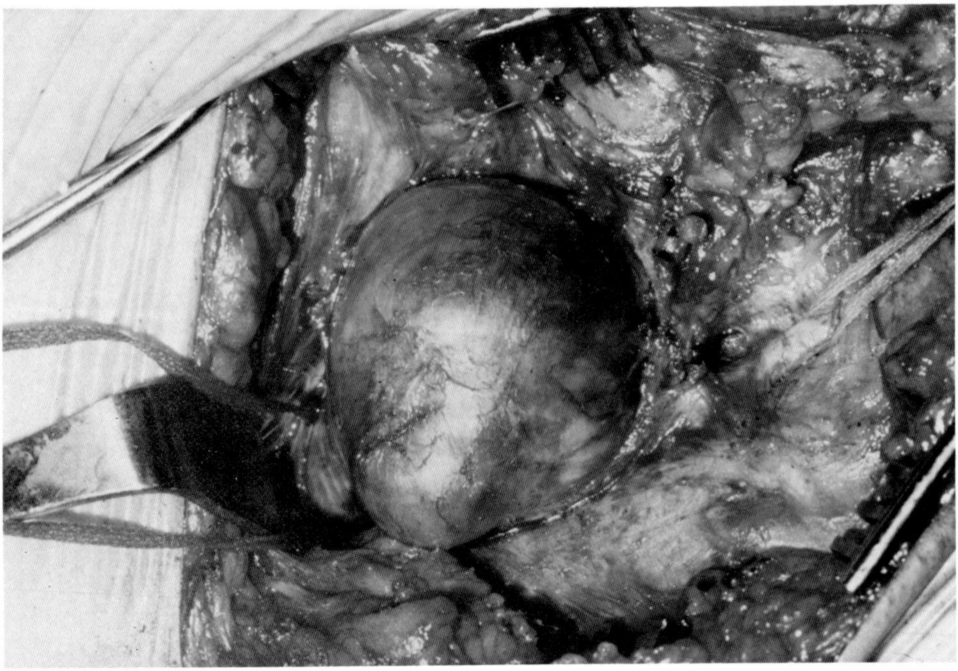

Figure 7.3. Anastomotic femoral pseudoaneurysm (the crimped Dacron graft is visible under the retractor).

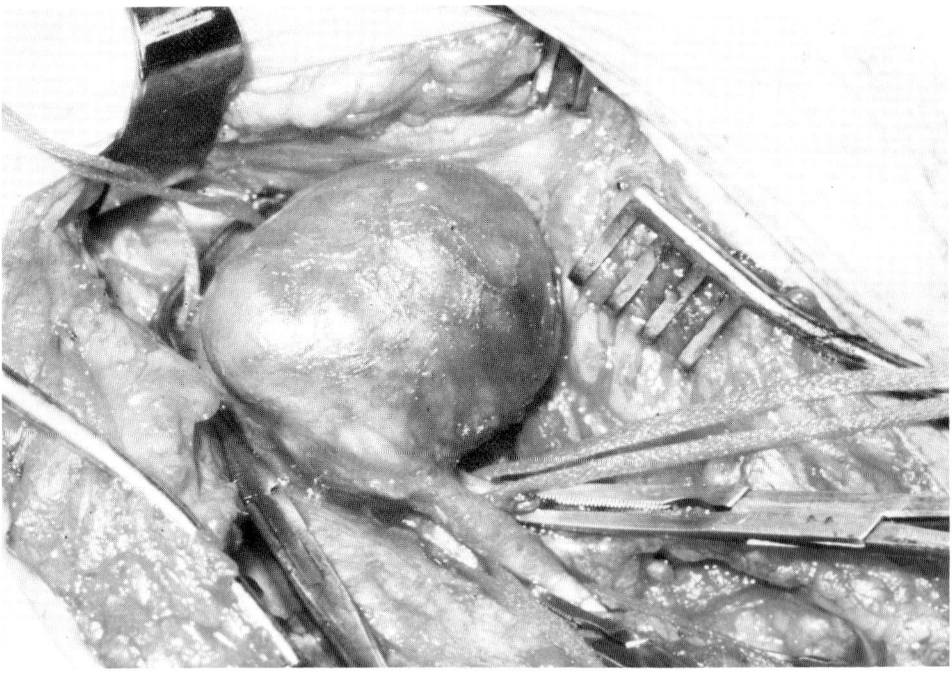

Figure 7.4. Control of inflow and outflow of a femoral pseudoaneurysm.

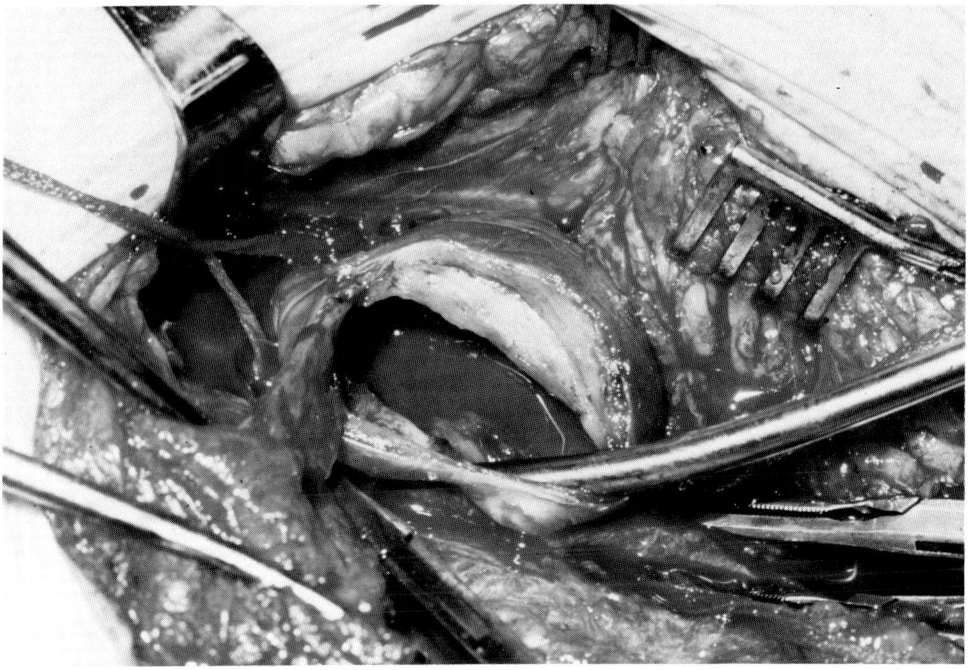

Figure 7.5. Femoral pseudoaneurysm opened to reveal fresh and organized thrombus.

now be occluded by a balloon catheter inserted into its orifice. The aneurysmal sac is then removed (Fig. 7.6). A flared tube of synthetic material is sutured to the stump of the aortoiliac graft proximally and as a "roof" patch to the common femoral artery distally (Figs. 7.7 and 7.8).

Non-infected pseudoaneurysms secondary to trauma or puncture wounds can often be treated by evacuation of the hematoma from the sac, identification of the arterial defect, and direct closure of the puncture site with removal of the sac of the pseudoaneurysm. Should the arterial injury be too extensive to permit direct closure without excessive narrowing of the lumen, division of the common femoral artery and re-anastomosis or graft interposition may be necessary. On occasion, the injury may involve the bifurcation of the deep and superficial femoral arteries. In this situation, a modified profundaplasty may be necessary to restore continuity of flow.

Infected pseudoaneurysms of the common femoral artery (Fig. 7.1) are, by far, the most difficult to treat of these lesions, partly because of the septic process itself and partly because of the high rate of failure in attempts to restore direct arterial continuity. Certainly, placing a synthetic graft in an infected field is doomed to failure. Even the use of autogenous vein, allegedly more resistant to infection, will usually result in dehiscence of the suture line and hemorrhage. In a review by Queral

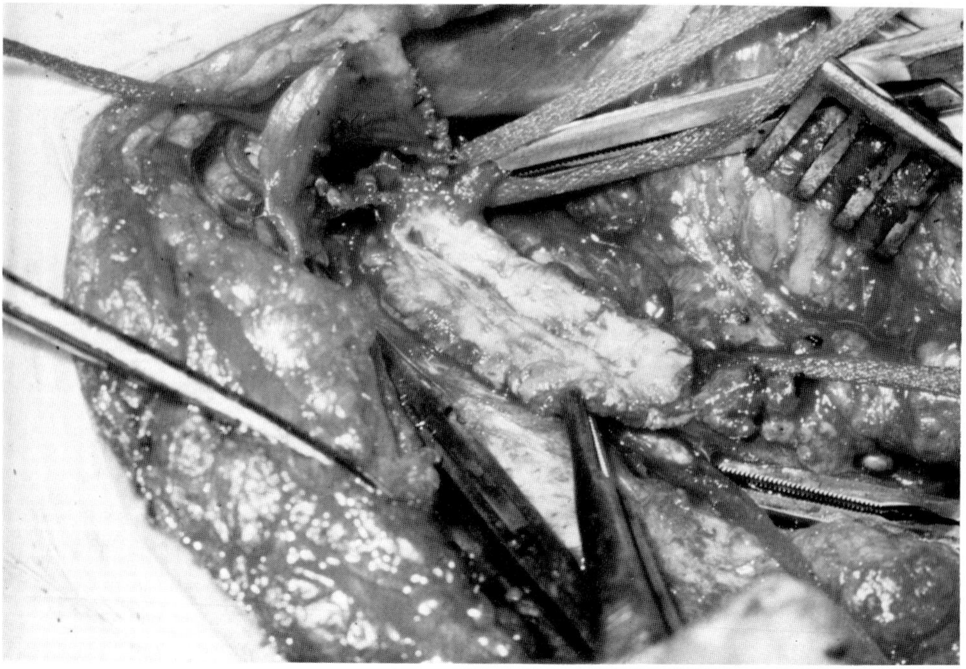

Figure 7.6. Sac of the femoral pseudoaneurysm trimmed to the margins of the common femoral artery.

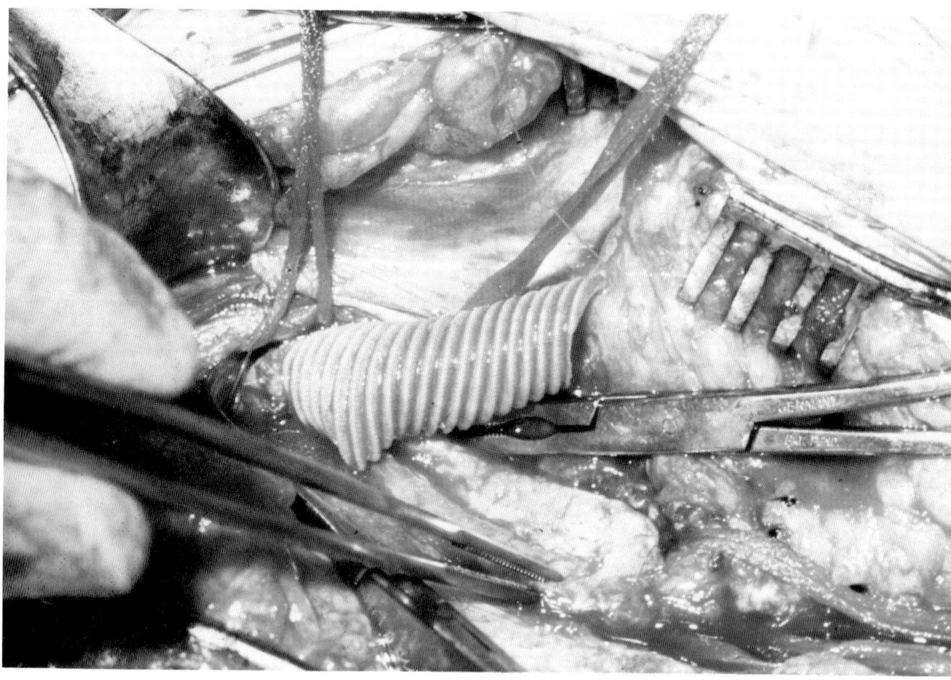

Figure 7.7. Dacron patch sewn to the distal limb of the aortobifemoral graft and being sewn to the native common femoral artery.

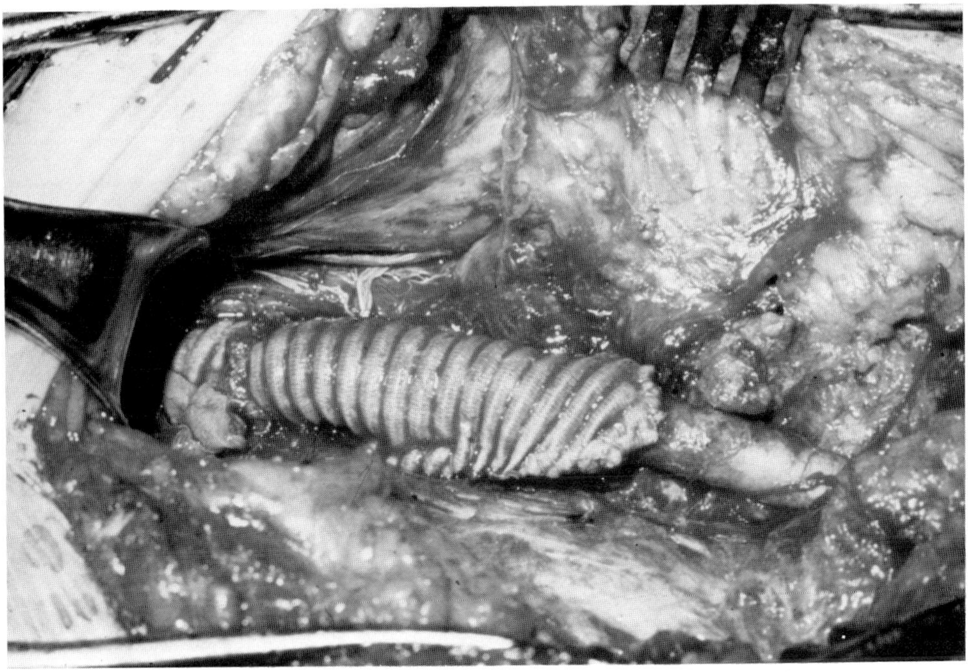

Figure 7.8. Repair of femoral pseudoaneurysm completed.

et al. (12), they stated that beginning with Ambrose Pare it has become apparent that these lesions are best treated by proximal and distal ligation, removal of the infected sac, open drainage of the wound, and appropriate antibiotic therapy. Figure 7.9 demonstrates the opened sac of an infected pseudoaneurysm of the superficial artery secondary to long-term intra-arterial balloon counterpulsation. Figure 7.10 demonstrates that the septic portion of the superficial femoral artery has been removed and the common femoral artery closed in such a manner that flow into the deep femoral artery is preserved. More often, however, it is the common femoral artery itself that is involved in the septic process. In this situation, the common femoral artery is debrided and ligated proximally; the deep and superficial femoral arteries are also ligated. No attempt is made to restore direct distal blood flow during the initial operation. In either situation, a layer of tissue is closed over the exposed vessels and the remainder of the wound is packed open. Postoperatively, the patient is observed carefully for signs of progressive ischemia of the limb using Doppler ankle pressures. If limb blood flow improves over the next 24 to 72 hours and the limb appears viable, reconstruction of the arterial circulation is delayed at least until the wounds heal. Reconstruction may be delayed indefinitely, depending upon the patient's general condition and degree of claudication experienced. Should observation or

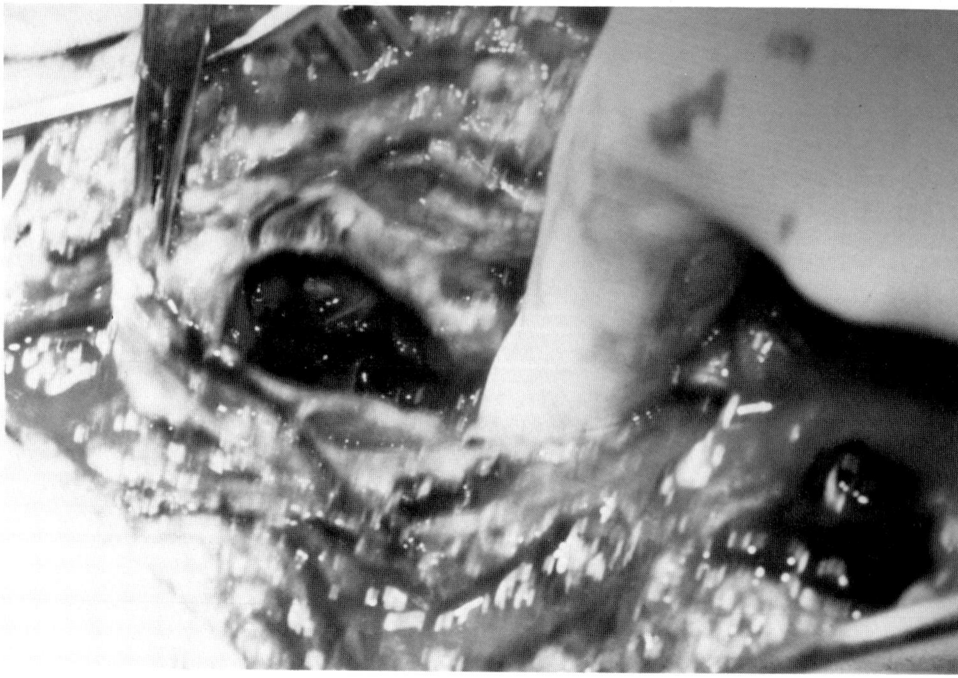

Figure 7.9. Sac of the infected femoral pseudoaneurysm shown in Figure 7.1 opened and revealing fresh clot.

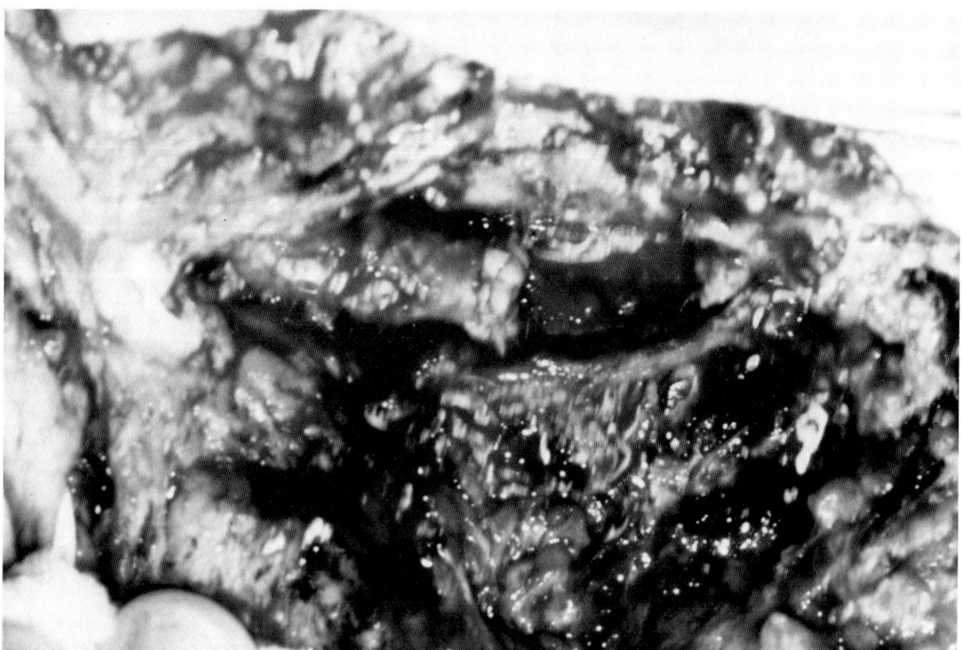

Figure 7.10. Infected femoral pseudoaneurysm debrided and stump of the common femoral artery closed, restoring flow into the deep femoral artery.

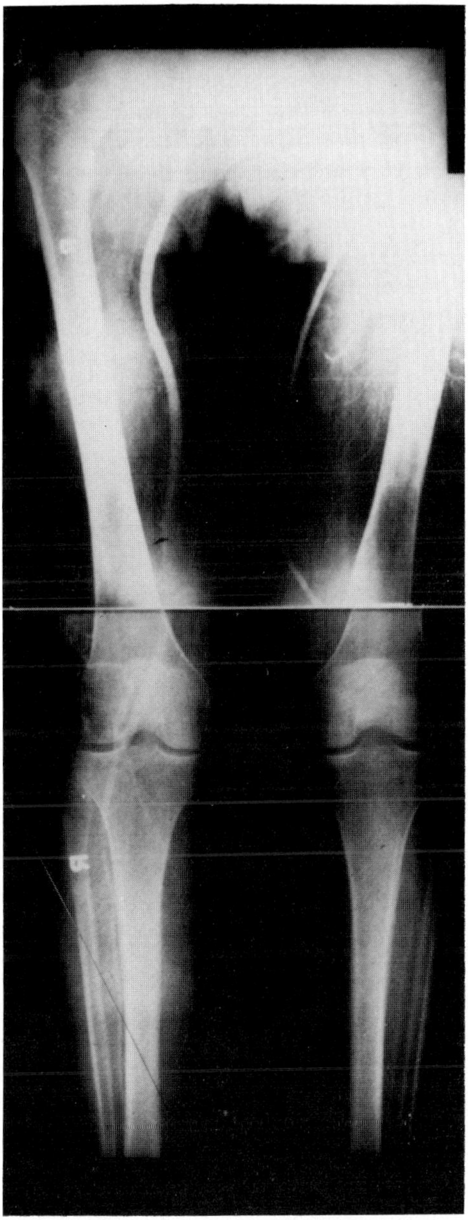

Figure 7.11. Angiogram taken one year following repair of an infected femoral pseudoaneurysm, showing a patent iliopopliteal Dacron graft placed when limb ischemia developed after ligation of the pseudoaneurysm (a patent left femoropopliteal vein graft is also apparent).

Doppler measurements indicate the limb is in jeopardy, restoration of the distal flow is undertaken, unless the patient's condition is so grave that it would seem prudent to settle for an amputation. If reconstruction is attempted, it is imperative the graft be placed in such a manner that the infected area is avoided. Figure 7.11 illustrates such a patient in whom a Dacron graft was sewn to the common iliac artery, led through the obturator foramen, and anastomosed distally to the popliteal artery far outside the area of infection. The angiogram taken one year later demonstrates the patent Dacron graft, as well as a contralateral femoropopliteal saphenous vein graft.

Ninety percent or more of popliteal aneurysms are fusiform enlargements secondary to arteriosclerosis. Excision of the aneurysm is the usual treatment, followed by reconstruction of the distal circulation using a reversed segment of the saphenous vein. Not infrequently, however, the size of the aneurysm or the reaction about it is such that complete removal of the popliteal aneurysm can result in serious injury to the closely associated popliteal vein or adjacent neural structures. In this situation, the aneurysm can be successfully treated by exclusion between ligatures and restoration of vascular continuity by a bypass graft using a

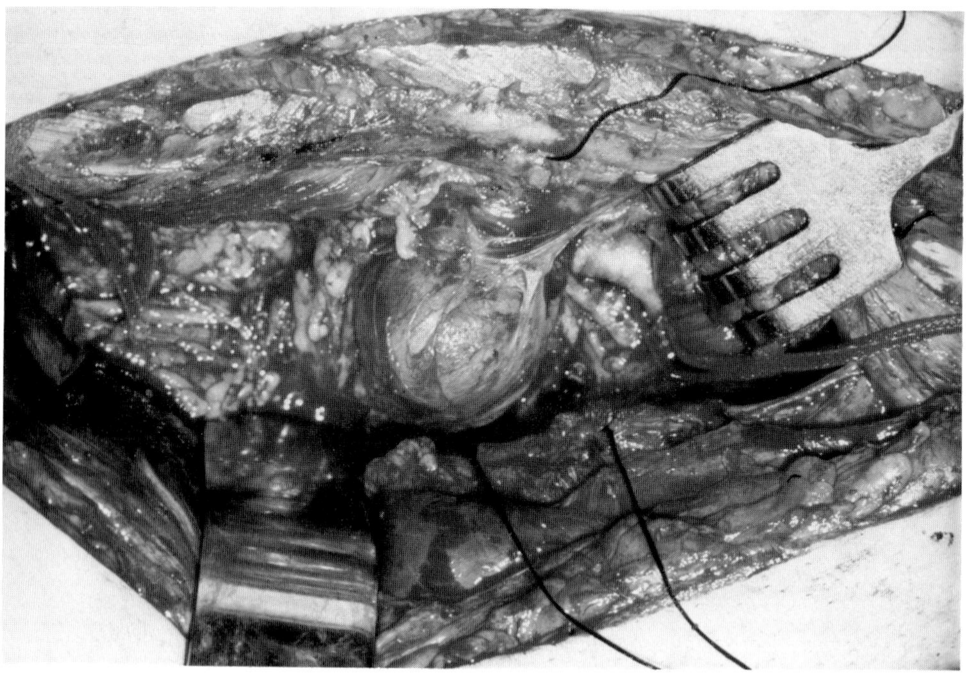

Figure 7.12. Popliteal aneurysm exposed revealing dense surrounding fibrous reaction.

reversed segment of the saphenous vein. Figure 7.12 depicts a patient in whom intense fibrous reaction surrounds the popliteal aneurysm. After proximal and distal control are obtained, the aneurysm is opened (Fig. 7.13), trimmed to reduce its bulk, and closed excluding the diseased vessel from circulation (Fig. 7.14). Continuity of circulation has been restored by means of a saphenous vein graft. In patients with a thrombosed popliteal aneurysm, the runoff vessels may also be partially occluded, necessitating extension of the distal graft into one of the tibial vessels. Delayed angiograms are essential in the evaluation of such patients for reconstruction. In some patients, the distal vessels may not be suitable for grafting even though the popliteal aneurysm remains patent. In this situation, ligation of the aneurysm with ipsilateral sympathectomy may be the only treatment feasible.

Pseudoaneurysms of the popliteal artery can also occur, primarily as a result of trauma to the area. As pointed out by Rich (13), gunshot wounds and blunt trauma are the most common wounding agents in the civilian population. Surgical repair of these lesions is indicated to prevent complications of the pseudoaneurysms (as described earlier).

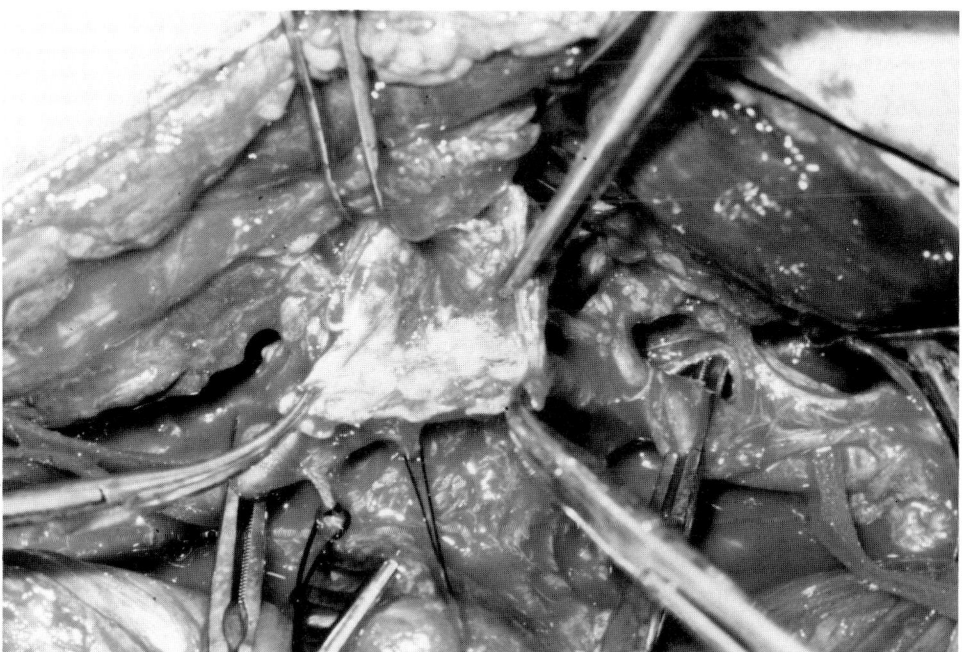

Figure 7.13. Popliteal aneurysm opened after proximal and distal control have been obtained.

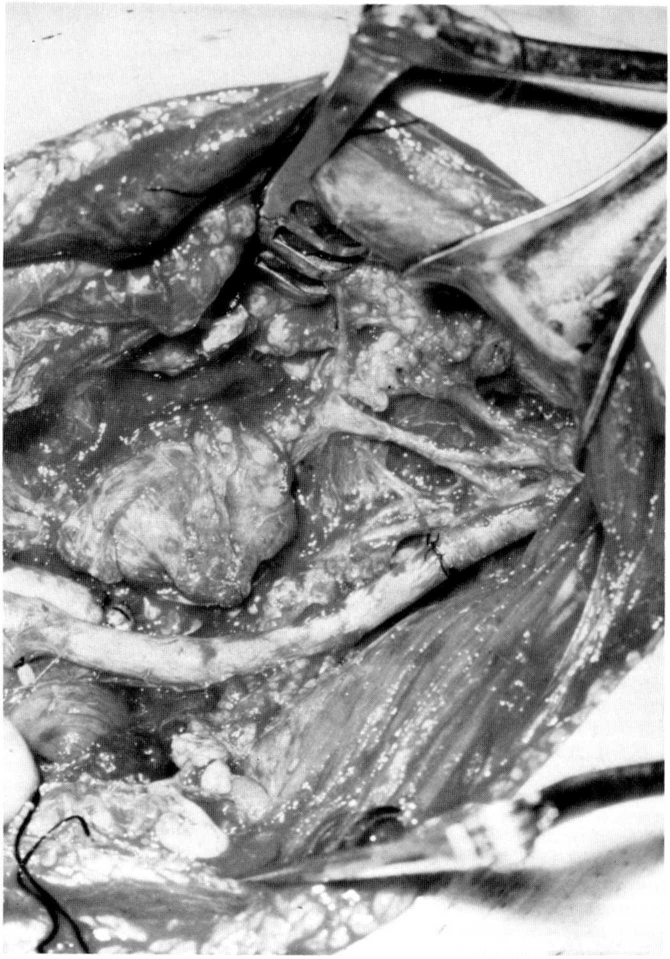

Figure 7.14. Saphenous vein bypass graft in place after exclusion of the popliteal aneurysm.

SUMMARY

The femoral and popliteal arteries are the most common sites of peripheral arterial aneurysms. Approximately 90% of the true aneurysms are arteriosclerotic in origin. One-third of patients with these lesions present with some surgical complication of their disease. Even when the aneurysm is initially asymptomatic, a high percentage of patients develop limb-threatening complications in the near future. Unless there is a cogent reason to avoid operation, femoral and popliteal aneurysms should be surgically repaired. While direct repair of the involved vessel is occasionally possible, replacement or bypass grafting are the procedures most commonly employed. In some situations, notably that of an infected pseudoaneurysm, urgent or emergent repair is indicated.

References

1. Barker, W. F. *Peripheral Arterial Disease*, pp. 431–432. W. B. Saunders, Philadelphia, 1975.
2. Bird, C. E. Sympathectomy as a preliminary to the obliteration of popliteal aneurysm. *Surg. Gynecol. Obstet. 60:* 926–929, 1935.
3. Blakemore, A. H., and Voorhees, A. B. The use of tubes constructed from vinyon-N cloth in bridging arterial defects—experimental and clinical. *Ann. Surg. 140:* 324–334, 1954.
4. Chitwood, W. R., Jr., Stocks, L. H., and Wolfe, W. G. Popliteal artery aneurysms. *Arch. Surg. 113:* 1078–1082, 1978.
5. Crichlow, R. W., and Roberts, B. Treatment of popliteal aneurysms by restoration of continuity. *Ann. Surg. 163:* 417–426, 1966.
6. Cutler, B. S., and Darling, R. C. Surgical management of arteriosclerotic femoral aneurysms. *Surgery 74:* 764–773, 1973.
7. Dubost, A., Allary, M., and Oeconomos, N. Aneuryme de l'aorte abdominale tracte par resection et grette. *Arch. Mal. Coeur 44:* 848–851, 1951.
8. Gifford, R. W., Hines, E. A., and James, J. M. An analysis and follow-up study of 100 popliteal aneurysms. *Surgery 33:* 284–294, 1953.
9. Matas, R. An operation for the radical cure of aneurysm based upon arteriorrhaphy. *Trans. South. Surg. Assoc. 20:* 396–434, 1902.
10. Osler, W. The Gulstonian lecture on malignant endocarditis. *Br. Med. J. 1:* 467–470, 1885.
11. Pappas, G., Janes, J. M., Bernatz, P. E., and Schirger, A. Femoral aneurysms. Review of surgical management. *J.A.M.A. 190:* 489–493, 1964.
12. Queral, L. A., Flinn, W. R., Yal, J. S. T., and Bergan, J. J. Management of peripheral arterial aneurysms. *Surg. Clin. North. Am. 59:* 693–706, 1979.
13. Rich, N. M. Vascular trauma. *Surg. Clin. North. Am. 53:* 1367–1392, 1973.
14. Tolstedt, G. E., Radke, H. M., and Bell, J. N. Late sequela of arteriosclerotic femoral aneurysms. *Angiology 12:* 601–602, 1961.
15. Wychulis, A. R., Spittel, J. A., and Wallace, R. B. Popliteal aneurysms. *Surgery 68:* 942–952, 1970.

CHAPTER 8

Primary and Secondary Sepsis in Aneurysms

THOMAS F. SWEENEY, M.D.
MORRIS D. KERSTEIN, M.D.

The concept of the interrelationship of emboli, infection, and arterial aneurysmal formation is not new. Osler (46) is generally credited with describing the pathophysiology of the mycotic aneurysm. He described its association with endocarditis and recognized the vegetations present on the heart valves. Others (65) earlier in the century had recognized the clinical entity. Tufnell (64) and Virchow (66) are credited with recognizing the importance of emboli in the production of aneurysms. Virchow (66) noted destruction of the inner and middle arterial coats and, in fact, found arterial dilatation and sac formation at the site of embolism. Tufnell (64) postulated the aneurysm was caused by pressure behind the embolus.

As reported by Wilson *et al.* (70), destruction of the arterial wall at the point of embolism was noted in 1873 by Ponfick, who felt this damage was a mechanical effect of blood pressure. It was Eppinger (17) who coined the term "embolomycotic" to signify the infectious relationship to arterial wall destruction. He proposed that infection was carried to the adventitia and spread inward. Unger (65) later showed that inflammation can start in the intima where the embolus lodges.

In 1909, Lewis and Schrager (34) introduced another etiologic classification for infected aneurysms. They presented a 12-year-old boy who developed a carotid artery aneurysm during suppurative osteomyelitis; thus, surrounding tissue served as the external source of infection. Crane (12) described a lesion not related to endocarditis, with no intravascular inflammatory focus, and without surrounding tissue inflammation. He called this lesion a "primary mycotic aneurysm," the route of infection being bacteria lodged into the wall by the force of blood. Revell (51) later postulated that the actual route of access to the aortic wall was through the vasa vasorum. Hankins and Yeager (27) demonstrated direct infection of intact intima would be unusual and intact intima is resistant to infection.

Given the numerous routes that can lead to infected aneurysmal formation, the term "mycotic aneurysm" can be misleading. A differentiation should be made between the pre-existing atherosclerotic aneurysm that becomes infected and the aneurysm that develops *de novo* as a result of infection in the arterial wall. The former will be referred to by the authors as an infected aneurysm, while the latter will be termed mycotic. The infected aneurysm usually occurs in the older patient and its walls are calcified, while the mycotic aneurysm rarely has calcified walls; it occurs in a somewhat younger age group. The latter also has a higher incidence in visceral vessels.

Patel and Johnson (49) have a simplified classification by source of infection: 1) infections from intravascular sources (i.e., embolism, septicemia, and extension of adjacent endocardial infection); and 2) infection from extravascular sources (e.g., spread from adjacent infection and iatrogenic).

Wilson *et al.* (69, 70) suggested a more descriptive classification which is somewhat more involved. *Mycotic aneurysm* is reserved for that aneurysm occurring in a normal or atherosclerotic artery resulting from emboli of endocardial origin. *Infected aneurysm* is an established atherosclerotic aneurysm infected by bacteremia. *Microbial arteritis* results from a bacteremia producing infection of normal or atherosclerotic vessels that may lead to rupture or pseudoaneurysmal formation. *Contiguous arterial infection* occurs by direct invasion of the artery from an adjacent focus. *Traumatic infected pseudoaneurysms* result from vascular injury due to trauma, iatrogenic insult, or injection (e.g., drug addicts).

AORTITIS

A related entity warranting discussion is non-aneurysmal suppurative aortitis. In the first half of the century, the most common cause of aortitis leading to aneurysmal formation was syphilis. Parkhurst and Decker (47), reporting on a 50-year experience prior to 1951, found 338 aortic aneurysms on autopsy; of these, 143 were syphilitic. Thirty-seven of these patients died of "internal rupture" or dissection of the aneurysm. They also noted three patients with infection in the aortic wall that produced erosion and rupture without aneurysmal formation.

In a later report, Bardin *et al.* (2) presented two patients with non-aneurysmal suppurative aortitis; one of whom died of an aortic rupture at the L-3 level. An atheromatous plaque was adjacent to this area and cultures were positive. Microscopic examination showed septic necrosis with micro-abscesses of the aortic wall in the area of rupture. The second patient developed distal aortic occlusion with positive blood cultures for *Salmonella enteritidis*. At surgery, he was found to have a beefy red distal aorta, but no aneurysm. This segment was resected and all layers of the aorta showed chronic inflammation and contained Salmonella.

In discussing aortitis with or without aneurysm, it should be noted both the source of the infection and the bacteria have changed over the years. In the pre-antibiotic era, it was extremely rare to find aortitis secondary to anything but endocarditis. There were a few cases attributed to osteomyelitis or pneumonia but, in general, the source was infected vegetation on the heart valve which emoblized (59). As a result, the bacteria most often implicated in aortitis were those causing endocarditis (e.g., streptococcus, staphylococcus, and pneumococcus) (32, 70).

MYCOTIC ANEURYSMS

Microbiology

During the antibiotic era, there has been a shift away from gram-positive organisms causing aneurysms, though some *Staphylococcus aureus* are still found. The majority now are gram-negative infections (13). Salmonella has emerged as the most common intruder (2, 71), even though Anderson *et al.* (1), in 1974, reported 16 cases of mycotic aneurysm in which most were caused by Staphylococcus and none by Salmonella.

The Salmonella pathogen usually causes a transient gastroenteritis. Cohen *et al.* (11) found that patients over 50 years of age with Salmonella bacteremia and clinical evidence of infection before hospitalization constitute a high-risk group for endothelial infection. Despite the fact that antibiotics are found to prolong fecal excretion of Salmonella and increase resistant strains, these authors suggest that patients over 50 years of age with acute Salmonella gastroenteritis should be treated with antibiotics to decrease their likelihood of developing endothelial infection. Zak *et al.* (71), in discussing 11 patients with ruptured large arteries secondary to Salmonella infection, proposed that the severe atherosclerotic change in these patients predisposed them to Salmonella arteritis during bacteremia (13).

INFECTED AORTIC ANEURYSMS

Microbiology

Saphir and Cooper (53) reported the first infected aortic aneurysm in 1927. Sommerville *et al.* (57) reported 6 infected aneurysms of 184 found at autopsy. In the antibiotic era, the source of infection is usually found in only 50% of cases. Bennett and Cherry (3), in their report of 11 secondarily infected aneurysms, make the differentiation that the inflammatory process is diffuse in the mycotic aneurysm; acute inflammation and necrosis are less extensive in the atherosclerotic aneurysm. Inflammatory response was found to be maximal at the point of rupture. Sixty-six percent of their positive cultures grew Salmonella species. Salmonella infection greatly increases the likelihood of rupture.

The type of bacteria also influences the likelihood of rupture. Jarrett *et al.* (32) suggest that gram-negative organisms are more likely to cause rupture than gram-positive ones. In their series of 16 infected aneurysms, only 1 of 10 gram-positive-cultured aneurysms ruptured, while 5 of 6 gram-negative-cultured aneurysms ruptured. They also noted that during surgery a particularly thin-walled aneurysm, prominent contiguous lymph nodes, or unusual surrounding inflammation should suggest infection.

Clinical Features

Although mycotic and infected atherosclerotic aneurysms are different pathologically, their clinical presentation and principles of treatment are the same. Seventy percent of these patients present with fever (32), often of unknown origin. A palpable mass and/or back pain are also common. Only after invasive testing can the diagnosis be made. However, any patient presenting with the combination of fever and pulsatile mass should be assumed to have an infected aneurysm.

Diagnosis

Diagnostically, 75% of patients will have leukocytosis greater than 10,000/mm^3 and 50% will have positive blood cultures. Flat plate of the abdomen may reveal a calcified aortic aneurysm. Mycotic aneurysms differ in that they are rarely calcified, while roughly 80% of atherosclerotic aneurysms can be identified on plain film. Ultrasonic evaluation can be helpful in delineating the aneurysm, but if this fails and suspicion is high, a computerized axial tomography (CAT) scan with contrast may be helpful; however, arteriography is rarely of help.

Once the diagnosis of an unsuspected infected aneurysm is made, surgical excision is indicated. Prolonged antibiotic therapy has not been successful in sterilizing the infected vessel (3, 46). Initial attempts at repair of such aneurysms were fraught with complications. It was soon found that, although the infected aneurysm was removed, reconstruction within the infected field yielded poor results (3). Graft thrombosis, recurrent infection, pseudoaneurysmal formation, and aortoenteric fistula were the most likely outcome (5).

Treatment

Extra-anatomic bypass, as suggested by Shaw and Baue (55), forms the main principle upon which successful care is based. Complete resection of the infected tissue, with drainage and ligation of the involved vessels, reconstitution within clean tissue planes, and intensive antibiotic therapy are the essentials of therapy. Various extra-anatomic routes are available for reconstruction, depending upon which vessel is involved. We prefer axillobifemoral grafts for the aortic aneurysm. Finseth and Abbott (19) reported successful repair of a Salmonella mycotic abdominal aortic aneurysm using a descending aorta-to-external-iliac-extrapleural, -peritoneal graft. Using this technique, they were able to avoid the infected retroperitoneal area. Davies *et al.* (13) reported a patient with a mid-infrarenal aortic aneurysm, which allowed them to resect the aneurysm and oversew the aorta above the bifurcation. A unilateral axillofemoral graft was placed with flow retrograde through the iliacs.

Distal aneurysms involving the femoral artery may be resected and reconstructed with saphenous vein through the obturator canal. Fromm and Lucas (21) reported several cases of femoral artery mycotic aneurysms in drug addicts and successfully employed the obturator bypass following resection of the infected area.

VISCERAL ARTERY ANEURYSMS

Although a relatively uncommon location for atherosclerotic aneurysms, visceral artery mycotic aneurysms do occur. A superior mesenteric artery aneurysm is most likely mycotic and should be treated as such (58). Olcott and Ehrenfeld (45) suggest that endoaneurysmorrhaphy is an excellent way to handle this problem. Though splenic artery aneurysms are the most common visceral artery aneurysms, only 1% are mycotic (54, 70); hepatic artery aneurysms are more likely to be mycotic.

In general, the diagnosis of visceral artery aneurysms is difficult to make. These aneurysms are not usually palpable and only if suspicion is high would one perform arteriography. The diagnosis is confirmed preoperatively by angiography, or intraoperatively by direct inspection. The dilated walls of the small vessel may be more effectively seen and evaluated by angiography than the larger vessels. Since it is common to have clot in the lumen of a larger aneurysm, one may misinterpret the column of dye and the interpretation may be a normal vessel. The smaller visceral vessels seem to have less calcium deposition and intraluminal clot. Both ultrasonography, the classic diagnostic tool, and CAT scan are more helpful than a contrast dye study in the larger vessel.

Although mycotic and infected aneurysms are rare, recent reports suggest that bacterial contamination of aneurysms is not. Williams and Fisher (68) found that of 68 aneurysms cultured during routine surgery, seven grew organisms; none of these patients presented with symptoms of infected aneurysms. Although prophylactic antibiotics were used pre- and intraoperatively, only 1 of 7 organisms was sensitive to the antibiotic used. All patients had Dacron grafts placed within the contaminated field and none developed infection. When positive cultures were obtained, antibiotics were switched to fit the sensitivities and used for two weeks. Ernst *et al.* (18) found 12 of 78 aneurysms grew positive cultures. Of 13 ruptured aneurysms, 5 had positive cultures. Two of 78 patients had graft sepsis problems, but only 1 of these had positive operative cultures.

CONTAMINATED ANEURYSMS

Microbiology

Contaminated aneurysms seem to differ from the full-blown picture of infected aneurysms; the bacteria appear to be dissimilar. The former tend to culture gram-positive organisms, mostly Staphylococcus, with very few gram-negatives; the latter are predominately gram-negative, with Salmonella accounting for a large number of cases. It appears that synthetic graft placement (in this unique situation) within a contaminated field, although worrisome, is safe, as only 1 of 19 patients developed graft sepsis. We suggest routine culture of all aneurysms with gram stains of any suspicious material. A gram stain with a large number of bacteria present might dictate an alternative approach (e.g., extra-anatomic bypass) to avoid infection developing in the vascular prosthesis.

INFECTED PROSTHESIS FOLLOWING ANEURYSMAL REPAIR

The placement of synthetic graft material within the arterial tree began roughly 50 years ago with the placement of paraffin-lined aluminum and glass tubes (8). Preserved arterial homografts (26) were tried briefly, but the first successful aortic aneurysm replacement was done by Hufnagel and Rabil (31) using Orlon cloth. Today's graft material is much more sophisticated; but placement of a foreign body is always accompanied by the possibility of infection.

That graft material is susceptible to infection was demonstrated nicely by Moore *et al.* (42). By placing Dacron grafts in the presence of septicemia, they were able to produce prosthetic infection in 100% of the animals. They later demonstrated that, with time, the graft becomes less susceptible to the bacteremic challenge (36, 38, 60). Four months after Dacron grafts were placed in the canine aorta, only 62% became infected from an infusion of 10^8 *Staphylococcus aureus*. At one year, none of the grafts developed infection with the same challenge.

Clearly, the prosthetic graft develops some form of protection from infection. Extensive work (36, 38, 41–43, 60, 61) has shown this protection develops as the graft becomes incorporated within its surrounding tissue. The graft surface is slowly covered and it is given the benefit of an endothelial intima that protects the remainder of the graft from recurrent bacteremic challenge. Sweeney *et al.* (61), in an experimental setting, demonstrated a graft may be replaced in a potentially infected bed with appropriate local care and systemic antibiotic coverage. Mackenzie and Lowenthal (37) demonstrated fibrous tissue ingrowth from the suture line which eventually endothelializes short-segment grafts. Most grafts are, of course, much longer than the 3-cm grafts used in the above studies. Berger *et al.* (4) were able to demonstrate this "pannus ingrowth" covered only 10 to 15 mm from each suture line.

Long-segment vascular grafts have other means of developing protection. Tissue ingrowth through graft wall interstices is the critical factor in longer grafts. Unfortunately, as shown by Sauvage *et al.* (54), man demonstrates the slowest rate of tissue ingrowth of five species tested. Wesolowski (67) demonstrated there is an optimal balance between rate of tissue ingrowth and risk of late hemorrhage—primarily determined by the size of the interstices.

Recently, work on endothelial cell seeding of prosthetic grafts has been presented by Graham *et al.* (25). Using 6-mm, double-velour, Dacron grafts 25 to 30 cm long in the dog, they were able to show 60 to 70% endothelial cell coverage at two weeks in grafts seeded with cultured autologous endothelial cells. At four weeks, 80% graft coverage was attained, compared to a maximum of 10% in the controls. Once developed, endothelial seeding may afford a means of achieving rapid protection of long-segment grafts.

As early as 1959, another aspect of graft infection was being considered—that of performance in the face of infection. Foster *et al.* (20) assessed the performance of freeze-dried homografts and synthetic nylon. Experimental infections were created around both types. All animals died, but the cause was different in each type. Eight of ten animals in the homograft group died of hemorrhage, whereas, in the synthetic group only three of ten hemorrhaged. The latter showed suture line breakdown due to failure of host artery to hold sutures. The former showed that either sutures had pulled out of the graft, or the homograft itself had broken down causing rupture. Other studies (29, 61, 69) comparing Dacron to bovine grafts have since confirmed these findings.

Although no graft material should be expected to perform well in the presence of infection, Moore *et al.* (39) found only one suture line rupture in 15 autogenous vein grafts placed in contaminated fields. Noting clinically that frequent, lethal hemorrhage occurred with the use of autogenous vein, Bricker *et al.* (7) showed vein graft dissolution experimentally. They also found Dacron grafts had a tendency to thrombose rather than hemorrhage. Their conclusion was that autogenous vein was superior to synthetics regarding patency, but the risk of hemorrhage was greater in the presence of infection. These findings might suggest that synthetic material is safer in a potentially contaminated field (e.g., trauma). Under the adverse circumstance of infection, thrombosis would occur in a synthetic graft but hemorrhage would occur with autogenous vein, the latter being more lethal.

Experimental work by Moore *et al.* (43) has shown that, with control of sepsis, graft placement may be successful. They placed canine common femoral auto- or allografts in contaminated femoral wounds while treating with antibiotics. As a part of the experiment, a third group had Dacron grafts placed under the same conditions. Twenty-one of 24 autogenous grafts remained sterile, while only 1 of 8 Dacron grafts was found to be sterile. Another group (48) placed Dacron grafts in canine infrarenal aortas during an induced staphylococcus septicemia. These grafts were later excised, wide debridement of the area carried out, and a second graft placed in the field during antibiotic therapy. Sterilization of these grafts was noted at time of sacrifice three weeks after placement.

Choice of graft material should be made with the knowledge that autogenous vein grafts afford relative resistance to infection but may break down. Secondly, once infection is established, stability and maintenance of graft integrity is a property of synthetic graft material. Thirdly, neointimal development is the main means of protecting the synthetic graft from a bacteremic challenge. Finally, porosity and length of graft determine the speed with which the protective cover develops.

The incidence of prosthetic vascular graft infections varies from 1.5 to 6%. The most likely area to become infected is the femoral anastomosis (40). Aortoiliac grafts have a low incidence of infection in all series; extending the graft to the femoral area, therefore, significantly increases the chance of infection. Moore *et al.* (40), however, feel long-term patency rates are improved in aortic grafts to the femoral region; they had only two infected grafts in 58 patients. The use of synthetic material in the femoropopliteal region reflects a somewhat higher rate of infection than those using autogenous saphenous vein (30, 62). Szilagyi *et al.* (62) noted only 2 graft infections in 445 autogenous vein grafts placed. Even more impressive is that 44 of these patients developed groin wound infections, but the underlying vein remained sterile. These data would appear to be somewhat contradictory to that of the work of Bricker *et al.* (7). The authors are more inclined to support the concept of autogenous material as the primary choice, particularly in the contaminated or potentially contaminated areas.

Although it is generally felt that infected lymph is a contributing source to femoral anastomotic infections, the literature varies on this point. Goldstone and Moore (24) found a high incidence of positive lymph cultures associated with infected foot lesions. Bouhoutsos *et al.* (6), however, were unable to correlate the two. Of 85 patients receiving grafts, 17 had infected foot lesions; 6 became infected, but only 2 of these had foot lesions. They were unable to obtain positive lymph cultures.

Care to ensure a tight suture line is also important. A perigraft hematoma is an excellent culture medium for possible contamination. Concomitant procedures should be avoided. Damage to the duodenum can lead to contamination of the aortic suture line, with resultant pseudoaneurysmal formation or aortoduodenal fistula.

Although most graft infections occur within the first 12 months, later graft infections have been reported (3, 44, 62). Defective tissue ingrowth and incomplete pseudointimal formation or intimal damage may leave the graft susceptible to infection. Ernst *et al.* (18) reported only a 2.5% infection rate, despite the fact that 15% of their patients had positive aneurysmal cultures. Perhaps it is this type of patient, who has a latent infection, that becomes evident several years later.

In their review, Liekweg and Greenfield (35) indicated *Staphylococcus aureus* to be the most common organism, accounting for approximately 50% of wound infections in vascular surgery. They found that, although slightly more common in groin wounds, Staphylococcus was also present in aortic infections and the difference was not significant. They also noted, along with Casali *et al.* (10), that gram-negative organisms are increasing in frequency, as are multiple isolates from the same graft. These authors postulated that widespread use of prophylactic antibiotics may be a major factor accounting for this change in flora.

Clinically infected prostheses can present insidiously as pseudoaneurysmal formation, or as frank hemorrhage, with catastrophic results. Fever, back pain, malaise, or septic emboli can be seen. The patient with fever of unknown source and a prosthetic graft should be assumed to have graft infection. Graft thrombosis may also occur. Once infected, suture line breakdown occurs. When the aortic suture line is involved, erosion into the duodenum may occur.

The diagnosis is suggested by positive blood cultures and is usually confirmed by arteriography. Suture line leak can sometimes be demonstrated. Although gallium scanning has not proven to be as useful as expected, a new technique is being developed which looks promising. Indium-111-labeled leukocyte scintigraphy is quite specific. The leukocytes are not taken up by either neoplastic lesions or uninfected healing wounds. Thakun (63) demonstrated this technique to be useful in identifying an infected vascular prosthesis.

Once established, graft infection carries with it very high morbidity and mortality rates. In most studies, aortic infections are associated with 50% or greater mortality. Femoral grafts, although carrying a lower mortality rate, have a very high morbidity with limb loss all too common. Like the infected aneurysm, prosthetic material, once infected, cannot be sterilized by intensive antibiotic therapy. Because of the high associated mortality, infected aortic grafts must be dealt with aggressively. Unilateral limb thrombosis may occur secondary to infection. Shaw and Baue (55) demonstrated that, if dealt with promptly, the limb of the graft can be excised, vascular continuity re-established around the contaminated field, and the remaining graft preserved. Diethrich *et al.* (14) had similar success by adding catheters for continuous antibiotic irrigation.

Propagation of sepsis occurs both in the patent and thrombosed infected vascular graft (10, 24, 67). Once proximal anastomotic aortic graft infection occurs, massive hemorrhage into the retroperitoneum or through a graft enteric fistula is the rule. Prompt action must be taken once the diagnosis is made. Total graft excision, with ligation of the aorta and iliacs, must be done and extra-anatomic bypass performed in those patients requiring limb revascularization (5). Vigorous, long-term (six weeks) intravenous antibiotic treatment is necessary. Even with aggressive management, mortality rates remain high. Casali *et al.* (10) found somewhat better results in those patients who underwent axillofemoral bypass first, followed by graft excision two to three days later. Goldstone and Moore (24) stated only one-third of their patients required immediate extra-anatomic bypass. They also noted much higher mortality in these patients than in those who could be revascularized several days later.

Ehrenfeld *et al.* (16) reported an alternative approach to extra-anatomic bypass grafting. Their study describes the use of autogenous reconstruction within the infected field, including endarterectomy and replacement of the infected graft, with arterial or venous autografts in 24 patients. They found that suture lines involving autogenous tissue healed, even when in an infected field. Three of 24 patients in their study died, for a mortality rate of only 13%, and there were 2 amputations.

In the femoral area, there is experimental evidence that long-term antibiotic irrigation of contaminated grafts can be successful (15). Carter *et al.* (9) and Smith *et al.* (56), employing both systemic and local antibiotics, were able to sterilize several prostheses in the groin. Conservative management of the femoral anastomosis as a proximal component of a limb graft, though not always successful, is infrequently associated with high mortality. In those that fail, graft excision with revascularization through the obturator canal may be a useful alternative (55).

Since graft infection is associated with high morbidity and mortality rates, despite the type of treatment, prevention is the best approach for the vascular surgeon. Although a few authors (22, 23, 43, 62) reported large series with low infection rates without the aid of prophylactic antibiotics, most surgeons employ them (10, 33, 49). There is good experimental evidence (36, 41) that perioperative antibiotics afford protection from bacteremic challenge. Parsa *et al.* (48) found only 1 of 16 canine Dacron grafts positive after antibiotic treatment during graft placement in the face of induced Staphylococcus bacteremia. DiGiglia *et al.* (15) demonstrated that continuous local antibiotic irrigation affords protection from experimental contamination. Soaking the graft in antibiotic solution may also prove a deterrent to prosthetic infection (20, 52, 61). Recent work by Harvey and Greco (28), studying the non-covalent bonding of antibiotics to a polytetrafluoroethylene benzalkonium graft, represents the forefront of research in preventing graft infection.

ANTIBIOTIC PROPHYLAXIS IN ANEURYSMAL SURGERY

Until recently, clinical experience dictated the preference for prophylaxis. Most surgeons used antibiotics in the hope they would afford some protection from graft infection, but no randomized studies were available. In 1978, Kaiser *et al.* (33) presented such a study. Comparing cefazolin to placebo in 565 arterial reconstructive procedures, they found a significant difference. Placebo, or antibiotic, was administered on call to the operating room and postoperatively every six hours for four doses. Infection rate in the placebo group was 6.8%, but only 0.9% in the antibiotic group. Of the 18 infections, 4 involved graft infection and all of these were in the placebo group. As an aside, it was noted that patients prepped with hexachlorophene-ethanol had a significantly higher infection rate than those prepped with povidone-iodine.

Szilagyi *et al.* (62) emphasized the importance of the groin incision as a source of graft infection. Location, lymphatic drainage, ischemic tissue, and frequent motion were all found to be contributing factors to the problem. Preparation with betadine must be carefully done and closure of the area meticulous to avoid dead space and hematoma formation. In another study, Pitt *et al.* (50) focused on prophylaxis and its effect on groin wound infection rate. They found that antibiotics administered topically or systemically afforded excellent protection from groin wound infection. There was no additional benefit from both therapies. In their study, the only risk factors contributing to increased infection were age greater than 70, obesity, and the presence of dry gangrene.

Two final sources of contamination are the aneurysm itself and the Lahey bag used intraoperatively. Positive cultures from the fluid (plasma) accumulated in the bowel bag were noted by Ernst *et al.* (18) and Fry (22). Studies mentioned earlier (18, 68) confirm the presence of bacteria in up to 15% of routine abdominal aneurysms. Since the prophylactic antibiotic used is frequently not appropriate for the organism cultured, the appropriate change should be made as soon as sensitivities are available. Long-term antibiotic administration in a patient with a positive aneurysmal culture is essential for uncomplicated graft placement (68).

SUMMARY

Infections in the vascular tree (whether mycotic, atherosclerotic, or prosthetic) have proven a most difficult challenge for the vascular surgeon. Morbidity and mortality rates remain high, despite technical advances, with the use of extra-anatomic bypass and newer antibiotics. New diagnostic methods (e.g., indium-111-labeled leukocyte scintigraphy and the CAT scan with contrast) may make the detection of such problems less difficult and time-consuming. Careful preoperative evaluation, prophylactic antibiotics, and meticulous surgical technique are essential to avoid life-threatening complications. Special attention must be paid to the groin wound because of its propensity to develop infection. If graft infection does develop, aggressive management is mandatory. Excision of the infected area, extra-anatomic revascularization, and long-term antibiotic therapy afford the best means of decreasing mortality and morbidity.

References

1. Anderson, C., Butcher, H., and Ballinger, W. Mycotic aneurysm. *Arch. Surg. 109:* 712–717, 1974.
2. Bardin, J., Collins, G., Devin, J., and Halasz, N. Nonaneurysmal suppurative aortitis. *Arch. Surg. 116:* 954–956, 1981.
3. Bennett, D., and Cherry, J. Bacterial infection of aortic aneurysms. *Am. J. Surg. 113:* 321–326, 1967.
4. Berger, K., Sauvage, L. R., Rao, A., and Wood, S. Healing of arterial prostheses in man: its incompleteness. *Ann. Surg. 175:* 118–127, 1972.
5. Blaisdell, F. W., and Hall, A. D. Axillary-femoral bypass for lower extremity ischemia. *Surgery 54:* 563–568, 1963.
6. Bouhoutsos, J., Chavatzas, D., Martin, P., and Morris, T. Infected synthetic arterial grafts. *Br. J. Surg. 61:* 108–111, 1974.
7. Bricker, D., Beall, A., and DeBakey, M. The differential response to infection of autogenous vein vs. dacron arterial prosthesis. *Chest 58:* 566–570, 1970.
8. Carrel, J. Permanent intubation of the thoracic aorta. *J. Exp. Med. 16:* 17–24, 1912.
9. Carter, S., Cohen, A., and Whelan, T. Clinical experience with management of the infected dacron graft. *Ann. Surg. 158:* 249–255, 1963.
10. Casali, R., Tucker, W., Thompson, W., and Read, R. Infected prosthetic grafts. *Arch. Surg. 115:* 577–580, 1980.
11. Cohen, P., O'Brien, T., Schoenbaum, S., and Mederios, A. Risk of endothelial infection in adults with salmonella bacteremia. *Ann. Intern. Med. 89:* 931–932, 1978.
12. Crane, A. Primary multilocular mycotic aneurysm of the aorta. *Arch. Pathol. 24:* 634–641, 1937.
13. Davies, O., Thorburn, J., and Powell, P. Cryptic mycotic abdominal aortic aneurysms—diagnosis and management. *Am. J. Surg. 136:* 96–101, 1978.
14. Diethrich, E., Noon, G., Liddicont, J., and DeBakey, M. Treatment of infected aorto-femoral arterial prostheses. *Surgery 68:* 1044–1052, 1970.
15. DiGiglia, J., Leonard, G., and Ochsner, J. Local irrigation with antibiotic solution in prevention of infection in vascular prostheses. *Surgery 67:* 836–840, 1970.
16. Ehrenfeld, W., Wilbur, B., Olcott, C., and Stoney, R. Autogenous tissue reconstruction in the management of infected prosthetic grafts. *Surgery 85:* 82–92, 1979.
17. Eppinger, H. Pathogenesis (histogenesis and aetiologic) der aneursman ein schliesslich des aneurysma equi verminosum. *Arch. Klin. Chir. 35:* 404, 1887.
18. Ernst, C., Campbell, C., Daugherty, M., Sachatello, C. R., and Griffin, W. D. Incidence and significance of intra-operative bacterial cultures during abdominal aortic aneurysmectomy. *Ann. Surg. 185:* 626–633, 1977.
19. Finseth, F., and Abbott, W. One stage operative therapy for salmonella mycotic abdominal aortic aneurysm. *Ann. Surg. 179:* 8–11, 1974.
20. Foster, J., Berzins, T., and Scott, H. An experimental study of arterial replacement in the presence of bacterial infection. *Surg. Gynecol. Obstet. 108:* 141–148, 1959.
21. Fromm, S., and Lucas, C. Obturator bypass for mycotic aneurysm in the drug addict. *Arch. Surg. 100:* 82–83, 1970.

22. Fry, W. Vascular prosthesis infections. *Surg. Clin. N. Am. 52:* 1419–1424, 1972.
23. Fry, W., and Lindenauer, S. Infection complicating the use of plastic arterial implants. *Arch. Surg. 94:* 600–609, 1967.
24. Goldstone, J., and Moore, W. Infection in vascular prostheses: clinical manifestations and surgical management. *Am. J. Surg. 128:* 225–233, 1974.
25. Graham, L., Vinter, D., Ford, J., Kahn, R. H., Burkel, W. E., and Stanley, J. C. Endothelial cell seeding of prosthetic vascular grafts: early experimental studies with cultured autologous canine endothelium. *Arch. Surg. 115:* 929–933, 1980.
26. Gross, R. E., Bill, A. H., and Pierce, E. C. Methods of preservation and transplantation of arterial grafts. *Surg. Gynecol. Obstet. 88:* 689–701, 1949.
27. Hankins, J., and Yeager, G. Primary mycotic aneurysm. *Surgery 40:* 747–756, 1956.
28. Harvey, R. A., and Greco, R. S. The noncovalent bonding of antibiotics to a polytetrafluoroethylene-benzalkonium graft. *Ann. Surg. 194(5):* 642–647, 1981.
29. Hermosillo, C., Parsa, F., Gordon, H., and Wilson, S. Infectability of dacron vs. bovine grafts by induced staphylococcus bacteremia. *Surg. Forum 25:* 256–257, 1974.
30. Hoffert, P., Gensler, S., and Haimovici, H. Infection complicating arterial grafts. *Arch. Surg. 90:* 427–435, 1965.
31. Hufnagel, C. A., and Rabil, P. Replacement of arterial segments utilizing flexible orlon prostheses. *Arch. Surg. 70:* 105–110, 1955.
32. Jarrett, F., Darling, C., Mundth, E., and Austen, G. Experience with infected aneurysms of abdominal aorta. *Arch. Surg. 110:* 1281–1286, 1975.
33. Kaiser, A., Clayson, K., Mulherin, J., Roach, A. C., Allen, T. R., Edwards, W. H., and Dale, W. R. Antibiotic prophylaxis in vascular surgery. *Ann. Surg. 188:* 283–289, 1978.
34. Lewis, D., and Schrager, V. Embolomycotic aneurysms. *J.A.M.A. 53:* 1808–1814, 1909.
35. Liekweg, W., and Greenfield, L. Vascular prosthetic infections: collected experience and results of treatment. *Surgery 81:* 335–342, 1977.
36. Lindenauer, S., Fry, W., Schaub, G., and Wild, D. The use of antibiotics in the prevention of vascular graft infection. *Surgery 62:* 487–492, 1967.
37. Mackenzie, W., and Lowenthal, R. Endothelial growth in nylon vascular grafts. *Br. J. Surg. 48:* 212–217, 1960.
38. Malone, J., Moore, W., Campagna, G., and Bean, B. Bacteremia infectability of vascular grafts: the influence of pseudointimal integrity and duration of graft function. *Surgery 78:* 211–216, 1975.
39. Moore, W., Blaisdell, F., Gardner, M., and Hall, A. Effects of infection on autogenous vein arterial substitutes. *Surg. Forum. 13:* 235–237, 1962.
40. Moore, W., Cafferata, H., Hall, A., and Blaisdell, F. In defense of grafts across the inguinal ligament. *Ann. Surg. 168:* 207–214, 1968.
41. Moore, W., Rosson, C., and Hall, A. Effect of prophylactic antibiotics in preventing bacteremic infection of vascular prostheses. *Surgery 69:* 825–828, 1971.
42. Moore, W. S., Rosson, C. T., Hall, A. D., and Thomas, A. Transient bacteremia: a cause of infection in prosthetic vascular grafts. *Am. J. Surg. 117:* 342–343, 1969.
43. Moore, W., Swanson, R., Campagna, G., and Bean, B. The use of fresh tissue arterial substitutes in infected fields. *J. Surg. Res. 18:* 229–233, 1975.
44. Najafi, H., Javid, H., Dye, W., Hunter, J. A., and Julian, D. C. Management of infected arterial implants. *Surgery 65:* 539–547, 1969.
45. Olcott, C., and Ehrenfeld, W. K. Endoaneurysmorrhaphy for visceral artery aneurysms. *Am. J. Surg. 133:* 636–639, 1977.
46. Osler, W. The Gulstonian lectures on malignant endocarditis. *Br. Med. J. 1:* 467, 1885.
47. Parkhurst, G., and Decker, J. Bacterial aortitis and mycotic aneurysm of the aorta. *Am. J. Pathol. 31:* 821–835, 1955.
48. Parsa, F., Gordon, H., and Wilson, S. Intraoperative antibiotics in the prevention of experimental dacron graft infection. *Vasc. Surg. 10:* 64–71, 1976.
49. Patel, S., and Johnson, W. Classification and management of mycotic aneurysms. *Surg. Gynecol. Obstet. 144:* 691–694, 1977.
50. Pitt, H., Postier, R., MacGowan, W., Frank, L. W., Surmak, A. J., Sitzman, J. V., and Bouchier-Hayes, D. Prophylactic antibiotics in vascular surgery. *Ann. Surg. 192:* 356–364, 1980.
51. Revell, S. Primary mycotic aneurysms. *Ann. Intern. Med. 22:* 431–440, 1945.

52. Richardson, R., Pate, J., Wolf, R., Ledes , C., and Hopson, W. B., Jr. The outcome of antibiotic soaked arterial grafts in guinea pig wound contaminated with E. coli or S. aureus. *J. Thorac. Cardiovasc. Surg. 59:* 635–637, 1970.
53. Saphir, O., and Cooper, G. Acute suppurative aortitis superimposed on syphilitis aortitis. *Arch. Pathol. Lab. Med. 4:* 543–545, 1927.
54. Sauvage, L., Berger, K., Wood, S., Yates, S. G., Smith, J. C., and Mansfield, P. B. Interspecies healing of porous arterial prosthesis: observations. 1960–1974. *Arch. Surg. 109:* 698–705, 1974.
55. Shaw, R. S., and Baue, A. E. Management of sepsis complicating arterial reconstructive surgery. *Surgery 53:* 75–86, 1963.
56. Smith, R. B., III, Lowry, K., and Perdue, G. Management of the infected arterial prosthesis in the lower extremity. *Am. Surg. 33:* 711–714, 1967.
57. Sommerville, R., Allen, E., and Edwards, J. Bland and infected arteriosclerotic abdominal aortic aneurysms. *Medicine 38:* 207–221, 1959.
58. Stanley, J., Thompson, N., and Fry, W. Splanchnic artery aneurysms. *Arch. Surg. 101:* 689–697, 1970.
59. Stengel, A., and Wolferth, C. Mycotic (bacterial) aneurysms of intravascular origin. *Arch. Intern. Med. 85:* 663, 1923.
60. Swanson, R. J., Moore, W. S., and Campagna, G. Effect of time on vascular prostheses susceptibility to infection of bacteremic origin. *Surg. Forum. 24:* 28–29, 1973.
61. Sweeney, T., Piorkowski, R., Ariyan, S., and Kerstein, M. An alternative in the management of vascular prosthetic infection. (Accepted for publication, *Angiology*, 1983)
62. Szilagyi, E., Smith, R., Elliot, J., and Vrandecic, M. Infection in arterial reconstruction with synthetic grafts. *Ann. Surg. 176:* 321–333, 1972.
63. Thakun, M. New radionuclide in the diagnosis of obscure infections. *Conn. Med. 45:* 302, 1981.
64. Tufnell, J. The influence of vegetations on the valves of the heart in the production of secondary arterial disease. *Dublin O. J. Med. Sci. 15:* 371, 1853.
65. Unger: Beits. Pathol. Anat. Allg Pathol. 51: 137, 1911.
66. Virchow: *Virchows Arch. (Pathol. Anat.) 1:* 272, 1847. As quoted in Stengel, A., and Wolferth, C. Mycotic (bacterial) aneurysms of intravascular origin. *Arch. Intern. Med. 85:* 663–671, 1923.
67. Wesolowski, S. A. Long-term behavior of tissue and prosthetic implants for arterial reconstruction. *J. Cardiovasc. Surg. 10(4):* 55, 1969.
68. Williams, R., and Fisher, F. Aneurysm contents as a source of graft infection. *Arch. Surg. 112:* 415–416, 1977.
69. Wilson, S., Hermosillo, C., Parsa, F., and Gordon, H. Experimental infection of dacron and bovine grafts. *J. Surg. Res. 18:* 221–227, 1975.
70. Wilson, S., Van Wogeman, P., and Passaro, E. Arterial infection. *Curr. Probl. Surg. 15(9):* 1–89, 1978.
71. Zak, F., Strauss, L., and Saphra, I. Rupture of diseased large arteries in the course of enterobacterial (salmonella) infections. *New Engl. J. Med. 258:* 824–828, 1958.

Index